ROUTLEDGE LIBRARY EDITIONS:
PSYCHIATRY

Volume 13

SOCIAL PSYCHIATRY

SOCIAL PSYCHIATRY

Edited by
ARI KIEV

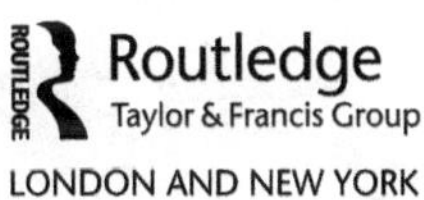

LONDON AND NEW YORK

First published in 1970 by Routledge & Kegan Paul

This edition first published in 2019
by Routledge
2 Park Square, Milton Park, Abingdon, Oxon OX14 4RN

and by Routledge
711 Third Avenue, New York, NY 10017

Routledge is an imprint of the Taylor & Francis Group, an informa business

British Library Cataloguing in Publication Data
A catalogue record for this book is available from the British Library

ISBN: 978-1-138-60492-6 (Set)
ISBN: 978-0-429-43807-3 (Set) (ebk)
ISBN: 978-1-138-32010-9 (Volume 13) (hbk)
ISBN: 978-1-138-32019-2 (Volume 13) (pbk)
ISBN: 978-0-429-45349-6 (Volume 13) (ebk)

Publisher's Note
The publisher has gone to great lengths to ensure the quality of this reprint but points out that some imperfections in the original copies may be apparent.

Disclaimer
The publisher has made every effort to trace copyright holders and would welcome correspondence from those they have been unable to trace.

SOCIAL PSYCHIATRY

VOLUME I

EDITED BY ARI KIEV, M.D.

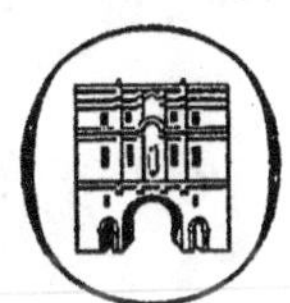

LONDON
ROUTLEDGE AND KEGAN PAUL LTD.

First published in Great Britain in 1970
by Routledge & Kegan Paul Ltd.
68-74 Carter Lane, London, E.C.4
Printed in U.S.A.

SBN 7100 6746 1

Acknowledgements:

Thanks are due to the publishers and organizations listed for permission to reprint the following:

Chapter 1—"Social Psychiatry: An Overview." Reprinted from the *Archives of General Psychiatry*, May 1965, Vol. 12, pp. 501-509. Copyright © 1965, American Medical Association.

Chapter 2—"Social Psychiatry: Vagaries of a Term." Reprinted from *Archives of General Psychiatry*, April 1966, Vol. 14, pp. 337-345. Copyright © 1966 by the American Medical Association.

Chapter 3—"Sociology and Mental Illness: Some Neglected Implications for Treatment." Reprinted from the *Archives of General Psychiatry*, December 1966, Vol. 15, pp. 635-648. Copyright © 1966 by American Medical Association.

Chapter 4—"Epidemiology and Mental Disorder: A Review." Reprinted from the *Journal of Neurology, Neurosurgery and Psychiatry*, 1964, 27, 277.

Chapter 5—"On the Social Epidemiology of Schizophrenia." Reprinted from *Acta Sociologia*, Vol. 9, fasc. 3-4, Copenhagen, 1966.

Chapter 6—"The Reliability and Validity of Measures of Family Life and Relationships in Families Containing a Psychiatric Patient." Reprinted from *Social Psychiatry*, Vol. 1, No. 1, 1966, pp. 38-53.

Chapter 7—"Emotional Disorders in an Israeli Immigrant Community." Reprinted from the *Israel Annals of Psychiatry and Related Disciplines*, Vol. 3, October 1965, No. 2.

Chapter 8—"An Experience with Sectorization in Paris." Reprinted from *International Trends in Mental Health*, edited by Henry P. David. Copyright © 1966, by McGraw-Hill Inc. Used by permission of McGraw-Hill Book Company, New York, N. Y.

Chapter 9—"Community Psychiatry: The Newest Therapeutic Bandwagon." Reprinted from the *Archives of General Psychiatry,* March 1965, Vol. 12, pp. 303-313. Copyright © 1965, by American Medical Association.

Chapter 10—"Psycho-social Forces and Public Health Problems." Reprinted from the *International Journal of Health Education,* Vol. IV, 1966, No. 1, pp. 3-11.

Chapter 11—"Maintenance Drug Therapy: The Schizophrenic Patient in the Community." Reprinted from *International Psychiatry Clinics,* October 1965, Vol. 2, No. 4, pp. 933-960. Copyright © 1965 by Little, Brown and Company.

Chapter 12—"British Experience in Community Care." Reprinted from *International Trends in Mental Health,* edited by Henry P. David. Copyright © 1966, by McGraw-Hill, Inc. Used by permission of McGraw-Hill Book Company, New York, N. Y.

Chapter 13—"Some Speculations on the Social Impact of Technology." Reprinted from *Technological Innovation and Society: Technology and Social Change,* edited by Dean Morse and Aaron Warner for the Columbia University Seminar on Technology and Social Change. Copyright © 1966, by Columbia University Press, New York, N. Y.

Chapter 14—"Housing and Mental Health in Developing Countries." Reprinted from Ciba Foundation Symposium *Transcultural Psychiatry,* edited by A. V. S. DeReuck and Ruth Porter, 1965.

Chapter 15—"Grieving for a Lost Home." Chapter 12 in *The Urban Condition,* edited by Leonard J. Duhl. Copyright © 1963 by Basic Books, Inc., Publishers, New York.

Chapter 16—"Theory of Human Behavior Based on Studies of Non-Human Primates." Reprinted from *Perspectives in Biology and Medicine,* Vol. 10, No. 2, Winter 1967, pp. 153-176, by permission of The University of Chicago Press. Copyright © 1967 by the University of Chicago Press.

Chapter 17—"On Aggression" Book Review. Reprinted from *British Journal of Psychiatry,* 1967, 113, pp. 803-812.

Chapter 18—"The Primate Socialization Motives." Reprinted from *Transactions and Studies of the College of Physicians of Philadelphia,* 4 Ser. Vol. 33, April 4, 1966.

Table of Contents

Part III—Community Psychiatry

Part IV—Social Problems

Part V—Animal Studies

Preface

The past several decades have wrought a revolution in psychiatry. A variety of new treatment programs ranging from sheltered workshop to crisis intervention therapy to around-the-clock telephone emergency services have been introduced. Increasing recognition has been given to the psychiatric aspect of a great range of social problems and special population subgroups.. Research efforts have also been given new impetus by recent developments in technology. A search for new methodologies, classifications, and ways of organizing into meaningful heuristic categories the mass of data being generated in numerous investigations has begun. Interdisciplinary investigations have multiplied as have the number of contributions relevant to psychiatry from ethology, sociology, biochemistry, community organizations, and other disciplines.

Increased specialization accompanying the information and publication explosion has made it impossible for most persons to keep abreast of relevant developments in areas other than their own. This is especially so in social psychiatry where substantive interests dovetail with a great number of fields of interest, such as community organization, political science, occupational psychiatry, and applied anthropology, and where methods derive from such diverse disciplines as social psychology and biology. It is for this reason that efforts must be made to organize important material from the expanding literature into some meaningful and useful form.

Several criteria were used in selecting the papers for this volume. First, of course, was their overall value in providing perspective on the questions, methods, trends, and new developments in social psychiatry and relevant disciplines. This criterion was established with the aim of facilitating, in one volume, the ready accessibility of these papers for those interested in social psychiatry.

More important than the interests of specialists, however, are those of medical students, residents, physicians, and those in auxiliary and related disciplines for whom a broad perspective and acquaintance with the aims and practices of social psychiatry is becoming increasingly important. In this sense, it is hoped that the volumes in this series will be used both for teaching purposes and as guidebooks while new issues and programs unfold in social psychiatry. With these considerations in mind, a second criterion used in selecting papers was that they be sufficiently well written to be comprehensible and stimulating to the nonspecialist.

It is extremely difficult to delineate satisfactorily all the diverse and multiple developments in the field of social psychiatry in recent years. Furthermore, to select the important contributions in the field for but three years is a formidable task. The literature is vast, and much of it reflects not only new developments, but also those begun in previous years. Given these limitations, we have selected, without attempting to be comprehensive, articles representing major trends, developments and viewpoints that were written in English and published in 1965 and 1967. The wider range of views and activities will, we hope, be gradually encompassed in subsequent volumes. To ensure wider coverage of developments in other parts of the world, we have established an international advisory board to assist in the selection of articles in subsequent volumes. We are especially fortunate to have their cooperation in this undertaking.

The preparation of this volume was supported by the Cornell Program in Social Psychiatry. Special thanks are due to Mrs. Ginger Ochsner, who assisted with the selection of articles and editorial work, and to the Payne Whitney Clinic librarians, Miss Mary Andresen and Mrs. Miriam Weissman who so generously gave their time in helping us to obtain the numerous articles and books from which the present ones were selected.

ARI KIEV

Social Psychiatry

Volume I

Introduction

ARI KIEV

SOCIAL PSYCHIATRY IS CONCERNED FUNDAMENTALLY WITH THE interrelationships between the sociocultural environment and the individual. While recognizing the contribution of heredity, physiology, and psychodynamic factors to the individual's personality and psychopathology, it focuses attention upon the impact of human environment on the individual and the effect of the individual on the environment. It is also concerned with the way in which environment affects form, distribution, frequency, treatment, management, and perpetuation of psychiatric disorders. It pursues these questions with the strategies and tools of such diverse disciplines as anthropology, sociology, social psychology, and epidemiology.

Much of the concern of social psychiatry has been in assessing the pathogenetic significance of broad social currents such as migration, acculturation, industrialization, poverty, discrimination, and automation. More recently with the hope of gaining new insights by focusing on the mechanisms involved in the interaction between social and psychological phenomena, attention has turned to more microscopic and experimentally manipulable situations such as sensory deprivation, the pathological family, and specialized hospital situations.

The methods of social psychiatry reflect its concern with the assessment of the individual and his environment. This, in its simplest form, entails a thorough psychobiological inventory of an individual, his life history and his total life situation. Such an inventory utilizes not only psychological testing, but also utilizes the clinical skills of the psychiatrist and, perhaps, those of the anthropologist or sociologist familiar with the ramifications of the patient's environment. These techniques are modified and diluted when one moves beyond the identified case in the clinic to the unidentified and subclinical cases that must be located in the community with the aid of case records, agency records, community leaders, and screening inventories. As the net is widened, one must rely on less definitive techniques, fewer skilled assessors, and, finally, less certainty about the representativeness of the population under study.

Research Obstacles

Investigators in social psychiatry labor under numerous handicaps. The lack of adequate, comprehensive case-finding techniques and objective diagnostic criteria are most prominent. In addition, investigators encounter problems in assessing attitudes towards the mentally ill. Patterns of hospital utilization often reflect not only the availability of beds, but also the attitudes, irrational fears, and traditional customs of populations and their physicians.

The specification of the environmental variables similarly becomes increasingly complex as inquiry extends beyond the clinic. The opportunities to comprehend the totality of an environment that are afforded those dealing with small and closed societies, become faint utopian wishes that can never be realized.

Methodological issues gradually predominate over interesting substantive questions as the study reaches beyond the confines of the self-selected and sometimes "captive" clinic population. Thus, the key problems in social psychiatry become increasingly the development of valid, reliable methods of measurement and the selection of population subgroups for study.

The complexity of studying the frequency and distribution of psychiatric disorders in particular in any community is underlined by the above as well as by the diversity of conclusions reached by various investigators. Most studies have been inconclusive because of methodological inadequacies. For example, without knowing hospital usage patterns, the number of untreated cases, and the kinds of alternative facilities or treatment methods available to a given population, those undertaking hospital studies have been unable to draw definite conclusions about the actual number of cases at a given time and the rate of inception of new cases at a given time.

Other problems in research occur when one compares various studies, for one is limited by the use of different criteria, of different definitions of psychological and demographic variables, and of different methods of investigation. Then, too, deciding just what constitutes a case is often particularly difficult. If only illness with conspicuous clinical manifestations is counted, many cases, such as the milder cases of schizophrenia, are lost. Other problems arise when one has to decide on the basis of time of occurrence of symptoms, which cases to include. For example, one must decide whether or not to count as cases those who have improved or recovered.

Case Registers

The value of comprehensive bookkeeping systems for solving some of the above problems has been demonstrated for a number of years in Scandinavia. Large scale epidemiological studies, especially those dependent upon follow-up, have been facilitated by national case registries of psychiatric patients and parish or municipal registration of in-and-out migrants. A case in point is Hagnell's recent survey of the "Lundby" population in Sweden studied ten years earlier by Essen-Moller.[1] Hagnell was personally able to interview 2,273 of the 2,550 survivors of the earlier investigation.

The increased use of the high speed computer has encouraged the development of comprehensive case registers of psychiatric patients in this country, the best known comprehensive registers are in Maryland and in Monroe County, New York.[2] Information on the age, sex, race, residence, diagnosis, mental state, and such in the records of patients admitted to psychiatric hospitals and outpatient departments are regularly recorded and provide much information on the working of the health services.

From such a register of information much can be gained. It is possible to obtain patterns of admission and readmission to hospitals and outpatient departments, characteristics of patients with recurrent hospitalizations, unduplicated hospital and patient utilization rates, and information about the special needs of particular diagnostic and population subgroups. By characterizing the patient population, one can more effectively determine the need for new facilities. Both retrospective studies of social factors such as events leading to psychiatric treatment, and prospective studies of the community adjustment of discharged patients are facilitated. Where good census data are available on the population, it is possible to compare samples of the patient population with the nonpatient population in terms of demographic and social factors, such as household composition, employment, medical care, and child care. The establishment of record linkage systems between the various medical and social agencies in the community will make possible the examination of the range of facilities used by selected groups of patients. It will also be possible to make more comprehensive studies of natural histories of various psychiatric illnesses.

Most importantly, etiological hypotheses can be formulated,

distinguishing between groups exposed to certain events and those not exposed to these events. Such studies are particularly valuable if the specific causes of the events are known. Knowledge of this sort is often particularly valuable, for one can follow cases that develop and study the natural history of the disease. Supplementary investigation may also be carried out to determine how groups of people are exposed to these causative factors and how these causative factors are distributed in the population. One can undertake such investigations by the use of epidemiological methods long ago established in the study of infectious diseases.

Community Surveys

A number of investigators have recently focused on the distribution and prevalence of psychiatric disorders in nonhospitalized populations. The results of several such long-term investigations in general medical settings have been reported in the past several years. Hare and Shaw found no marked differences between the mental health of those who had moved to a new housing estate and those who had remained in the older district; this is an important finding in view of the previously held notion that on new housing estates mental health is often poor.[3] Studying a large number of general practices in London, Shepherd and his co-workers found a total prevalence rate of 140 per 1,000 persons at risk and an inception rate of 52 per 1,000 at risk, for all types of psychiatric disorders combined—these figures "place psychiatric illness among the commoner causes of consultation in general practice."[4]

To plan for more effective preventive and action programs, other surveys have sought to determine rate differences in different population subgroups or ecological zones. Such surveys have often suggested lines for subsequent etiological studies.

In their assessment of psychiatric morbidity many clinicians have been critical of survey instruments that focus on selected symptom patterns rather than on specific psychiatric diagnoses. Unfortunately since it has been difficult to engage sufficient numbers of psychiatrists in field-interviewing one is unable to rely on perhaps the most sensitive of instruments, a psychiatric interview by a trained psychiatrist. For the study of the epidemiology of symptoms, there may be, however, considerable value in such instruments. Indeed symptoms may not be distributed in the population in accord with the distribution of diagnostic groupings; instead, they may be present in the absence of significant clinical conditions and, moreover, in conditions with which they are not traditionally associated. Since symptoms may be learned and thus affected by social and cultural factors, they may have a particular epidemiology of their own and may be studied from the point of their distribution in given populations. A consideration of ways for improving case-finding methods for assessing symptoms is particularly urgent at the present time. For example, the National Health Survey has an ongoing survey, but utilizes no psychiatric questions.[5] It would be of great value to be able to incorporate certain questions into the National Health Survey to determine the distribution and prevalence of particular symptoms throughout the United States or throughout various subgroups of the population.

Much still remains to be learned of the response bias of different subgroups to screening inventories; measures of the intensity and duration of these symptoms must be established. There also is a need to develop valid and reliable questions regarding other psychiatric phenomena such as schizoid and paranoid thinking and the behavior disorders. Such questions are not included in most of the screening instruments now in use. Validation of different patterns of responsiveness to different questions and a method of distinguishing psychiatric symptoms from what might be considered reasonable adaptations to modern life are other areas in need of study.

Social Change and Mental Illness

An important question that has intrigued social psychiatrists for years concerns the psychological disruptive effects of social change. The recent work of the Cornell groups in both Nigeria and Nova Scotia has been of considerable interest. They have both found that the prevalence of psychiatric disorders was reduced in a previously surveyed area that over time had become more socioculturally integrated. Speaking at a meeting on psychiatric epidemiology and mental health planning in Maryland in 1966, Leighton said:

> A disintegrated community is basically one that is no longer a community, being crippled with regard to most of the processes upon which group survival depends. Their general property is manifest in a plurality of specific malfunctions such as defective communication among the members of the group; lack of leadership and followership; inability to arrive at group decisions; defective child rearing, training and education; deficiencies in work and productivity; lack of reactions and weak control of hostile impulses.
>
> The importance for mental health is that epidemiological research reveals a much higher prevalance of psychiatric disorders in the disintegrated groups than in others. This is probably a good example of multiple factors at work, much as was the case with regard to typhus in Upper Silesia. It is also very likely that the relationship of behavior, mental health, and sociocultural disintegration is reciprocal—each to some extent causing the other. There are, however, theoretical reasons and some evidence to suggest that raising and

lowering the level of disintegration can raise and lower the prevalence of psychiatric disorders. In one particular instance, under study a community was seen to change over a ten year period from an extreme of disintegration to a level of integration that approaches its regional average. The fact that mental health moved clearly in the predicted direction suggests that sociocultural disintegration is a salient cause of psychiatric disorder.[6]

Community Psychiatry

Progress in improving research methodologies and in gaining "hard" data has encouraged the development of numerous new programs in community psychiatry. The Community Mental Health Center Act of 1964 allocated $150 million for the construction of new treatment facilities throughout the country—the ultimate goal being the construction of 1000 community mental health centers. Since that time, a number of programs have been undertaken.

The new atmosphere in the United States has encouraged many to look at various pragmatic programs to care for large numbers of people. Attention has been focused on the experience of the Soviet Union, for example, where an elaborate asylum system never developed and where the emphasis has been instead on outpatient clinics, sheltered workshops, and domiciliary visits that provide specialized care.[7] Different techniques in use in other countries are also of relevance to community psychiatry. The mental welfare officer of the United Kingdom, who is duly authorized to seek out disturbed patients in the community and arrange hospital admission for them, is a type of person who might usefully be developed in our own society where the physician, to arrange for the temporary observation of disturbed patients, must frequently rely on the police force. The use of the family and the native healer as key supports in the village treatment system in Abeokuta, Nigeria suggests still other resources that might usefully be adapted.[8]

Storefront psychiatry utilizing indigenous or neighborhood personnel in "first aid stations" linked to mental health clinics at Lincoln Hospital in the Bronx is one novel approach that has been successfully developed. Crisis intervention along the lines of the program in Amsterdam, Holland is yet another approach that is being developed.[9] Additional approaches include the use of mental health aides, neighborhood service centers, mental health counsellors, housewives, student volunteers, day hospitals, night hospitals, and rehabilitation centers.[10]

Increased contact with impoverished groups in new treatment settings has also had a significant impact on traditional concepts of psychotherapy and has led to renewed interest in short-term psychotherapy, group therapies and various forms of supportive influence. The psychotherapist's value system has been seen as having major significance in his selection of cases, his style of treatment, and his treatment objectives.

The initial impetus for the developments came from the dramatic successes obtained with the new psychopharmaceuticals and the open door revolution in psychiatry in England. The resulting progress underscored the harmful effects of long-term hospitalization and the beneficial effects of community based and continuous care.

Attention is now being shifted to a careful consideration of the question as to whether these new facilities will really make obsolete the need for a state hospital system for custodial care or whether they will simply provide care for new groups of patients attracted to newer, closer, and more pleasant clinics. The questions also arise as to whether sufficient personnel will be available for such centers and whether the paramedical auxiliaries who are already functioning in some settings will be adequate substitutes for psychiatrists.

Burden on the Community

A number of investigators have begun to examine the magnitude of the problem involved in caring for the mentally ill at home, i.e., the burden on the community. In Brown's recent study, the key relatives of 29 per cent of first admitted patients and 60 per cent of previously admitted patients who were not in hospitals at the time, attributed one or more current problems, such as poor health and economic hardship, to having the patient at home.[11] Although the most severely disturbed patients (28 per cent of those who were at home) were causing severe distress, they were well tolerated by parents. Parents often made little complaint even when they felt great distress, and a number developed skilled methods of managing disturbed behavior and subtly adjusted their expectations of the patient. The overall impression was that most patients who were neither hospitalized nor severely disturbed showed signs of remarkably little strain, even when they were unemployed. The one exception to this, however, was during periods when their condition relapsed.

In a recent study of 410 families with a mentally ill member, Sainsbury and Grad found that two-thirds of the families had recognizable problems that they attributed to the patient's illness and that one-fifth had a burden that they rated as severe.[12] More than one-half ascribed symptoms of emotional disturbance to worrying about the patient, while one-fifth of them attributed neurotic symptoms such as insomnia, headaches, irritability, and depression to concern about the patient's behavior. Social and leisure time activities were restricted in a third of the families and children were adversely affected in a third. Twenty-nine percent had their domestic routine upset. A quarter of the families had their income reduced by at least 10 percent, and 9 percent of the families had their income cut to less than half its usual level.

Three to five weeks after referral to community or hospital care, the burden on families had decreased significantly. Chichester (community) had a reduced burden in 62 percent and Salisbury (hospital) in 61 percent of the families. When the whole sample was analyzed, 44 percent of the families in whom any adverse effect had been recorded were relieved in Salisbury and 35 percent in Chichester. While the relief in different diagnostic groups was not significantly greater in one service than in the other, patients with depression did cause more hardship if they were treated in the community than if they were treated in the hospital. In spite of the community service's admitting 50 percent fewer patients, the overall burden on the family one month after referral was not reduced significantly more in one service than the other, except for certain types of patients and certain social circumstances where home care left the family with more problems.

In a recent study Pasamanick found that when the family was economically disadvantaged, the burden of the patient's illness was even greater and often led to a reluctance to accept patient's return home after short periods of hospitalization.[13] Pasamanick's study also showed that among state hospital patients there was from intake to the sixth month, a significant lessening of patient's problems; after this period of time there was, however no significant lessening. Once the more acute symptoms and signs which primarily contribute to the perception of the patient in the household as a burden, had been relieved, there was little possibility of other gain. There were no significant differences between the two categories of patients —ambulatory and state hospital—nor, within the home treatment group, between the drug and placebo cases. The "significant others" on an item-by-item basis indicated that they were hard pressed by the demands of having a sick patient at home—they expressed greatest concern in regard to the welfare of the patient and household, the physical strain imposed, the patient's need of an excessive amount of attention, the bodily symptoms and complaints of the patient, and the patient odd ideas and speech.

Rogler and Hollingshead in a study of schizophrenic families in Puerto Rico, described a heavy burden on the mentally healthy spouse in terms of sexual tensions, and domestic chaos, moreover, their findings indicate that when the wife is the patient, there is additional stress upon the children.[14] More specifically they found that schizophrenia in husband or wife impairs a husband's capacity to provide for his family. Conflict with the spouse over economic hardships occurs, however, only when the wife is schizophrenic. They also found that:

> Organized patterns of cooperation between relatives observable in the well families break down in the sick families. Sick persons are not woven into closely knit family groups that include both sets of relatives. The problems experienced by a person's own relatives are not referred to his in-laws for solution. The husband-schizophrenic families are drawn into the wife's family group and away from the husband's. In families with sick wives, each person turns to his family or origin for emotional support. Thus, the conflict and isolation rupture the extended families of sick persons.[15]

A number of other studies of the post-discharge experiences of mental patients make inferences about the observed differential adjustment of patients in different family settings, in terms of differing role expectations that exist within these varied settings.[16] It is assumed that conjugal families are less burdensome and less burdened than are parental families—but no data has been forthcoming to demonstrate observed differences in these settings. On the basis of general cultural ideas about normal behavior, certain assumptions are made to explain some of the findings, but no data are yet available to document patterns in normal homes.

Thus recent investigations raise many important questions.

Is the burden on the family related to the severity of the disorder? Is it something that fluctuates with the clinical state of the patient as Wing and Grad have suggested, or is it related to certain long-standing structural features of the family that make it unable to tolerate extremes of behavior? Are there important social class and cultural factors that bear directly on the extent to which the burden is perceived, tolerated, and managed?

The recent investigations provide a number of leads for further research. In view of the finding that the patient is more of a burden where economic problems already exist, it appears to be important that future investigators establish controls for this and other socioeconomic variables that may influence the results of such inquiries. In addition, in view of the difficulty of distinguishing subjective complaints about the patient from the objective burden on the family, it would be more useful to focus on general patterns of family life than on problems directly associated with the patient, for a focus upon the patient alone tends to heavily weight the data with subjective accounts of distress. This more general approach has been found useful in current investigations of patterns of perception of household roles and tasks in "psychotic" and "normal" families, and in Brown and Rutter's study of the children of disturbed parents.

Social Breakdown Syndrome

Recent studies of the social breakdown syndrome have also indicated that the severe patterns of social disability associated with psychiatric disorders are the very kinds of things that lead people to come to the hospital. The social breakdown syndrome that is characterized by withdrawal, anger, and hostility, all associated with varying degrees of severe destruction of the affected person's social relationships, was first described by the Program Area Committee on Mental Health of the American Public Health Association, and cited as a major target for public health and preventive measures.[17]

The social breakdown syndrome has much heuristic value for psychiatry insofar as it focuses on the disability in psychiatric disorders as distinct from the illnesses themselves. It also suggests a number of important and objectively measurable questions about the natural history of psychiatric disorders, both in the hospital and in the community, in addition to the fact that it suggests questions about the patterns of social performance in the different disorders. It reminds us that we must learn more about the spontaneous recovery rate of untreated psychiatric patients, about the various social and cultural, as well as psychiatric, factors contributing to disability, and about the extent of disability in psychiatric patients from cultures with different attitudes towards the mentally ill. Although the manifestations of social breakdown appear to occur most frequently in chronic hospitalized schizophrenics, this group is not the only group affected. We must know more about such patterns in the psychoneurotic, psychopathic and depressive disorders, furthermore, we must know how disability is manifested in different age and sex groups. This knowledge is particularly important, for the prognostic significance of the different disorders is likely to change with the advent of new treatments. Indeed much remains to be done to assess the relative contributions of new medicines and new attitudes to the prevention and modification of psychiatric disability.

The Developing Countries

A word is in order about the implications of these new developments for the countries of the third or developing world. These countries contain rapidly expanding populations and have little hope of adequate resources or personnel to handle now, or in the future, the psychosocial disorders that predictably should increase as industrialization and urbanization are progressively introduced. Given these conditions, it is imperative that approaches be developed that multiply the effects of limited existing psychiatric resources through increased use of technological and personnel resources not now in use.

The psychopharmaceuticals have created new opportunities for the community mental health center form of treatment in these countries. They have provided a rapid, effective, and inexpensive way to treat many patients on an outpatient basis and to reduce the time spent in hospitals. Use of medicines can be effectively taught to general practitioners, who are often the first to encounter the psychiatric patients. The monitoring of symptomatology, side effects, and dosage requirements can be taught to various types of paramedical personnel such as nurses, social workers, and occupational therapists.

There are undoubtedly other models yet to be developed that will extend the range of the physician's network; one example is closed circuit TV networks between hospital units and satellite clinics in underpopulated rural areas. It will also be valuable to find ways of integrating new programs with school or factory programs to reduce the costs and maximize the use of existing personnel and bookkeeping practices.

Much attention has been paid to the role of culture in the development of personality; values; culture-bound syndromes such as koro, latah, amok, and windigo; and the role of culture in influencing the incidence and prevalence of disease in various societies. Further cross-cultural inquiries should prove valuable in differentiating the universal features of psychiatric disorders from those features or symptoms which are culturally determined. Cross-cultural differences in the symptoms of schizophrenia are a case in point. In a worldwide questionnaire survey conducted by Wittkower and Murphy of McGill University, Indian schizophrenic patients were commonly reported to be catatonically rigid and negativistic, often displaying stereotyped movements; Southern Italian patients were typically aggressive and expressive. African patients, on the other hand, showed a tendency to be quieter than those of the Western world.[18] The withdrawal of Indian schizophrenics was seen to relate to the formal, hierarchical Indian culture that has high regard for introversion and emotional control. The barrenness of the clinical picture in preliterate Africans was tied to the paucity of their culture and intellectual resources and their difficulties in dealing with abstractions.

More important than these reported differences that suggest a tie-in between symptoms and culture, was the finding that four of twenty-six symptoms and signs were consistently reported as characteristics of schizophrenia in these various societies. These were social and emotional withdrawal, auditory hallucinations, delusions, and flatness of affect. These findings suggest that there are nuclear features of the illness of schizophrenia that are not culturally determined and that may be distinguished from culturally determined symptoms.

Interest in the etiological role of social and cultural factors in psychiatric disorders leads to a consideration of incidence and prevalence rates in the developing countries. In most developing areas, it is difficult to ascertain information such as age and sex of the total population. Without such simple census information it is extremely difficult to know what the actual rates are for a given population and therefore impossible to compare adequately rates for two different groups, even within the same country.

Two major international efforts currently underway are Program B of the World Health Organization and the study of diagnosis of mental disorders in the United Kingdom and the United States. These studies are being undertaken by a joint team of investigators from the Maudsley Hospital in London and Columbia University in New York. These teams are concerned with the development of methods and instruments for case identification that can be used meaningfully and reliably in different cultural settings. These studies are primarily methodological ones and may, in time, provide instruments of some usefulness to large scale epidemiological studies.

Animal Studies

Social psychiatry has obvious links with new trends in services, family studies of schizophrenia, and psychopharmacology. It has a less obvious relationship to ecological and ethological studies of animal behavior.

What is the relevance of the recent animal studies to social psychiatry? Harlow's experimental deprivation of monkeys, Calhoun's work on "behavioral 'sinks,' " and other such studies provide new perspective on certain characteristics of group behavior in all species, including man.[19]

A case in point is Lorenz's work on aggression.[20] According to Lorenz, species inclined to bond formation exhibit the most aggression. As the capacity for affective bonds increases so, too, does the capacity for destructive emotions toward these same objects. This notion is consistent with knowledge of transference and with data on homicide victims who are in the great percentage of cases related to their murderers.

According to Lorenz, man has no built-in inhibitory mechanism for handling his aggressive impluses as do a number of carnivorous species. Unlike the wolf, man cannot bare his neck to his attacker to set in motion or release some built-in inhibitory mechanism of the attacker's aggression. Man has only his reason to use for defensive purposes or for the threat of counteraggression.

These observations and speculations suggest the importance of a search for new ways to channel those aggressive instincts that cannot be contained by biological mechanisms.

The excitement attendant upon these ethological studies has

distracted attention from ecological studies that clarify relationships among the levels of organization of functions, the changing environmental requirements, and the way animals and humans behave. The study of caged animals may help us to understand the behavior of long-term institutionalized mental hospital patients who also live in conditions of limited space and arousal. Zoo animals have long been known to exhibit stereotyped movements when chained or too narrowly confined. Thus in captivity, bears will constantly nod, elephants move their heads back and forth, tigers trot back and forth, and hyenas make figure eights. The parallels to the regressive behavior of some mental patients are too striking to ignore and suggest the value of further experimental work on both animals and humans in altering space and arousal dimensions of various living situations.

As the world population rapidly explodes beyond the upper limits of the technological resources necessary to sustain it, it appears reasonable to ask whether this rate of increase will be controlled through the operations of factors similar to those that limit population in the animal world. There are species that automatically reduce their reproductive and sexual activity when conditions of crowding develop. Patterns of territoriality and pecking order also probably contribute to the regulation of numbers in the animal world and may have relevance for mankind as well.

Data on territoriality among animals has also added a new dimension to our understanding of identification. An instinctual need for territory may account for much of the difficulty encountered by immigrants, especially those who do not retain those traditional symbolic rituals that bind them in spirit to a homeland—this need is no doubt related to the great incidence of disorder among those who too rapidly (and hence unsuccessfully) attempt to acculturate themselves to new lands.

The recent work of Calhoun and others challenges the notion of fixed instinctual or imprinting patterns. Experimental changes in environment have produced marked shifts in behavior of some animals. The same species of animal may learn different things at different times in the course of its development. The kind of learning an animal does and the role this learning plays for the animal are, in part, dependent on the situation in which the animal learns. Thus Calhoun's notion of a learned self-cycling mechanism in lemmings emphasizes that environmental influences operate in progressive stages and that previous experiences play a role in determining how the behavior of an animal will develop. Such a mechanism may not only not operate for all species, but also it may not operate for all of a given species. This view is supported by the fact that lemmings in different locales adjust to population densities by different behaviors.

Whether or not humans behave more like lemmings than like other species, the concept of ecological traps proposed by Calhoun has much heuristic value in examining human situations. One need only turn attention to the crowded urbanizing areas of the developing countries to see such traps being set up daily, where migration from rural areas to cities depletes the rural working force and produces large overcrowded urban slums. These slums are effectively behavioral sinks with their high rates of morbidity, delinquency, and technological unemployment, and they invariably parasitize the economy of the country and slow its development.

PART I

Social Psychiatry: Definitions and Parameters

Introduction

THE ARTICLES IN THIS FIRST SECTION HAVE BEEN SELECTED because of their value in outlining the range of activities encompassed by social psychiatry. As Ruesch notes, studies in social psychiatry are concerned with the structure of the community, the significance of groups, individual functioning, and the mechanics of communication. Thus legal, military, educational, governmental, religious, and hospital institutions are all relevant areas for concern and may be approached through disciplines such as sociology and anthropology, which concentrate on describing social organizations, and epidemiology and ecology, which concentrate on the distribution and frequency of various disorders within social environments. There is room too, for focus on preventive measures and techniques for influencing legislatures, social organizations, and social institutions.

Bell and Spiegel review the history of social psychiatry and add further perspective to the evolving nature of the field that continues to be concerned with three major etiological questions: to what extent is mental illness caused by the stresses of the social environment, to what extent are social problems caused by psychiatric problems, and, to what extent are both mental illness and social problems the result of interaction of both.

In the last decade, social psychiatry has benefited from increasing cross-fertilization with the social sciences. A case in point is the insightful article by Zusman, a psychiatrist who discusses sociological approaches useful in understanding and treating mental illness. The sociologist studies mental illness as a social phenomenon. This is exemplified by the process of labeling. According to Zusman, attitudes towards the mentally ill may reinforce existing symptoms or produce new ones. Labeling someone as mentally ill (when he might only be temporarily manifesting certain symptoms in an intolerable situation) sets up a situation of expectancies for the individual that may lead to his permanent adoption of the role of mentally ill.

Most important is the notion that some psychiatric illnesses are the product of social forces that operate upon a person in a self-fulfilling way. The individual who is treated as if he is disturbed may increasingly become disturbed. While further investigations should look at whether this process occurs only in susceptible individuals, there is evidence that much of the disability associated with chronic psychiatric disorders is the result of faulty management of the symptoms of social deterioration such as withdrawal, negativism, incontinence, self-destructiveness, and apathy. These behavioral patterns therefore may not be indicative of schizophrenia or chronic psychiatric disorders, but rather may be secondary symptoms grafted onto the underlying disorder by social and interpersonal factors in certain hospital settings.

Chapter 1

Social Psychiatry

An Overview

JURGEN RUESCH

PSYCHIATRY DEFINITELY HAS PASSED THROUGH ITS INFANCY and, after a somewhat hectic adolescence, has come of age. Signs of maturity can be observed in many ways. While at the beginning of the century Kraepelin, Bleuler, Freud, and Jung still hoped to find universal laws of normal and abnormal functioning, contemporary psychiatrists have become more cautious. Id psychology has been replaced by ego psychology; the search for universal dream symbolism and for the collective unconscious has given way to phenomenological and existential approaches.[1] The bitter disagreements about high-level theories and dogma are on the wane, and what remain are personal and organizational rivalries of professionals. Furthermore, the shrinkage of space and the spread of science over the four corners of the earth have cautioned psychiatrists not to generalize from small samples or from local conditions. The period of sweeping generalizations is over, and the field has become more pragmatic and relativistic, and the psychiatrist more modest.

The life cycle of a discipline follows a well-established pattern.[2] First, there are the casual observations that induce scientists to declare that there is a topic worthy of further exploration. Once the subject has been identified, a period follows in which observations are systematically collected and an attempt is made to arrive at some empirical generalizations. The really exciting phase of a discipline arrives when the basic discoveries are made. If hypnotherapy went through this phase in the second part of the 19th century and psychoanalysis at the turn of the century, social psychiatry has reached this stage of development in the 1960's. Once the generalizations are worked out, there come the founding of associations, the organization of conventions, and the establishment of university chairs and departments. In these stages, scientists concentrate upon refining their theoretical systems and on improving their methods.[3] As the university teachers formalize training, the students have to wade through established curricula, stand for exams, and obtain degrees. Once they have complied with all these demands, they are usually admitted to membership in the established organizations or they are licensed by the state. This type of institutionalization contributes to the stagnation of the field until a new discovery revolutionizes thinking or a younger and more pertinent discipline displaces the old field altogether.

At the present time, psychiatry is developing in three distinct directions. In the area of psychological psychiatry fragmented studies of thinking, feeling, or dreaming and speculation about what goes on inside the person have been replaced by an attempt to understand the individual's total experience. In the domain of biological psychiatry, which received a great boost from advances in electronics, biochemistry, and pharmacology, the focus has veered away from anatomical and physiological studies of the central nervous system and toward considerations of the organism as a whole as exemplified in studies of sleep, food, and sensory deprivation. Social psychiatry, finally, focuses upon the structure of the community, the significance of the group for the individual, and the mechanics of communication. Although each of these major directions has its own theories and methodologies, the subspecialties are no longer separated into air tight compartments, and information from neighboring fields is permitted to seep in. In keeping with the trends of the time, universities now have departments of behavioral science comprising psychology, sociology, economics, and anthropology, and departments of molecular biology including biochemistry and genetics. And departments of psychiatry are made up of psychological, biological, and social subdivisions. The last is the youngest and newest, and perhaps deserves special consideration.[4]

What Is Social Psychiatry?

According to Leighton,[5] social psychiatrists engage in a variety of activities that are related to but not identical with those of the clinical psychiatrists. The social psychiatrist deals with the law,[6] the military,[7] education,[8] industry,[9] government,[10] religion,[11] hospitals,[12] and other social institutions that are concerned with health. But social psychiatry is not unified by a set of activities[13] as much as by a point of view.

1. *The Sociological and Anthropological View.*—This is exemplified in the study of social functions of people and institutions participating in psychiatric transactions.[14] In these studies the uninvolved observer does not wish to alter the existing situation and he simply describes social organizations and values as he sees them.

2. *The Epidemiological and Ecological Point of View.*—More specifically medical, this approach attempts to relate the overall social and environmental conditions to the occurrence of disorders of behavior.[15] The observer is somewhat more involved in that he has to pass a judgment on who is sick and who is well and how illness relates to the social setting.

3. *The Preventive Point of View.*—The steering of legislatures, organizations, and institutions towards action designed to further mental health requires personal commitment and political know-how on the part of the participants. Rarely are

data on mental health so self-evident that they need not be backed by unfaltering conviction.[16]

4. *The Therapeutic Point of View.*—The social management of patients, ex-patients, would-be patients, and their relatives requires medical, psychotherapeutic, and group therapeutic skills. In the therapeutic situation the psychiatrist is no longer an observer but an operator who wishes to bring about certain changes in individual as well as group behavior.[17]

The *information* that the social psychiatrist seeks refers to the following:

> First, to the characteristics of the persons participating in a social situation in terms of their age, sex, occupation, education, cultural orientation, expectations, and skills.
>
> Second, to the context which governs their interaction. The context defines the nature of the situation, specifies the prevailing rules, and lists the rewards that are available, and the opportunities and limitations for action.
>
> Third, to the processes of communication and physical action that interconnect the participants.

The *abstractions* used in social psychiatry, which invariably refer to two or more people in interaction with one another,[18] indicate that the field is characterized by a point of view rather than by the nature of its operations. The focus of study is not, as in psychoanalysis, the intrapsychic events or the consideration of an individual in isolation from others[19] but the social process that connects person with person and person with large-scale events. Such interaction does not take place in a vacuum but occurs in a specific context that significantly influences whatever people do with each other. A context may be described in situational terms—combat, funeral, or classroom—where the participants are all in one place; or it may be embodied in a system characterized by the sharing of values or the participation in social organizations. In this latter case, the members are scattered but nonetheless interconnected over distance and time. The context thus pinpoints the membership in a group, indicates the roles[20] and functions that the participants may assume, and specifies the game that is to be played. Scientifically speaking, the context defines the parameters of the system; pragmatically speaking, it furnishes the participants with a frame of reference.

The aims of social psychiatry do not include the development of simplified, straight-line generalizations. When psychologists generalize about intelligence and ability, or psychoanalysts about the nature of the ego, they imply that the feature in question is present all the time. When sociologists generalize about urban or rural societies, they again imply ever-present characteristics. The social psychiatrist's emphasis, in contrast, is directed at establishing under what conditions and at what times certain features appear or disappear. The "lock and key" analogy of modern enzyme theory, which indicates how certain variables fit together, is also applicable to the theories of social psychiatry. The match of character to situation, personality type to type of context, individual to group, group to physical environment, and endogenous characteristics to external circumstances determine the level of functioning. Knowledge concerning the "who," "with whom," "when," "where," and "in pursuit of what," all embedded in a general pattern, constitutes the basis for therapeutic intervention.

Areas of Inquiry

Social psychiatry is the issue of the union of social disciplines with psychiatry. The original contributions of the parent disciplines are still visible: social science and psychoanalysis offered theories; clinical medicine contributed somatic therapies; medical psychology added empirical generalizations; nursing introduced personal care; social work emphasized economics and group functioning; public health and epidemiology added the preventive point of view. All of these approaches have contributed to the understanding of mental health and to the development of psychiatric treatment methods.[21]

But if we wish to advance social psychiatry as a field, we cannot be content with individual skill or speculative interpretations. We have to collect a cumulative body of knowledge. Although up to now the scientific method has yielded little useful information about mental disease, we nonetheless have to continue the search. Perhaps we have used the wrong methods. Scientific analysis is based upon the breaking up of complex events into smaller and smaller units, and in the course of this process the original pattern gets lost. The laws of physics and chemistry are based upon the observed mass effects of anonymous particles, their number being in the neighborhood of 10^{23}. The laws of the social sciences are based on the responses of people, their number being in the neighborhood of 10^4 to 10^7. The laws of the life sciences, including social psychology, animal psychology, and clinical psychiatry, are based on the observation of identified individuals, either alone or in smaller groups. Their number is in the neighborhood of 10^0 to 10^2. At the level of abstraction of the gas laws (10^{23}), individual contexts and variations of particles cancel each other out. At the level of abstraction of economics (10^4 to 10^7) contexts begin to matter and can be neglected only under certain circumstances. At the level of abstractions about people, either alone or in small groups (10^0 to 10^2), the contexts always influence the responses. Therefore social psychiatry supplements generalizations about the behavior of individuals and groups with information about contexts.

In contrast to the social scientist, who is inclined to study one aspect of behavior at a time—for example, roles, intelligence, or value orientations—the social psychiatrist investigates patterns. The emphasis upon patterns as opposed to single aspects is dictated by the necessity for remedial or preventive intervention. When professionals have to act they have to know all there is to be known at the moment of the intervention. Time and timing, therefore, is a dimension that all operating disciplines share in common and that distinguishes them from the basic sciences. It follows that when the social psychiatrist wishes to utilize information contributed by the nonapplied sciences he has to simplify the information and add a time dimension.

From the anthropologists the social psychiatrists learned the appreciation of preferences and *values*.[22] These are reflected in intellectual, scientific, and artistic products, in social organizations, or in action behavior.[23] Data on ethnic values[24] and social status[25] are most relevant for psychiatry because remedial help is the more effective the better it fits into the value orientation of the family.[26]

The investigation of *people* characterized by some feature in common has led to the study of age,[27] sex, social, occupational,[28] and recreational groupings. Although these people are distributed fairly evenly in the normal population, they become a problem when they emerge in large quantities, have difficulties in adaptation, or congregate as a group. As a result, disciplines such as geriatrics,[29] child psychiatry,[30] and criminology, including the study of delinquency,[31] have emerged.

The sociologists' studies of *social order*[32] led to investigations of agricultural, urban, primitive, technological, authoritarian, and democratic societies.[33] These sociological studies have opened our eyes to the fact that what was believed to be specific or pathological for one group could also be found in other groups and that measures that were effective in one group did not necessarily work in another. Again, it has not been proved conclusively that any kind of organization or society has a significantly higher rate of mental disease or that any kind of remedial organization is therapeutically more effective.[34]

A somewhat different emphasis is exemplified in the studies of *social and cultural change.*[35] Geographical mobility,[36] social mobility,[37] ethnic acculturation,[38] change of economic conditions[39]—all have been assumed to be a potential source of stress.[40] A quickening rate of change relative to the tolerance limits of the individual is in many instances associated with emotional instability or mental disease. But the tolerance limits for social change show great individual variation, and what causative role social change plays in the etiology of mental disease has not been clearly established.

Investigations of *small groups* such as families, military units, or gangs reasserted the observation that a group is held together by some feedback process, interference with which either strengthens the bonds or leads to disintegration.[41] The group to which an individual belongs apparently exerts a far more powerful influence than is commonly assumed.[42] Modern group therapists,[43] family therapists,[44] and military psychiatrists[45] all emphasize that if the patient can be kept within his group rehabilitation proceeds much faster.[46] As of today we must conclude that rehabilitation of the mentally ill over the long-term is a social rather than a psychological task. Apparently the specifics of the social situation in which the patient lives spell the difference between invalidism and functioning or hospitalization and living at home.[47]

Studies of *routine situations* have been concerned with the analysis of the mental hospital,[48] the prison,[49] the factory,[50] the ship, or the military situation. Recently the weekend, after-work hours, and vacations have come under scrutiny.[51] The lesson from these studies seems to point out three facts:

> First, that situational factors such as isolation, boredom, or fatigue are significant in contributing to nervous breakdowns.
>
> Second, that individual or group factors bearing upon motivation, skill, intelligence, or morale significantly

> may counteract the situationally or structurally unfavorable conditions.
>
> Third, that people's relationship to each other, or the "how" of communication, is usually more significant than the formal organization prevailing on the spot.[52]

Studies of *unusual situations* as they arise in disaster,[53] war, and famine, and under experimental conditions,[54] have indicated that quantitative deviations in intensity and timing of external stimuli can tax the tolerance limits of the individual to such an extent that he may break down.[55] These limits, however, vary somewhat with the individual's expectations on the one hand and his ties to the group on the other. Also it has become obvious that behavior during catastrophes[56] has many similarities with brainwashing procedures and religious conversion.[57] These findings raise some interesting questions. If behavior becomes disorganized and subsequently is most easily changed under extreme conditions, are we psychiatrists, with our pleasant, middle-of-the-road techniques, missing an opportunity to change behavior? Are other hospital and office techniques stabilizing the pathology of our patients, in part at least?

Communication and interaction have been studied under many different headings. Social perception, social learning, role interaction, language and codification, speech, networks of communication including the mass media of communication—all have come under observation.[58] The unit of study in all these approaches is the message and not the person.[59] In this manner, a message may be followed from its origin to its destination and the conditions that alter the message may be studied. For psychiatry, several conclusions are warranted:

> First, that verbal communication forms only part of man's transactions with man and that nonverbal communication and action are particularly relevant for the sick and for their rehabilitation.[60]

> Second, that interaction and communicative behavior seen over the short-term are not necessarily predictive of behavior over time.
>
> Third, that the way the communicative behavior of one person is matched to the communicative behavior of another person can become the source not only of satisfaction and frustration but also of social conflict and disorganized behavior.[61]

In matching character with situation or personality type with social organization it became obvious that certain *character features* manifest themselves in specific situations only. Compensation neuroses, for example, can only arise if there exists financial liability or insurance; and delinquency becomes rampant when unemployment or lack of leisure time activities idle the young.[62]

The epidemiology and ecology of mental disease,[63] formerly the province of public health, have become central concerns of social psychiatry.[64] The epidemiological approach enables us to ascertain where disease and dysfunction exist, to determine how many people are afflicted, and to check the effectiveness of therapeutic procedures. In this connection, the sociology of institutions and their way of procedure[65] have over and over been the subject of critical analysis. The data from epidemiology combined with the suggestions of insiders (psychiatrists) and the social criticism of outsiders (sociologists and social psychologists) today constitute one of the powerful steering mechanisms of the field of psychiatry.

The Social Therapies

The social therapies are based on a number of *observations and assumptions* that can be summarized as follows:

> 1. Man is a herd animal and distinct separation from the group is painful to him.

2. Every individual strives to prevent separation from the group at the same time that he attempts to remain a distinctly separate entity within the group.

3. The perception of excessive social differences between self and other people produces tension, indicating that the perceiver may be rejected as a member of this particular group.

4. Equalization of differences is achieved through:

(*a*) Selective and standardized exposure of people to things, persons, and situations, thereby giving them an equal opportunity of experience (training).

(*b*) Social interaction, thereby establishing correspondence of information and behavior (communicative exchange).

(*c*) Explanations which have to be shared to explain existing differences (interpretation).

(*d*) Coercive action, thereby threatening the individual in case of deviance (positive exclusion, imprisonment, hospitalization).

5. If differences cannot be resolved by any of the above methods, the ensuing tension usually gives rise to new group formations.

The social therapies are designed to alter existing conditions and they approach this task by influencing both the social system and the individual. The *social system* can be modified as follows:

By introducing new organizational structures or removing obsolete ones. Agencies, committees, associations, laws, and regulations can be created to take care of social needs as they arise.

By altering the networks of communication. The flow of messages, the place of decision-making, the checks and balances—all can be changed. This is a task of management.

By adapting treatment methods to the prevailing social order. Treatment methods can be adapted to fit the local political, economic, and ethnic values and practices.

The *individual* is approached with the following aims in mind:

> To increase his awareness of himself and of the ways he fits into the existing social and cultural patterns.
>
> To help him acquire communicative skills and the ability to get along with people.
>
> To help him abandon unnecessary assumptions which restrict his effectiveness.
>
> To influence his attitudes in the direction of understanding and tolerance of behavioral differences.

Social and individual efforts may be combined, always with an eye on the restitution of self-corrective processes. If this can be achieved without restructuring the group, all the better. But frequently an individual does not wish to remain a member of a given group, as might be the case with a schizophrenic or a rebel. Here the question arises as to whether the patient can find another suitable group, and often only patient or marginal groups will accept a sick individual. By working with both the patient and the new group, the psychiatrist can help each to learn to tolerate the other.

In practice, the social therapies are known under a number of different names:

> The concept of *community psychiatry*[66] refers to a complicated set of operations that are aimed at changing the attitudes and tolerance limits of a given group to insure the best treatment of their sick members. Once this goal has been achieved, psychiatric treatment methods and procedures can be adapted to that particular community (rural, metropolitan, military, industrial, college, etc.) and the necessary resources and facilities can be mobilized.[67]
>
> The term, *therapeutic community*,[68] refers to carefully managed relationships between patients and staff in an institutional setting, whereby the patients have time-

limited and often controlled contact with the area and the people surrounding the hospital.

Group therapy, group psychotherapy, analytic group psychotherapy,[69] and psychodrama all utilize the group setting for therapeutic purposes. Depending upon the particular methods, the main efforts are directed towards guidance, counseling, or lecturing, towards inspiration and exhortation, towards activity and play, or towards the acquisition of insight.

Family therapy involves the treatment of an entire family by the same or by different therapists.[70] The family members may be interacting with each other in the presence of the psychiatrist or the therapeutic team, or they may be seen separately.[71]

Occupational therapy and work, play, music, drama, or dance therapy are oriented towards skilled activities and personal expression whereby human interaction is subordinated to the physical task at hand.[72]

Social programming refers to the discussion of specific social tasks individually or in groups. Reduced to step-by-step operations, the technical aspects of how to get a job, how to behave at a social gathering, or what side effects to watch for when taking drugs can be taught to the patient and his relatives.[73]

The Psychiatrist as Arbiter of Mental Health

In every society the desirable and the undesirable social patterns are a matter of public knowledge. On the American scene, for example, early parental deprivation, maternal over-protection, broken families, repeated change of foster homes, authoritarianism, withdrawal, and dependence are mentioned among the undesirable patterns. But if one attempts to relate an early pattern—for example, material deprivation—to deviant behavior observed later in life,[74] one runs into methodological difficulties. The cause and effect relationship of any two behavior patterns that are separated by a span of 20 or 30 years cannot be demonstrated because of the enormous number of intervening factors.[75] Scientific proof therefore is usually missing and these relationships are better classified as hunches. Nobody, for example, has ever been able to show that an authoritarian family structure produces more deviant behavior than a democratic one. But in practice lay people and physicians treat hunches as if they were based upon scientific proof.

Behavior patterns at variance with cultural norms attract attention, and when they occur the social and medical disciplines are called upon to take charge. If the causes of certain conditions are known and effective remedial measures are available, the situation can be easily rectified; but if the causes are unknown and effective measures are not available, as in the case of schizophrenia or crime, people tend to turn to normative control. The first step towards normalization consists of inventing satisfactory explanations that will permit acceptance, toleration, or rejection of a given deviant pattern. While at one historical period these explanations may emanate from the church and at another from the state, at present this task has been assumed by psychologists, social scientists, and psychiatrists.

The explanation of abnormal behavior patterns is known also as interpretation. The psychiatrist's interpretative explanations serve to satisfy the patient's and the public's quest for certainty. Explanations, even if they prove to be false, appease anxiety; and contemporary explanations are just as effective as those given at the time of Hippocrates. Even if explanations given in 1960 will be considered archaic if not outright false a few decades from now, it would be foolish to deny their usefulness. It is likely that the therapeutic value of medical or psychiatric interpretations is not a function of their truth at all. If perceived differences in behavior create anxiety, people attempt to get together on the basis of explaining these differences. If agreement cannot be reached on the first level of explanation, higher order abstractions may bring about consensus. The feeling engendered by sharing explanations may be more relevant for social cohesiveness than the truth of the statement under discussion. In this sense, explanations have a leveling and normative influence upon the population.

But the normative role of social scientists and psychiatrists embodies certain dangers. Just as the political scientist has been accused of not being scientific but of reflecting the affairs of the day, so is the psychiatrist in danger of reflecting present sociopolitical trends. Through the process of reification, he mistakes conjecture for established scientific truth, and in so doing he really speaks as a normative agent and not as a scientific expert on mental health.

An example may illustrate the point. One hundred years ago the care of the aged presented no social problem because the elderly lived within the circle of the family, if indeed they reached the age to require care at all. But with increasing longevity, large-scale migration, the breaking up of families, and the trend towards small apartments, the care of the aged has become a national problem.[76] At present some overzealous organizers are inclined to separate the young, the middle aged, and the old in such a way that mutual identification and historical continuity are interfered with. The construction of retirement communities is motivated by financial profit and practical considerations. Nobody really knows whether old people fare better in homogeneous or in heterogeneous age groups, or whether society benefits from isolating the aged. But some professionals already have labeled these procedures as desirable and mentally healthy.[77]

Changing the ethics of human conduct or planning large-scale social reforms does not fall into the domain of social psychiatry. Neither collectively nor as individuals have psychiatrists been endowed with greater intelligence or characterized by more enlightenment than any other group of people. If, however, scientifically valid information points out a needed course of action, professional associations may take the initiative to bring about a change. But the task of social planning has to be shouldered by representatives of all occupations.

Summary

The elimination of infectious and deficiency diseases, the triumphs of surgery, and other advances in medicine have made it possible to prolong life and to maintain man as a kind of metabolic machine. Through a variety of verbal approaches, man's secret and unconscious desires, his thoughts, and his feelings were explored in the belief that increased knowledge of self improves the individual's ability to cope with his problems. To this basic tenet of the insight therapies has to be added the dictum of the social therapies: the more accurate and reliable information a person has about the physical and social setting and the more social skills he possesses, the more successful his actions become. If clinical medicine, psychiatry, psychoanalysis, and individual psychology aim at improving the individual's functioning, social psychiatry attempts to better the functioning of the group as a whole. This emphasis shifts the focus of therapy away from abnormal behavior and towards communication and interaction.

Theoretically speaking, the social psychiatrist does not attempt to develop sociological abstractions—he leaves these to the sociologist; nor does he look for psychological abstractions—he leaves these to the psychologist and the psychoanalyst. Instead he attempts to match person to person and person to situation. His abstractions refer to fit, which is determined by whether or not the person in question can function satisfactorily within a given social context. The social therapies then are designed for patients who are seriously ill, who do not function socially and perhaps never did, whose condition may require long-term care, and with whom the short-term somatic and psychological therapies have been exhausted or are ineffective or inapplicable.

The field of social psychiatry thus has the following distinguishing characteristics.

It is a point of view rather than a mode of operation.

It focuses upon people's social functioning rather than upon their psychopathology.

It deals with individuals in groups rather than with persons seen in isolation from one another.

It attempts to influence not only persons but also social organizations, communication networks, and situations.

It advocates treatment and prevention of mental illness through a broad approach which in addition to the patient involves his relatives and coworkers and the institutions that affect his life.

And finally it strives to influence the everyday life attitudes of citizens that are conducive to human satisfaction and mental health.

The appplication of the principles and methods of social psychiatry is not confined to the mentally ill. Problems such as morale, social isolation, segregation, violence, working conditions, or population density all affect the mental health of millions. By consultations with key persons and agencies and by teaching and public discussion, a better understanding of these problems can be achieved, which, if it is effective, may be followed by legislative or executive action.

Chapter 2

Social Psychiatry

Vagaries of a Term

NORMAN W. BELL AND JOHN P. SPIEGEL

IN THE SHIFTING SANDS OF PROFESSIONAL INTERESTS, MANY new ideas and concepts are issued under the banner of "social psychiatry." Despite the conjunction of the traditional opposites (*socius* and *psyche*), the term has become accepted through usage. It appears in the names of institutes, professorships, learned journals, and numerous books; a few people even identify themselves as "social psychiatrists." Such widespread usage suggests that a special field has come into existence, one that needs distinguishing from clinical psychiatry by the addition of the adjective "social" and from social psychology (or sociology) by the inclusion of "psychiatry." Yet the coherence (if there is any) of this field (if it is one) is notably difficult to discover.

It may be replied that social psychiatry is too young and developing a field to have acquired precise definition, which would only constrict it and stunt its growth. And indeed, if one consults bibliographies and footnoting habits, one gets the impression of recent origin. But modernity can be illusory. This paper is an act of disinternment, an attempt to trace the origins and usages of the term social psychiatry, concentrating on the period before 1940.

The pedigree of the term does not, of course, do justice to the general notion that social factors influence the form or prevalence of illness. That idea is at least as old as Hippocrates' concept of the "epidemic constitution."[1] and every age, at least since the 1700's has bemoaned the increase in mental illness produced by the pace and strain of "modern life." But tracing how the term "social psychiatry" has been used, with what denotations and connotations, may allow us to see what is old in the new and to come to a more inclusive, and hopefully more satisfactory, idea of what social psychiatry is or is not.

So far as we have been able to determine, it was E. E. Southard, Director of The Boston Psychopathic Hospital from 1912 to 1920 and founder of its pioneering Out-Patient Clinic, who first used the words "social psychiatry." In the first volume of *Mental Hygiene* in 1917[2] Southard presented a classification of specialties in the field of psychiatry. Social psychiatry along with metric psychiatry, was listed as a "new and promising" specialty. His discussion of the concept proceeded by drawing an analogy to social psychology.

> Social psychiatry (developing from a conjugation of social and psychiatric concepts, as social psychology has already developed from a conjugation of social and psychological concepts)—employing modern methods of social service investigation and care and aiming to make use of characterological and ethological categories and the available facts of the psychology of the instincts, behaviorism, vocational psychology, and the like.[3]

Southard went on to present a new disclaimer.

> Concerning 5. *Social psychiatry,* it may well be claimed that a good portion of it is nothing but pious wish. At any rate, it might be maintained, should we not separate the comparatively certain fields of psychiatric social service (in which, e.g., several American clinics are getting solid results) from that darkling portion of social psychiatry that lies next to social psychology? Perhaps.[4]

He also introduced here the idea of a differentiation from "psychiatric social service," itself a new field at the time. Specific indication of what is contained in social psychiatry was conspicuous by its absence.

By the next year, 1918, Southard had carried his ideas a good deal further. In the meantime he had given courses in "social psychiatry" to social workers at the School of Social Work in Boston (Simmons College).* In a 1918 article[5] his interest in classifying fields and professions was evident—social work was identified as applied sociology, the relations of social workers and sociologists being analogous to the relation of the nurse to the physician. The analogy was extended; just as in medicine the public health nurse and the medical social worker have become differentiated, there should be a differentiation of nurses and social workers in the field of psychiatry. The discussion continued with an extensive table of the differences in point of view between social work and mental hygiene. Although the point was not made explicit, social psychiatry appeared to be an attempt to bridge these two fields, which have fundamentally different, but not conflicting, viewpoints and sentiments. The bridging was to be accomplished by case study.

> In order practically to bring out the individualism of mental hygiene as contrasted with the family-groupism and community-groupism of social work, the technique adopted in the course on social psychiatry here discussed was to demonstrate . . . intensively studied social service cases. . . .[6]

The idea that social psychiatry is an area lying between two established fields (today we would call it an interdisciplinary area) was supported by the further statement that:

* A course had also been given under the sponsorship of the Boston Red Cross Society, but we have been unable to locate any documents regarding its organization and content, or to identify any participants other than one social worker.

> The psychiatric social worker was thus taught to see what the mental hygienist starts with knowing, namely, that a large number of problems in social psychiatry cannot be left to the management of the social worker, since the heavy hand of organized government and administration, and the filigree psychic interior of many a personal situation interpose.[7]

This conception was reinforced by Southard's concluding remarks that a course on social psychiatry should include applied sociology (including techniques of social investigation), social psychology, neuropsychiatry, supervised case experience, and psychological testing.

Southard's ideas were evidently popular and received a considerable boost in the crash program for training psychiatric social workers in 1918. On relatively short notice a summer program was organized at Smith College in anticipation of the many problems developing as a result of the Great War and its anticipated end. Southard and his co-workers at Boston Psychopathic played a prominent part. The program, first described by Edith Spaulding, was seen as a course in social psychiatry and for the first time a relatively specific definition was given.

> The course in social psychiatry endeavored to show to what degree abnormal and antisocial behavior result from the inability to make such adjustment [of primitive instincts to modern civilization].[8]

While this definition was more specific than any Southard had given, it may be noted that it is virtually indistinguishable from the major starting point of psychoanalysis, which was at this time also receiving considerable attention from psychiatric social workers. Spaulding went on to give the outline of this course, which included the physical causes of mental disease, slides of brain lesions, history-taking and mental and neurological examination of patients, epilepsy, personality in general, hysteria, constitutional inferiority, psychopathic personalities, psychoneuroses, manic-depressive psychoses, alcoholism and alcoholic psychoses, dementia praecox, paranoid states, and war neuroses and psychoses. In this list there is nothing that would suggest that the content of social psychiatry was different from that of clinical psychiatry. The list of participants suggests the importance accorded to psychoanalysis—James Jackson Putnam and A. A. Brill were among the lecturers. In addition to those with strong psychoanalytic interests, Southard and Adolph Meyer participated. However, the increasing influence of sociology was manifest in the activity of F. Stuart Chapin and Seba Eldridge, both members of the Smith College Department of Sociology. Prof. Eldridge taught courses in sociology and social psychiatry during the years 1918 and 1919 in the psychiatric training program of the Smith College School for Social Work; after participating in an evaluation of this program, Prof. Chapin was appointed director of the School for Social Work during the period 1919–1921. In addition, he taught courses in social organization.

Despite Southard's emphasis on applied sociology as one of the sides of social psychiatry, and despite the apparent correspondence of interests between social psychiatry and psychoanalysis, the term was not used in the pioneering Roundtable Discussion between sociologists and psychoanalysts at the meetings of the American Sociological Society in 1920.[9] Even Edith Spaulding, who participated with E. R. Groves, W. A. White, Phyllis Blanchard, C. C. Robinson, and Iva Peters in this Roundtable, did not use the term.

The term reappeared, however, in 1924. In that year, Southard and Mary Jarret published *The Kingdom of Evils,* a book which had only a brief influence. Southard had died three years before its publication, and the influence of psychoanalysis in schools of social work soon overwhelmed the social psychiatric directions initiated by Southard and his associates. In it, however, social psychiatry was defined extensively, if not precisely.

> . . . "social psychiatry" is not used as an alternate for "psychiatric social work." Psychiatric social work is the special form of social work in which psychiatric knowledge is particularly required. Social psychiatry is an art now in the course of development by which the psychiatrist deals with social problems. Social psychiatry is a branch of psychiatry and a special kind of medical art. That part of the knowledge of psychiatry which has a bearing upon social problems is given to social workers in courses named social psychiatry—that is, the essentials of psychiatry from the standpoint of social work. The special preparation of the psychiatric social worker should consist not only of courses in social psychiatry but also of practice in social work with psychiatric cases. The inclusive term mental hygiene is used to cover the activities of psychiatrist, psychologist, the psychiatric social worker in promoting mental health wheresoever.[10]

The inclination of Southard to see social psychiatry as an interdisciplinary body of both knowledge and practice was still present in this passage. Another significant element was the definition of social psychiatry as a part of medicine, rather than of some other profession.

In the same year, 1924, the American Psychiatric Association held a roundtable discussion of social psychiatry. Unfortunately, the proceedings of this discussion, chaired by William Healy, were not published, so the dawning conceptions of social psychiatry among clinical psychiatrists cannot be determined. The participants are similarly unknown, although the list of persons attending the meetings as a whole does not include known social scientists. However, the next year, Clinton P. McCord, a psychiatrist, presented a paper on social psychiatry. In it, he recorded that he and a Dr. Amsden had been teaching a course in social psychiatry at Albany Medical School. McCord's discussion referred mainly to the demands of community organizations—courts, schools, businesses, welfare agencies, and prisons—on psychiatry. The course in social psychiatry he outlined was largely oriented to giving physicians an acquaintance with such organizations and with available treatment facilities.

It is highly relevant to the theme of disinterment and historical restoration which motivates this paper that the content of McCord's course on social psychiatry of 1925 corresponds almost precisely with the content of contemporary discussions of planning for community mental health programs and for the training of "community psychiatrists."[11]

The place of the dynamic conceptions of psychoanalysis is also clear in McCord's outline, and in his concluding statement.

> . . . it is the special province of Social Psychiatry as a specialty that the newer formulations [seeing mental mechanisms and emotional conflicts are related to conduct disorders] are being widely tested and further developed and clarified.[12]

For McCord, social psychiatry appeared clearly as a specialty within medical psychiatry; other professions did not appear to be involved in the practice of social psychiatry.

For no discernible reason after 1925 the term social psychiatry dropped from use for some years. It does not appear in the index of a volume of the *American Journal of Psychiatry* again until 1939. Even though not in the index, the term was used at least once. In a 1929 article, James S. Plant, a psychiatrist and a student of Southard, referred to social psychiatry as a set of mass measures to prevent the causes of poor mental hygiene.[13] The emphasis was still on practice, but now on a scale much broader than the individual. For the first time social psychiatry signified the treatment of such social units as the neighborhood, the community, and the society.*

* In the interest of historical accuracy, it should be noted that the term, social psychiatry, was actually used twice. It was included in the name of the foundation established by Trigant Burrow in 1927, "The Lefwynn Foundation for Laboratory Research in Analytic and Social Psychiatry," to pursue his work which was outside of the main stream of psychiatry.

But by the late 1920's the term "social psychiatry" has apparently lost its appeal to psychiatrists while at the same time it had become popular in the social sciences, especially sociology. It appears in the index of *Social Science Abstracts,* a short-lived project of the Social Science Research Council (1928–1932). In 1929, panel discussions of social scientists and psychiatrists began to be held again, though now at meetings of the American Sociological Society. They were repeated, without being labeled as social psychiatry, in the next four annual meetings. In 1932 Ernest Groves, a sociologist, published a review of the field,[14] in which he gave no definition of social psychiatry, but mentioned that it had been advancing among psychiatrists, sociologists, and in the field of mental hygiene. He also made the following statement, which reflects the psychoanalytic notion of the repressive nature of society, an idea which was stimulating to sociologists.

> The psychoanalytic pioneers in the field of psychiatry had been forced from the first to recognize the sociological aspects of their problem. In spite of the confusion resulting from Freud, Adler, Jung, Kempf, Burrow, and others, coming forward with their specialized methods of attacking neurosis, the sociologist could detect in all of them the recognition that the problem of the patient was a product of the process of socialization and that the neuroses revealed the hazard of the individual's attempt to adjust to collective behavior.[15]

By 1934 the term had been wholly appropriated by sociologists, apparently in default of any further interest in it among psychiatrists.

> The field of social psychiatry embraces all abnormal forms of social adjustments, made by individuals and groups as well.
>
> Like social psychology, social psychiatry is a division of sociology.[16]

Brown also discussed the therapeutic side of social psychiatry.

> On the therapeutic side, social psychiatry needs to give psychoses, neuroses, and other mental emotional adjustments a proper social definition. The public needs to be informed concerning the true nature of the adjustments. They are not conditions to be ashamed of any more than pneumonia.[17]

Although Brown did not specify who was to provide this therapeutic aspect, his mention of the public's needing to be informed suggests that the practice of social psychiatry was not conceived as exclusively a medical responsibility.

In this same volume, Joseph K. Folsom contributed a chapter on "The Sources and Methods of Social Psychiatry." Folsom did not supply an explicit definition of the term, but included within the scope of his review were 150 studies, each of which dealt with a sociological and a psychiatric variable. These included a wide variety of empirical investigations, such as epidemiological and ecological studies, correlational studies of a personality variable or symptom with a social and demographic variable, with attitudes, or with social conditions such as change and mobility. Folsom noted[18] that, in most of these, the psychiatric variable was the dependent variable, and that studies in which it was the independent variable were much less frequent. Nevertheless, he did cite studies of psychiatric problems as they affect delinquency, criminality, and marital conflict. In this review it is apparent that sociologists used the term social psychiatry in a broad, eclectic way, extending it, at least by implication, to any aspect of psychiatry which had relevance for sociology. Similarly, the identification of social psychiatry as an interdisciplinary area in which both the clinical and the social science professions are interested was apparent again in the bibliography on social psychiatry appended to the May 1937 issue of the *American Journal of Sociology* devoted to Freud* and in Dunham's review of the field.[19]

On the other hand, in the same year (1934) that Folsom published the review referred to above, he also published a textbook on the family, using the expression "social psychiatry" in the subtitle.[20] There, as in his text on social psychology of 1931,[21] which contained a chapter on social psychiatry, the term was not defined but it was clear that it was based on psychoanalytic theories of personality development and functioning.

After a ten-year absence, the term "social psychiatry" again made an appearance in the *American Journal of Psychiatry* in 1940.[22] As usual, no definition was given, but it is apparent that Hartwell had in mind a type of practice. Hartwell referred, as McCord did, 15 years earlier, to the demands being made on psychiatrists for aid†[23] in a variety of social situations and proceeded to speak bluntly about the question of whether social work was to become an independent profession or was to be led and controlled by psychiatry.

After 1940 the term "social psychiatry" became increasingly accepted and talked about by psychiatrists, while it fell among disuse among sociologists. It appeared with such frequency in the indexes of the *American Journal of Psychiatry*, in *Excerpta Medica*, in *Index Medicus*, in *Index of Modern Literature*, and in *Psychological Abstracts*, that it is impossible to give a complete cataloguing. By the 1950's the term was well institutionalized, although it still does not appear in standard psychiatric dictionaries and was not used until quite recently in *Sociological Abstracts*.

A good example of the more recent usage of the term is to

* This bibliography was a compilation of suggestions by both sociologists and psychiatrists, and lists the items as suggested by one, the other, or both professions.

† It is interesting to note that Hartwell includes, in addition to many of the same type of persons McCord listed, sociologists and medical clinicians.

be found in the writings of Thomas Rennie and his coworkers. The year 1955 marked something of a flowering of social psychiatry, at least in America.* In that year, the first issue of the *International Journal of Social Psychiatry* appeared. Its first article was an essay defining social psychiatry, by Thomas A. C. Rennie, who was listed as "Professor of Psychiatry (Social Psychiatry) Cornell University Medical College." Like all who had written on this subject, from Southard on through the years, Rennie commented on the many groups of people in the community who seek the advice of the psychiatrist and on the interdisciplinary response required to meet the need.[24] What he particularly focused upon, however, was the novelty of the approach. He wrote as if he were in the act of launching a new movement, and, since he was writing the lead article in a new and international journal, there was some reality to this assumption, even though the content of the article contained nothing essentially new.

> Growing evidence accrues that the interdisciplinary approach to some problems of mental health and illness has brought about a *new development in psychiatry* worthy of the name "social psychiatry." . . . Social psychiatry is concerned not only with facts of prevalence and incidence, it searches more deeply into the possible significance of social and cultural factors in the etiology and dynamics of mental disorder.[25]

Rennie went to considerable lengths to give a precise definition of this "new development in psychiatry" while keeping in view its broad sweep and its ambitious aims.

> Social psychiatry, by our definition, seeks to determine the significant facts in family and society which

* By contrast, in Great Britain and Europe social psychiatry appears to have acquired much earlier a more stable meaning centering on a type of psychiatric practice which kept the social aspects of illness and treatment in view. Maxwell Jones' book, *The Therapeutic Community* (New York: Basic Books, 1953), was originally published in Britain under the title *Social Psychiatry*.

> affect adaption (or which can be clearly defined as of etiological importance) as revealed through the studies of individuals or groups functioning in their natural setting. It concerns itself not only with the mentally ill but with the problems of adjustment of all persons in society toward a better understanding of how people adapt and what forces tend to damage or enhance their adaptive capacities. . . . Social psychiatry is etiological in its aim, but its point of attack is the whole framework of contemporary living.[26]

He also emphasized the necessity of developing new methods, theories, and concepts for a field of this magnitude.

> To forge tools and instruments to accumulate systematically such data on psycho-biological and socio-cultural integration of man on cross-sections of the population is the task of social psychiatry . . . social psychiatry must concern itself also with persons who never seek psychiatric therapy.
>
> Social psychiatry is, therefore, the study of etiology and dynamics of persons seen in their total environmental setting.[27]

In spite of the vagueness and excessive generality of the last sentence, Rennie clearly made many advances over early attempts to define (or avoid defining) social psychiatry. In his definition, social psychiatry is not an area in which both social sciences and psychiatry are mildly interested; rather it is one to which they mutually contribute methods, theory, and substantive findings. No longer does it consist of the speculative application of psychoanalytic principles and concepts to social and cultural phenomena, nor is it to be construed as an eclectic resort to various psychiatric theories to account for these phenomena. Instead, Rennie envisaged a distinct area, one with its own interdisciplinary methods, its own focus, and its own data, in short, a specialized field.

There is another way in which Rennie stands distinct from

most of his professional forebears. He nowhere implied that social psychiatry is something to be practiced.* It is a field of knowledge, which, whatever the implications may be for practice, is not explicitly tied to practice itself.

Since Rennie had a relatively clear vision of the field and since he wanted not merely to gaze upon, but actively enter the field, it is instructive to look briefly at some of the work which he began or inspired. An example is the attempt to conceptualize the field and its modes of collaboration presented in the work of Leighton et al.[28] In the "Preface" to their book, the author-editors describe the history of the discussions sponsored by the Committee on Research in Psychiatry and the Social Sciences of the Social Science Research Council. They state:

> After some time devoted to discussing concepts, the committee agreed that initial emphasis should be placed on phenomena that had both individual and group aspects. At first these were defined in terms of the research foci of existing projects in social psychiatry. Following some experimentation, however, this did not prove workable and it was decided better to have a wider framework of ideas from which to make a selection. Topics were then chosen to serve as "portals of entry." . . . The approach, in short, was problem oriented. . . .[29]

Several pages later (p. 4) the editors present, in a footnote, an explanation of social psychiatry which speaks of what the term "brings to mind," and of what "the field can contribute." The editors of this volume also reintroduce the notion of speaking of "guides to action in dealing with mental illness"

* This view was not shared by Rennie's British colleagues. In his "Introduction" to the same first issue, Lord Johnson coupled social psychiatry and group therapy as promising methods (*ibid,* p. 3). Bierer, (*ibid,* p. 30), also referred to the therapeutic aspect of social psychiatry, though with a viewpoint much more extensive—and more nebulous than Lord Johnson's. In the same issue a lay contributor, John Custance, gave an almost philosophic definition of the term: "Social psychiatry is the psychiatry of human relationships—i.e., each one of us is involved in it." *ibid,* p. 66).

p. *vii*), and of "a rich field of research and practice." The volume as a whole contains a variety of essays and reports of clinical and research undertakings. The "exploration" produces many nuggets, but no charting of the region.

In recent years, the idea endorsed by Rennie that social psychiatry is a field of research, with no specialized techniques of application, has steadily receded from view. Its place has been taken by increasing demands for social psychiatry techniques which can be put immediately into practice. "Action for Mental Health," "planning for mental health centers," "programs in community psychiatry," are slogans supported not only by organized psychiatry but also by the national administration which has voted large sums of money for their implementation. There is an expectation that sufficiently intense planning for instant social psychiatry and convertible mental health will sooner or later produce a marketable product. In the current atmosphere of haste, attempts to conceptualize the field, to elaborate theories, and to devise new methods of research have largely fallen by the wayside.

Comment

This tracing of the usages and connotations of the term "social psychiatry," particularly in its early life, shows that the basic idea is hardly the ". . . new development in psychiatry . . ." which Rennie noted. Indeed most of the central elements in the concept seem to recur several times over, each time being seen as new.* In this cyclical process of death and rebirth few changes have taken place. The enterprise began in the dialogue between clinical psychiatry and the new profession of social work. After a decade and a half it was seen as an integral

* In a future publication we hope to show that this "Columbus complex" (as Sorokin has called it) is characteristic not only of general conceptions but also of the specific interests and ideas.

part of sociology. Again after a brief flowering there it receded only to be adopted later by psychiatry and in the last decade by a combination of psychiatry and the social sciences. Correspondingly, institutional adoption moved from schools of social work to the American Psychiatric Association to the American Sociological Society. Latterly, after a fallow period, in which it was unclaimed by any profession, it has come to have its own institutional forms, including a new International Association.

It is easy enough to ascribe the current popularity of social psychiatry to the typical American attitude: "Don't stand there mumbling; do something!" Even if we don't know what to do, there is the national assumption that some action is better than none at all. Once an idea has been identified as both new *and* scientific, there is an insatiable demand that something be done about it. And if the new, scientific idea also promises amelioration of such vast public problems as mental illness, crime, delinquency, alcoholism, and a good many others, then the demand reaches a programmatic intensity corresponding to the fitful enthusiasms that reduced "Prohibition," "The New Deal," "The Square Deal," and "The New Frontier" to slogans which became empty and passed away after playing a brief part on the national scene.

Quite apart from the national appetite for social and political programs, our review of the vicissitudes of the term "social psychiatry" reveals an inherent and as yet unresolved scientific problem which, concealed behind the scenes, has inhibited the many attempts to define the field and to determine what is to be done within it. This is the etiological problem—the question of causal sequence. In its simplest terms the question can be stated in three forms: (1) Are mental illnesses (and other forms of deviant behavior) caused by stresses and strain in the social environment? (2) Or are social problems caused by the psychological instabilities of individuals, instabilities which can be traced to essentially psychobiological causes? (3)

Or are both mental illness and social problems the result of interaction between social and psychobiological forces?

What many of the authors of the past have responded to is the fact that the answers to these questions are not yet known. This is why they have attempted to define a field of knowledge and to search for methods by means of which the answers could be evolved. When the winds of intuition have blown in the direction of the first form of the question, then the social scientists have attempted to appropriate the field. When the prevailing opinion leaned toward the second alternative, then psychiatrists seized the helm. In the most recent era, the third alternative has been in the forefront. But the fact is that to the present we have only opinions or presuppositions to put in the place of firm answers. The findings are equivocal.

Obviously, if the answers are not available, there is little rational support for any type of practice whatsoever. But the traditions of empirical medicine have never accepted such a strictly rational and negative position. Lacking certainty, the physician still is obligated to do the best he can to relieve suffering. This responsibility, not carried by the social scientists, produces the vacillation among the psychiatrists as to whether social psychiatry is exclusively a field of research, or whether it also includes a type of practice.

The type of practitioner required, however, would still depend upon which of the three positions outlined above was thought to be correct. If mental illness and social deviance are caused primarily by social conditions, then the practitioner would have to be an applied sociologist. If social problems are caused by personality disturbances, then—and logically, *only* then—would the practitioner be a social psychiatrist. If the essential, etiological process is the result of interaction between social and psychological factors, then a new type of practitioner—let us say, a psychosociologist—is required. It is the unknown functions and techniques of such an interdisciplinary practitioner which are currently under investigation in the planning for comprehensive, community-oriented, mental health programs.

There are some, however, who would claim that the etiological questions outlined above have been raised in an erroneous form. Such persons, among whom we include ourselves, hold that just as the mind-body dichotomy had to be given up as unfruitful, so the individual-society distinction needs to be reexamined. Within the past decade and a half, new and more comprehensive models for viewing the behavioral world have developed. Under various names—general systems theory, transactional theory, a general theory of action, a unified theory of behavior, and existentialism—a conceptual revolution has been taking place. Involved in this revolution is the presupposition that physical, biological, psychological, social, and cultural phenomena are all interrelated and interdependent within a field of behavior. No one of these sectors of behavior, it is held, is prior to or more real than another, nor is one the *cause* of another. The levels which we see and define as independent variable-dependent variable relationships are conveniences of the mind, devices which help us to approach scientific problems, but which do not provide us with final or general conceptions.

In a schematic way, this model envisions a series of ever-broadening and always interrelated systems, from the somatic systems, through psychological systems in the individual, to small groups (such as the family), to large groups (such as an industrial organization), to the whole society, the system of cultural values and beliefs, and ultimately the universe. Between the extremes of atomic particles and the whole universe, any point of reference can be treated *as if* it were a system with its own structure, processes, and functions, or *as if* it were a subsystem or a suprasystem. How it will be viewed will depend upon the problem and purposes at hand but the choice of any one formulation must be recognized as involving a partial and biased picture.

Viewed from the presuppositions of this model, the etiological questions stated above dissolve into new formulations, and the term, "social psychiatry," becomes one among many possible combinations. In place of the old formulations, one finds new questions about the interrelations (or transactions) between systems.[30] Answers to these questions require constant research collaboration between scientists of all persuasions: biochemists, geneticists, physiologists, psychologists, pediatricians, psychiatrists, sociologists, political scientists, anthropologists, and indeed, scholars such as historians and philosophers.

Such far-flung research combinations require labels for different kinds of training for professional collaboration. Thus the label, "social psychiatrist" could be applied to a person whose basic training is in clinical psychiatry, but who wishes to be trained for collaborative research with a sociologist. The term, "cultural psychiatrist," would be applied to the same kind of person who seeks training for research with a cultural anthropologist in the area now called "transcultural psychiatry." Similar descriptive adjectives may be elaborated for the research training counterparts in the collaborating disciplines, e.g. "psychiatric sociologist" or "psychiatric anthropologist" for those persons already trained in sociology and anthropology who wish to be further trained for research collaboration with psychiatrists. At the present time, it is not clear that such a refined system of classification for research training is necessary, although the new subdisciplines already instituted, such as "medical sociology" and "psychological anthropology" suggest that it may be desirable.

Apart from its usefulness as a label for a certain type of cross-disciplinary research training and research procedure, the term, "social psychiatry," would appear to have no logical meaning. There is little merit in applying it to the many and heterogenous methods of practice and prevention in the area of community mental health now being elaborated in an experimental fashion. In order to preserve the technical meaning of the word, "psychiatry," the term, "social psychiatry," had best be reserved to differentiate the research activities of psychiatrists interested in the social area from those interested exclusively in intrapsychic or biological factors. Undoubtedly there are, and will continue to be, attempts to use the term as an umbrella under which to assemble a wide variety of "the helping professions" involved in community mental health programs: psychiatric social workers, psychiatrists, clinical psychologists, educational or school psychologists, criminologists, parole and probation officers, youth and group workers, and personnel in public welfare organizations of all sorts. But, for these manifold activities, the inclusion of the word, "psychiatry," in the general designation does an unjustice, both to the medical profession and to the many nonmedical professions involved in such an extensive enterprise. It is not the purpose of this paper to propose the new terminology that is needed for the area of community mental health practice and prevention. But it is our prediction that if a more adequate terminology is not instituted, the term, "social psychiatry," will continue to be subject to the vagaries which we have outlined above.

Chapter 3

Sociology and Mental Illness

Some Neglected Implications for Treatment

JACK ZUSMAN

SOCIOLOGY PROVIDES A POWERFUL TOOL FOR UNDERSTANDING and treating mental illness. Recent work is making it increasingly clear that sociological theory and techniques are valuable additions to the biochemical, genetic, and psychological approaches. Yet sociology is relatively neglected by psychiatrists both in treating of patients and training residents. Few residencies provide any sort of introduction to the sociological study of mental illness, and sociology is not usually considered one of the basic sciences essential for psychiatry. In examining and treating patients it is common practice to devote much attention to constitutional or psychological factors associated with the onset of the illness. Less consideration is usually given to the social situation in which the symptoms occurred and to the chain of social events that can result, for example, in the formation of a group of persons, one labeled as a patient and the others as staff. Evaluation of new forms of treatment is frequently concerned with measuring physical, biochemical, or psychological changes produced in patients by the application of physical, biochemical, or psychological forces. The social impact of the new treatment upon both patients and staff, or the interaction between the physical, biochemical, and psychological effects of a treatment and its social influence, is often forgotten. Advanced training for psychiatrists in fields such as genetics, biochemistry, or psychology (psychoanalysis) is quite common. The number of psychiatrists who have advanced training in sociology is small.

The purpose of this paper is to call attention to this neglect and to provide examples of some of the ways in which a sociological approach to mental illness can be useful for treating patients. A number of social treatment techniques are currently successfully in use. However, for the most part these techniques have been developed empirically, and little effort has been devoted to theoretical analysis in order that the effective elements be isolated and applied in other situations.

An attempt will be made here to present some general principles regarding mental illness and treatment that seem fruitful for further development of current techniques and discovery of new ones. Much of the material to be discussed has been drawn from studies that are impressionistic and preliminary. In some cases the material comes from a field other than psychiatry, notably criminology and penology.

No claim is made for the originality of the ideas gathered here. Indeed, some of them have appeared in so many places that it has not been possible to find the earliest or most important reference. Nor has it been possible to include all of the forms in which the ideas have been expressed. Often the particular example offered has been chosen simply on the basis of convenience or familiarity, and represents many other references that could have been cited.

The sociologist is interested in investigating the prevalence of mental illness in relation to the occurrence of social factors. Internal physiological or psychological organization is only of secondary importance. This does not mean that the effects of traumatic past events upon an individual's psychological status, or his genetic and biochemical constitution, are unimportant in understanding his mental illness. These are simply put aside in this context to concentrate upon social factors.

This approach is not concerned with mental illness in the

abstract. Mental illness is operationally defined when two people come together, and as a result of their interaction one person comes to call the other mentally ill. The encounter is of particular interest when the person who calls the other mentally ill has been designated by society to officially apply such labels, i.e., a psychiatrist. The sociologist is interested in examining what happened in the interaction between the two persons that led to one of them labeling the other. Mental illness as a social phenomenon can be examined through this encounter. Without the encounter there is no socially recognized illness.

There are many ways in which social forces can act to influence an individual's chances of being labeled as mentally ill. Six of them will be discussed here. *First,* many different forms of socially deviant behavior occur. Which of these deviations is considered to reflect mental illness and which results in the application of some other label (deviations can be labeled favorably or unfavorably) or is accorded no social recognition at all depends upon socially determined convention. *Second,* the special considerations and exemptions from responsibility that our society accords to the mentally ill are very important and even lifesaving for some persons. The fact that these exemptions are available only to those exhibiting the symptoms of mental illness tends to lead desperate people in the direction of mental illness. *Third,* membership in a subcultural group may lead an individual to act so that in the course of functioning normally in his subculture, he violates the standards of the larger culture. This deviation is often diagnosed by representatives of the larger culture as mental illness. *Fourth,* the application of the label of mental illness to an individual is likely to influence how other people regard him and how he regards himself. In several ways, being considered mentally ill exerts pressure upon him to act to fulfill the common stereotype of mental illness. This will either reinforce the diagnosis or lead to a new one. *Fifth,* some of the treatment prescribed for the mentally ill is so severe and disruptive to normal functioning that it leads to appearance of new symptoms and new forms of mental illness. This has been known for many years. The persistent popularity of such treatment must in large part be based upon its usefulness and value to society rather than its helpfulness to the mentally ill. *Sixth,* the absence of a coherent social structure and associated stable standards of behavior can lead to an increase in the occurrence of deviant behavior. This in turn is likely to be associated with an increase in the number of persons considered to be showing symptoms of mental illness.

Each of these points will now be elaborated.

Mental Illness Is One Name for Deviant Behavior

Every social group must deal with deviance to insure continued existence and stability. There must be some way of promoting compliance with accepted standards of behavior. One way our culture has of doing this is to call a person exhibiting deviance mentally ill, and then apply special methods for controlling the deviance.

It is important to recognize, however, that standards of deviance and acceptability are relative. No single bit of behavior (or symptom) can be considered to be inherently deviant or inherently mentally ill. The crucial factor is the social context in which the behavior occurs. The same behavior may, depending upon the situation, be considered socially acceptable, mentally ill, or criminal (indicating the application of another method of social control).

For example, an adolescent who commits a car theft may confess to a policeman, be called a juvenile delinquent, and be jailed. He may instead consult a psychiatrist, and then he is likely to be labeled mentally ill and receive psychotherapy. Or he may tell only his friends and be considered a hero. The label and the social reaction to the deviant behavior depend greatly upon who observes the deviance.

Even the occurrence of such traditionally symptomatic behavior as responding to hallucinations or producing nonsensical speech may be considered admirable deviations under the proper circumstances—e.g., in a lysergic acid diethylamide (LSD) session or in a church where speaking in tongues is practiced.

In making a diagnosis the psychiatrist often measures the reported or observed behavior against his own standards of social appropriateness, although he may be unaware that this is what he is doing. Similarly, the patient may be unaware that he often has a good deal of control over whether he will be labeled mentally ill by choosing to whom and the context in which he reveals his deviant behavior.

A related example of the possible importance of social context in determining the response to deviance occurs in the interaction between the patient's behavior and the patient's social class. Psychiatrists tend to diagnose lower-class people more frequently than upper- and middle-class people as schizophrenic.[1] Psychologists interpreting Rorschach tests consider a lower-class person to be sicker than a middle-class person on the basis of the same test results.[2]

There is some evidence that merely by placing himself in a particular context a person may get himself labeled as mentally ill regardless of the extent of his deviance. In a study of the use of prepaid insurance coverage for psychiatric treatment it was found that "nearly every patient who takes the trouble to go to a psychiatrist's office is likely to be treated."[3] Possibly every one of us has engaged in some deviant behavior or experienced some symptom which, when described in the appropriate context, such as a psychiatrist's office, leads to a diagnosis. Quite likely if many of these "symptoms" had been described to a clergyman or a policeman, the label of sinner or minor criminal would have been applied instead.

Finally, a survey of the mental health of the aged population of the city of Syracuse, N. Y., found that only a minor portion of the people who where "certifiable"—who met the criteria for involuntary admission to a mental hospital because they were dangerous to themselves or to others—were in mental hospitals. Most such persons were in other institutions or in the community.[4] The difference between being hospitalized and not being hospitalized obviously was not in the presence or absence of symptoms alone, but depended also upon social circumstances.

To sum up, the diagnosis of mental illness is a social process occurring when two persons interact and one of them applies the designation to the other. The diagnostic operation seems to depend upon two factors: (1) social deviance, and (2) the social context in which the deviance occurs or is revealed. Deviance is always relative to the standards of a group. Our society controls certain forms of deviance by calling them mental illness and treating them in a special way to alter or eliminate them. Most, if not all, people have engaged in enough deviant behavior so that in the proper context, some sort of psychiatric diagnosis can be made.

Narrowing the Definition of Mental Illness

The usefulness of the recognition that diagnosis of mental illness is only one way of dealing with social deviance requires considering what are the most effective ways of controlling social deviance. It may be that in cases presently called mental illness, it would be more effective to call them something else and deal with them in another way.

For example, minor sex deviations are customarily treated as either criminal acts or symptoms of mental illness. If considered to be criminal, then an offender is sent to prison or put on probation. If mentally ill, he is sent to a mental hospital or given outpatient treatment. There are no data available on which form of treatment is more effective in controlling the deviation, and there are proponents on both sides. Both treatments stigmatize their recipients. Both treatments can lead to confinement under difficult and damaging conditions, which can then lead to social disability. Both treatments can also be carried out under humane conditions with an emphasis upon rehabilitation. The decision as to which type of treatment is best for a person caught engaging in a sexual deviation should depend upon a number of individual factors. Quite possibly in some areas of the country and with members of some social groups, it is more effective and more humane to treat sexual deviation as a criminal act and eliminate it from the category of mental illness.

A review of all the deviant acts presently considered to be symptoms of mental illness with a goal of removing many of them from the list would be more than a matter of shuffling names. As will be seen, there are a number of harmful side effects of psychiatric treatment and a number of harmful effects of a person's being considered mentally ill. These effects can in themselves lead to new forms of mental illness or worsen preexisting ones. In addition, once a person has been designated as mentally ill, then by a carefully guarded tradition his treatment can be directed only by members of a very expensive, very limited group: psychiatrists. This has often meant that he could receive no treatment at all. Had his deviation been called something else, members of other professional groups whose time is not so expensive or limited and whose effectiveness is possibly as great could be more easily made available to him.

In general, one maneuver in preventing or treating mental illness is to define the deviation as outside of the boundaries of mental illness. Several projects presently in existence have taken this approach. Such groups as Synanon,[5] Alcoholics Anonymous,[6] and the Black Muslims[7] have taken areas of social deviance often dealt with by psychiatry, stated emphatically that their areas of concern are not within psychiatric competence (whether this is correct or not is beside the point), and attempted to deal with deviance by nonpsychiatric methods. Results are supposedly good. If this is true, the saving to the community in psychiatric time and human suffering is considerable, and the stigma and other negative aspects of mental illness are avoided for the deviants involved.

Even within psychiatry and its related professions, movement in this direction can be seen. Referral of selected patients by psychiatrists to clergymen has been discussed.[8] There has been increasing use in mental hospitals of nonprofessional personnel to provide treatment[9] (although often it is called remotivation, rehabilitation, or some other name). In outpatient clinics nonprofessional personnel are being used as therapists and in other traditionally professional roles.[10] Even in cases where such personnel are being used as direct substitutes for psychiatrists, they are likely not to have the same illness-oriented approach to deviance as medical training provides, and they do not carry the same authority to designate someone "ill," as the physician does.

Patients can be taught to control where and how they reveal their deviance. One method of treatment that has been used with chronic schizophrenics is to emphasize to a patient that most people may think some of his ideas or his actions are strange. Therefore, if he wants to avoid misunderstandings with people whose reactions he is not sure of, he must not talk about his voices or must not argue about his idea that he is being pursued by the FBI. A psychiatrist may choose to deliberately ignore some of a patient's symptoms or tell the patient they are not appropriate for discussion. In this way he avoids making these symptoms a focus of attention and an important part of the illness. They may fade into the background while the doctor concentrates on other symptoms he feels are more important or less easily discouraged.

Mental Illness as a Demand for Privileges

Persons who are ill are traditionally given special treatment in our society, particularly exemptions from customary responsibilities. This has been pointed out by Sigerist[11] and Parsons.[12] The mentally ill receive exemptions even broader than those accorded to the physically ill—many of the mentally ill are considered to be unable to assume any responsibility at all, even for the most elementary aspects of personal care. Our courts provide an extreme example of how this tradition tends to increase the number of people who are considered mentally ill. Accused persons plead insanity to escape being held responsible for their actions and being punished. A similar process can occur less obviously in other situations. Artiss has described how the symptoms of mental illness can be considered as communications, sometimes as requests for relief from unpleasant responsibilities.[13] Berne has pointed out how the knowledge that one has been diagnosed as mentally ill can be used by the ill person to avoid the demands of others.[14] Although there are little adequate data, clinical experience suggests that in some cases of mental illness, the only escape from an unbearable situation has been for the person involved to become ill.[15]

On the surface, the tradition of relieving a mentally ill and suffering person of responsibility is a humane one. Mental hospital patients are not called upon to function in any way. They do not have to take responsibilty for self control, for participating as members of a social group, or for supporting themselves.

It has come to be recognized, however, that this type of treatment is damaging for mental patients, especially when it is prolonged.[16] It leads to disuse and consequent loss of the social skills that are necessary for the patient to function outside of the hospital, and thus tends to prolong hospitalization. In some cases it can contribute to making the illness chronic and incurable. It then becomes the opposite of the humane practice it is intended to be.

Minimizing Exemptions for the Mentally Ill

The experience in many modern mental hospitals that have successfully unlocked all doors and required that all patients take responsibility for themselves and work productively has demonstrated that patients can carry out these functions.[17] It has been found that loss of self control and development of social disability need not accompany mental illness.[18] Many of the facets of the deterioration seen in chronic functional psychoses, long felt to be inevitable, now seem to be a reaction to long-term hospitalization and not to the illness.[19]

In working toward prevention of disability from functional psychoses, it seems useful to consider psychoses as similar in some ways to rheumatoid arthritis. Except during occasional acute flareups, bed rest (or its mental equivalent) is absolutely contraindicated lest joints and muscles (or affected social skills) be frozen and atrophy from disuse. No matter how great the pain the patient must continue to function as best he can, since the instant he relaxes his efforts the inherent tendency of his disorder to disable him can become overwhelming. Treatment must be oriented toward teaching him how to live with his illness and make the best use of his intact abilities, rather than toward complete recovery which rarely, if ever, occurs. Despite his illness, with the proper training and support the patient can be expected to function fairly normally with temporary setbacks during periods of acute exacerbations.

Steps in the direction of elimination of special privileges for the mentally ill have returned in a number of programs. Some mental hospitals are operated with the expectation that every patient will be assigned to a job shortly after admission and that he will work in a job as long as he is a patient.[20] Many psychiatric treatment facilities now have extensive industrial operations and work programs for their hospital and outpatients.[21] The Veterans Administration has operated a program where long-term patients who are able to work but not be discharged from the hospital are made hospital employees and given special quarters at the hospital.[22] Military psychiatry provides a notable example. During World War II soldiers who became mentally ill were rapidly evacuated to large treatment centers far removed from the battle or their normal duty stations. Few of these soldiers ever recovered to the point where they were able to return to any sort of military duty. The present practice is to provide brief treatment for mentally ill soldiers as close as possible to their duty stations, and as soon as possible after the onset of the symptoms. Evacuation is done only as a last resort. This serves to prevent the soldier from getting the idea that mental illness will result in his being sent away from his unit and his duties. It probably also communicates to the soldier the expectation that recovery will take place rapidly and he will shortly be returning to his unit. With such a program there has been a remarkable increase in the number of mentally ill soldiers who recover and are able to return to duty.[23]

Future developments may lead in the direction of entire mental hospitals built around a work program. The principal activity of both patients and staff in such a hospital would be the operation of a number of business establishments during the day. Only after working hours would some of the more traditional hospital activities—psychotherapy, recreation, etc., take place. Patients would be partly or completely financially self-supporting, and might even be able to contribute something to family support when necessary. The diagnostic skills of the psychiatrist would be focused upon judging at what level patients are capable of functioning, what sorts of social demands can safely be made upon them, and what areas of social functioning require attention before the patients are capable of being accepted in the community again. Work is possibly the most important area of social functioning in keeping a person integrated into society, and so a great deal of emphasis must be put on that area. One major portion of the staff would be assigned to finding jobs outside the hospital and placing patients in them.

A change in the custom of relieving the mentally ill of responsibility would have several major repercussions. Persons in need of a socially accepted means of escaping a difficult situation would not be able to use mental illness. There is a need for such a social escape mechanism, however, and presumably some other method would appear to take the place of mental illness. The quality of the care for the mentally ill could be expected to greatly improve as the mentally ill earned enough money to pay for good care and became purchasers rather than merely recipients. Their opinions and complaints regarding treatment would be more likely to be taken seriously, and their financial contributions could help to pay for the improvements they would want. Some of the commonly held fearful and rejecting attitudes toward the mentally ill might change. Many of these attitudes seem to be based upon fear of irresponsible behavior in the mentally ill. When the mentally ill are no longer considered typically irresponsible, some of the basis of the stigma will be gone. Finally, our understanding of the natural courses of all of the serious mental illnesses might be radically altered. Almost all of what we know of the course of psychoses is based upon study of patients being treated in conventional hospitals. Treatment of patients under radically different conditions is likely to produce a change in the course of the illness.

Mental Illness From Membership in a Deviant Subculture

Many subgroups in our society, particularly those that are relatively isolated, have developed standards and customs quite different from the majority. Such practices as speaking in tongues, handling poisonous snakes, or walking naked in the street, while accepted or admirable to members of certain groups, can easily be considered symptomatic of mental illness. The regular occurrence of such blatant symptoms as hallucinations or delusions may be normal and indeed expected in members of some groups.

It is not uncommon for psychiatrists to take some aspects of social background into account when examining patients. A person who comes from the backwoods of Kentucky and who handles poisonous snakes is not likely to be judged psychotic on the basis of this alone. However, there are other cases where the social context of symptoms is rarely taken into account. The foremost example of this occurs when an individual is examined and found mentally ill, without any consideration of the subculture of the group to which he is closest—his family. Customs that seem bizarre or indicative of severe illness to an outsider may be part of everyday functioning within the family. Can they then be taken as signs of psychopathology in the individual family member?

Only relatively recently has attention been devoted to the families of the mentally ill. It has been found that when one member of a family is diagnosed as psychotic, the other members of the family are often just as socially deviant. The "Identified Patient" may differ from his family not necessarily in severity of illness, but in social circumstances.[24]

Another area where membership in a deviant subculture is important and often neglected is examination of patients who are in a mental hospital. A number of authors have pointed out that when patients are admitted to a mental hospital a good deal of pressure is exerted upon them to conform to typical patient behavior.[25] This typical behavior is severely deviant from the point of view of life outside the hospital and is usually interpreted to indicate the presence of the chronic form of psychosis. Little attention has been given to the norms of the patient group as an explanation of the presence of symptoms.

For hospitalized patients acceptable behavior can include for example, apathy, untidiness, and passively obeying orders.

This is understandable, considering that patients often live under conditions where they have no clocks, calendars, mirrors, or clothes of their own. Their illnesses are considered hopeless and their opinions and desires are considered worthless by the staff, and often by the patients themselves. Any patient who does not conform to the patient norm and develop the usual "symptoms" is indeed deviant, and likely to be subject to pressure from both patients and staff to conform.

A third area where allegiance to deviant norms results in deviant social behavior, much of it considered to be symptomatic of mental illness, is among "culturally deprived" persons. Such persons are likely to have grown up under conditions where drug addiction, promiscuity, physical violence, school failure, and chronic unemployment were common. Participation in some of these activities, far from being abnormal, was considered one of the signs of adulthood.[26] It is very doubtful, therefore, that the occurrence of such symptoms or others like them has a meaning in any way comparable to their meaning when they occur in a middle-class person. From the point of view of the majority culture these symptoms may be undesirable traits, but it seems very questionable to attempt to deal with them as medical problems.

Changing Cultural Allegiance

When social deviance results from conformity to a deviant set of norms, the logical way of dealing with it is to change the norms to which the deviant individual adheres. For many years attempts in this area have been part of the treatment programs of certain mental hospitals (although not described in such terms) that have insisted upon isolating the patient from his family as much as possible.[27] There is a great deal of folklore in mental hospitals about how patients get worse after visits with their families and how some patients do well once they are separated from the family and have adjusted to the hospital. (The problem is, of course, that once the patient returns to his family he either has to give up the norms he has acquired in the hospital and conform once again to those of his family, or the family is likely to reject him.)

Family therapy may be looked upon as an attempt to modify the norms of the family group. The therapist interacts with the family members so that the family norms become obvious, and then uses skill and authority to bring about a change. This change often seems to be in the direction of adhering to the norms of the majority culture. In this way the source of conflict between the new norms of the patient and the norms of the family is eliminated.

In hospitals there have been many changes to eliminate development of a deviant hospital subculture. Doors have been unlocked, allowing patients to move about freely; patients have been urged to visit and work in the outside community; and social barriers between patients and staff have been lowered.[28] All of these tend to increase the interaction between patients and normal people—the carriers of the majority culture—and lead the patients to adopt the norms of the majority. This has been brought even further by the institution of a new type of volunteer program in some hospitals. In the traditional program the volunteer is used to replace a staff person so that the staff person can perform some duty requiring a higher level of professional skill. In the new programs the volunteers are used simply to provide the enthusiasm, point of view, emotional reaction, and social influence of normal people on the wards.[29] Informal socializing and participation as a member of ward groups is quite possibly a more important contribution for a volunteer than substituting for a staff member.

Finally, within the last few years several massive attempts have begun in the United States to integrate entire deviant subcultures into the majority. These programs include such things as Project Headstart and the other programs of the

Office of Economic Opportunity, Mobilization for Youth, Haryou-Act, and similar projects. One of the ways in which they operate is to attempt to change the norms of their participants from those of the "culture of poverty" to those of the majority culture. They do this through direct teaching of the new norms, through providing new experiences for participants in the expectation that new norms will develop in response to experience, and by attempting to insure that participants will be able to successfully find places in the majority culture.

It seems likely that major advances in prevention and treatment of mental illness will be made in this area in the future. Since a set of deviant norms can develop and persist when a group is segregated from the majority,[30] it may come to be recognized that the best way to change the behavior of a mentally ill person (or a criminal) is to place him in the midst of a group of normal people rather than in a segregated group of fellow deviants. Most mental hospitals and prisons as we presently know them may disappear, to become an administrative office that controls the whereabouts and treatment activities of scattered patients or prisoners. Patients or prisoners would come together only for group meetings at designated times when all interaction and group pressure can be observed and controlled by staff. At other times the deviants would be at work in selected jobs and living with selected families or in hotels and dormitories.

Greater efforts are likely to be made to eliminate segregated minority groups within the country. Improvements in mass communication, education, and mobility are likely to be helpful in this direction because they increase interaction with isolated groups. Elimination of racial segregation and of substandard working conditions such as those of the migrant farm workers will tend to lead to disappearance of major deviant subgroups into the majority culture. Intensive efforts to eliminate poverty are likely to have a major effect. Poverty apparently is one of the biggest limiting factors to the uniform experience and communication among groups that leads to uniform norms. The increasing influence of mass communications, particularly television, may make it more difficult for deviant norms to develop even within individual families. The frequent portrayal of family life in these media tends to set a uniform national standard and exert pressure for conformity.

Mental Illness as a Self-Fulfilling Prophecy

Patients admitted to a mental hospital with symptoms of an acute illness, e.g., hallucinations, delusions, excitement, etc., often develop entirely new symptoms after a period in the hospital, e.g., apathy, uncommunicativeness, untidiness, etc.[31] These latter symptoms have been attributed by a number of authors to conditions within the hospital and not to the natural course of mental illness. One explanation offered is that the second set of symptoms, previously considered to be a manifestation of "chronic psychosis," is a part of a new illness called the social breakdown syndrome.[32] The social breakdown syndrome occurs in mental hospitals as well as in other places where the mentally ill are considered and treated by those around them as if they are hopeless, helpless, and dangerous. This manner of treatment of the mentally ill seems to act as a self-fulfilling prophecy to induce a new long-term, severely disabling mental illness in those made susceptible by an acute illness.

The means by which popular misconceptions of the behavior of the mentally ill can lead to the development of new symptoms is uncertain. One possibility is suggested by some related work. Orne has reported that by telling a psychology class that the typical behavior of hypnotized subjects included spontaneously raising one arm, he was able to elicit this (atypical) behavior "spontaneously" from members of this class who were hypnotized.[33] He enlarges upon this and similar work to discuss how the "demand characteristics" of a situation—"implicit and nonverbal cues," "mutually shared expectations"—

influence behavior in that situation. There are many demand characteristics of the mentally ill situation. Through folklore, reading, movies, television, and watching other people we all learn what these are. Every one of us has developed some conception of how a mentally ill person acts (inaccurate though it may be), and are thus equipped to play this role should we ever find ourselves in the appropriate situation.

When an acutely ill patient is hospitalized he brings with him his conception of the mentally ill. Before this conception can have any effect on his behavior, however, he must come to see himself as mentally ill. His previous image of himself as a normal person must be severely shaken. The turmoil of his acute illness is often sufficient to do just that. The experience of seeing things or hearing things and then discovering that other people are not perceiving them or the experience of losing ability to think and communicate so that other people understand or the experience of suddenly losing self-control and doing something previously inconceivable, all tend to make the patient doubt the very existence of the world as he has always constructed it. He just does not know any longer who he is or what he can trust. His experience as a social being that has developed over the years has suddenly become undependable in guiding him.

As a result he desperately searches for clues for the appropriate way for him to act in the new situation. One set of clues is his conception of how a mentally ill person acts. Another set is the way the people around him seem to regard him and treat him. If he is brought into court or into the hospital in handcuffs or in custody of a policeman, if he is taken away from his family, not permitted to take part in making major decisions regarding his future, and finally locked behind bars, he is in effect told that he is dangerous, incompetent, and unwanted. (It is important to note that this communication takes place regardless of contradictory verbal communication taking place at the same time. In this case action speaks louder than words.) This application of negative labels through actions further disrupts the patient's previous image of himself and makes him even more susceptible to the long-term effects of the labels. He begins to see himself as unfit for life in ordinary society and not able to exert the self-control and judgment expected of normal people.

Arrival on a ward of a mental hospital can step up this process even further. Goffman has referred to the stripping process,[34] where the patient is divested of all of his personal possessions, his clothing, his privacy, his individuality, his identity. He is told strongly in word and deed by both staff and more experienced patients that socially appropriate behavior for him is to be passive, to do what he is told, accept what he is given, and to fall into step with the patients around him. Alternatively, it is acceptable for him to react violently and struggle against the bars, locks, physical restraints, and alert and powerful attendants, all communicating their readiness to deal with his violence. The only avenues of communication open to the patient are as a passive, accepting person or as a violent, completely rejecting person. These are the expectations that his surroundings communicate to him as the only acceptable roles.

On the other hand, should the patient attempt to communicate as a rational adult and, for example, ask that he be allowed to make decisions for himself or that he see his physician when he requests it, that he be given his own room and be treated with the respect he is accustomed to, he will have great difficulty making himself understood. His requests are likely to be considered symptoms of his illness. Those around the patient do not expect him to act as a normal person and have trouble taking normal behavior at face value. A patient will have great difficulty in maintaining such behavior, since he will not receive a pertinent response. Instead, there will be a great deal of pressure upon him to conform to expectations. Over a period of time his conformity to expectations is likely to become automatic, and he will even tend to impose the same pattern upon new patients who come after him.

Changing the Popular Picture of Mental Illness

The pressure of expectations—the self-fulfilling prophecy—upon the mentally ill can be a force for recovery as well as for deterioration. Patients can be influenced toward greater self-control, more rapid recovery, and less apathy and passivity. Use of the pressure of expectations however, requires bringing about a change in attitudes in those in contact with the mentally ill. If this is taken to mean the public at large, then, of course, this is an impossible task.

It is possible, however, to make a change in the attitudes of patients and staffs in mental hospitals. These people are the ones who exert the greatest influence upon hospitalized patients, and it is this latter group that we are most concerned with.

In general, the attitude that seems most therapeutic for those in the mental hospital to take is that mental illness is an acute episode from which complete recovery frequently can be expected. During the course of the illness patients are able to fulfill most of their normal responsibilities and take part in normal activities, and it is therapeutic for them to do so. Most of their capabilities will not be limited by their illnesses. Although individual patients will be deficient in one area or another of social functioning, as a group patients are capable in all areas and can assist one another. The job of the staff is to provide expert advice in areas where they are expert, and exert no more control than this. (Even though many of these assumptions are uncertain or unproved, it seems to be therapeutic to act as if they are true rather than to assume they are not true. There is a precedent for this in psychoanalysis, where, as a therapeutic maneuver, the patient is often asked to assume personal responsibility for occurrences whose causes are very uncertain.)

Concrete steps to dramatize this therapeutic attitude that can be taken include elemination of all forms of physical security and restraint devices; elimination of special service and recreational facilities in hospitals (e.g., libraries, barber shops, theaters, etc.) so that patients get the message that they are capable of using and are expected to use public facilities; provision of clocks, calendars, and newspapers for patients so that patients see that the staff considers the patients' time and contact with the outside world as important; emphasis on discharge planning and vocational training so that the patients see that the staff believes they are likely to recover; emphasis on neatness and cleanliness among the patients with provision of nice-looking clothes, toilet articles, etc., so that patients are encouraged to maintain normal standards of dress and personal hygiene; encouragement of communication among patients and staff on a person-to-person level so that patients are encouraged not to seek a dependent relationship with the staff, but rather continue to see themselves as independent adults; and placement of responsibility for control on patients by giving them access to knives, razors, scissors, glass, etc.

As an example, in one hospital, staff members are deliberately not given training in methods of physically controlling patients and are instructed never to use force on a patient. It is felt that by training the staff to use force, even if only in emergencies, the attitude of the staff as a result of the training may tend to increase the need for force. In the rare case where a patient is out of control, the police are called to use force. There are many other ways in which a change in attitude toward the mentally ill can be put into effect.

The question of how an administrator who has determined to bring about such a change can influence his staff to put it into practice needs further discussion. It is simple to tell the staff they are to change their methods of dealing with patients, and even to get them to give lip service to the principles, but getting them to change the tone of their interactions with patients is another matter. Recently several authors have written of techniques by which administrators can put into practice some of the principles of leadership and influence learned from small-group research.[35]

Generally it seems that staff will tend to treat patients in a manner similar to the way they themselves are treated by their supervisors. If staff members are treated as responsible adults, given a good deal of freedom in the way they do their jobs, and are approached with consideration for their individual needs, they are likely to react the same way with their patients. In addition, they must not be held responsible for behavior of patients nominally in their care, when under the open hospital system they have no real authority to control that behavior.

Iatrogenic Mental Illness

Some of the most popular forms of psychiatric treatment are capable of producing new symptoms and additional illnesses. The clearest example of this is mental hospitalization, particularly custodial care, as has already been discussed. There is little, if any, evidence that hospitalization is an effective treatment for mental illness. Even before Pinel in 1798, there were those who recognized the harmful effects of hospital treatment for the mentally ill. Yet hospitalization persists as a major form of treatment. One obvious explanation for this contradiction in the medical tradition of careful evaluation of treatment is that hospitalization is serving a social function more than a medical function. Although its medical value has always been doubtful and continues to be so, its social usefulness is so great that this overrides all other considerations.

Szasz has pointed out that the modern psychiatrist, in carrying out his functions, serves more than one master.[36] Although the psychiatrist usually talks in terms of observing the interests of his patients before all others, he also frequently must act in the interests of society, sometimes to the detriment of his patient. Since a major social value is that society be protected from the unpleasant sight and disordered actions of the mentally ill, the psychiatrist may be forced in protecting this value to do some harm to some of his patients. (Many patients, of course, must be hospitalized for their own good.)

Similarly, within the hospital when the physician prescribes heavy doses of sedatives, tranquilizers, or shock therapy to quiet an agitated or unpleasant patient, he may be doing so for the sake of the comfort of the staff or the orderliness of the hospital—all important social values—and not for the sake of the patient who is left semistuporous or confused. In the course of carrying out some of the duties set down for him by society, the psychiatrist can prolong an illness in some cases, or produce a new one.

"Above All Do No Harm"

The ancient admonition to physicians, "Above all do no harm," prescribes an ideal that is difficult for the psychiatrist in particular to follow all the time. Caught as he often is between conflicting demands, the psychiatrist must inevitably take an action that, while helping one person, injures another. It is important for him, however, to be aware of the effect of his actions so that he can rationally decide upon a course. He must attempt to keep in mind which of the treatments at his disposal are founded upon careful research and demonstrated effectiveness and which are based upon years of tradition and no research. He must recognize that the effectiveness and the harmfulness of a treatment varies individually from patient to patient, and he must attempt to increase his diagnostic skills in order to be able to take this into account. He must try to keep constantly in mind that he is in the midst of conflicting interests, that his treatment has great power to harm as well as to help, and that a significant amount of what he has been taught is based upon social utility and not medical science.

Mental Illness and Social Disorganization

Durkheim was one of the first to point out clearly the relationship between the state of the social group and the deviant behavior of its members.[37] In his view there was an increase in deviant behavior (suicide) when the norms of the group no longer controlled its members' behavior. This he called anomie, or normlessness.

This concept has been built upon by many workers in the field. For example, attempts have been made to specify the various patterns by which individuals respond to anomie, and to account for some forms of juvenile delinquency in terms of anomie.[38]

There have been numerous explanations of the occurrence of mental illness in terms of social disorganization, disruption of social values, or social stresses.[39] Little evidence is available regarding the accuracy of any of the various theories, and their details will not be gone into here. Suffice it to say that many sociologists and psychiatrists agree that the coherence of the social structure of a group strongly influences the susceptibility of group members to mental illness. One way of decreasing the amount of mental illness would be to increase the protective influence of the group.

Cloward and Ohlin's detailed explanation of the occurrence of delinquent gangs[40] and the plan for control of delinquency that was based on it[41] provide an example of what could be attempted in the area of mental illness.

Controlling Anomie

Cloward and Ohlin start with Durkheim's view that anomie occurs when men's goals become unlimited rather than socially regulated—any man can aspire for any position in society. They point out Merton's refinement that anomie results not from a lack of regulation of goals alone, but from disruption of the relationship between goals and socially legitimate ways of attaining these goals. Thus the problem of anomie becomes not that men aspire to goals unattainable for most of them, but that they aspire to goals that are not attainable by means within the bounds of social acceptability.

Cloward and Ohlin then point out that this theory permits distinctions to be made among segments of society regarding degrees of anomie. In those segments where access to attainment of goals is relatively free by legitimate means there will be less deviance than in segments where legitimate access is limited. In the case of our society where the principal goals—economic, educational, and vocational—have tended to become uniform through all groups, but where legitimate access to these goals is very limited for the lower socioeconomic groups, it can be predicted that most deviance will be found in the latter groups. Cloward and Ohlin call this a "differential opportunity" explanation for deviant behavior. Thus an individual's chances of becoming socially deviant depend upon the organization and rules of the social milieu in which he finds himself.

Cloward and Ohlin do not deal with mental illness. Their interest is in juvenile delinquency. However, they point out that the form which deviance takes depends in part upon the opportunities available for deviance (e.g., it is impossible to be a drug addict when no drugs are available). Many forms of deviance are possible, and it is conceivable that their formulation applies to certain forms of mental illness as well as to juvenile delinquency.

A later publication with which Cloward and Ohlin were associated presents a program for combating anomie. Its title, "A Proposal for the Prevention and Control of Delinquency by Expanding Opportunities," summarizes the approach.[42] By increasing access to goals through legitimate means for those whose access is otherwise limited, it is hoped to reduce anomie and thus prevent deviance. Access would be increased through education, vocational training, and assistance in job-hunting. Community organization efforts would increase political power in the community and increase access to the benefits that go with power.

Projects such as this one are being set up throughout the country. Still remaining to be examined is the effect of these programs upon mental illness, as well as the design and evaluation of similar programs specifically aimed at mental illness.

When specific predictions are made regarding results, as in the above example, it then becomes possible to test the hypothesis. Again, this is a goal toward which psychiatry could profitably orient itself.

Summary

Sociology is relatively neglected as a basic science of psychiatry and as an approach to developing new methods of treatment. Social factors influence the occurrence and the nature of mental illness in many ways. Mental illness is socially defined only in the encounter between two individuals, one socially labeled psychiatrist, and the other, patient. Some persons are influenced toward mental illness by its availability as an escape from intolerable situations. Other persons come to be called mentally ill when they function normally within a subculture that is deviant by majority standards. Social attitudes toward the mentally ill can reinforce existing symptoms or produce new ones. The disorganization of a social group can lead to mental illness among its members. Each of these concepts provides a suggestion for a method of dealing with mental illness. Some of these methods are already in use, having been developed empirically. Others can be seen to be developing. Theoretical understanding speeds up and makes development more effective.

PART II

Epidemiology

Introduction

THE ARTICLES SELECTED FOR INCLUSION IN THIS SECTION ENcompass a wide range of methods and issues using the epidemiological approach to psychiatric problems. Shepherd and Cooper's article is an extremely good review of the epidemiological method which includes studies of causation, illness expectancy, expansion and completion of the clinical picture, delineating clinical syndromes, community diagnosis, historical trends, and the workings of health services. The various examples of these applications of epidemiology which are cited certainly indicate the tremendous strides that have taken place in recent years.

Of particular significance in this review is the obvious emphasis given to studies of health services and of community diagnosis that to date have predominated over other uses of epidemiology. This emphasis makes sense when one considers the complexity of pursuing the search for causes and discerning genuine historical trends. This survey indeed points to the harsh realities of the field that require that some of the most interesting substantive issues be given a lower order of priority than the more answerable questions.

The major effort of the epidemiologist is to study the distribution and frequency of illness in the population and the factors contributing to its disposition. Such knowledge supplements clinical experience and points to possible etiological factors. In the course of time a number of epidemiological findings have come to be generally accepted about the distribution of schizophrenia; one notion, in particular, is that the highest rates of schizophrenia are to be found in the central area of cities and that they are associated with low status occupations. Kohn, in his comprehensive review, questions these findings and raises numerous issues for further investigation. He wonders whether these findings are peculiar to particular cities. While he concludes that this is not so, he does note that there was no correlation of the above in small towns with 36,000 people or fewer. Therefore, the above is probably valid only when considering larger urban environments. He also notes that the simple "drift hypothesis," which asserts that schizophrenics drift to lower socioeconomic levels as their illness progresses, no longer holds in the light of new findings. The important question remaining is whether in lower socioeconomic levels, the stress of schizophrenia leads to migration, or whether the stress of migration leads to schizophrenia.

Kohn also questions the adequacy of hospital rates as measures of the incidence of mental illness, for such rates measure only the number of people hospitalized at a specific time, i.e., prevalence, rather than the number of new cases, i.e. incidence.

Other areas of debate arise when one considers studies done in the community, diagnosing representative samples. How valid can this information be, as there is still a great need for good diagnostic scales? Then too, Kohn questions the dynamics of social class affecting the probability of an individual's becoming schizophrenic. Is it a function of the socioeconomic status or some other correlated variable, such as the stress of early childhood experience, that accounts for the fact that more schizophrenics are found in the lower socioeconomic levels?

Finally, Kohn notes the similarities *increasingly found* between the families of schizophrenics and families of lower economic status. There is, thus, in a search for the etiology of this illness, great need to examine the interactive effect of variables such as social class, early family relationships, genetics, and stress.

Another of the major objectives of epidemiological investigation is to determine whether certain individuals are more susceptible or vulnerable to specific disorders. This is the study of individual risk. To determine variations in susceptibility, it is desirable to be able to ascertain whether specific groups delineated by age, sex, race, occupation, migration status, or by other biological or sociological characteristics suffer more often from a particular disorder than do other groups. Ideally in such determinations one would want to be able to survey as comprehensive a group as possible, including not only obvious cases in treatment, but also subclinical cases in the community. The determination of greater risk in one group might not only lead to the development of special services for the group, but might also contribute information in search for etiological factors that may be concentrated in the personal experience or living circumstances of individuals in this group.

The survey of Hoch and Moses is an example of this kind of inquiry. They report on emotional disorders in a lower class immigrant housing development in Israel where one in five was found to be suffering from an emotional disorder. Young women and middle-aged men who had immigrated from the Afro-Asian countries and the European women who were in the 50- to 65-year-old age group had the highest percentage of mental illness and may be taken to be the groups with the greatest vulnerability to disorder in this society. This type of finding points also to the nature of epidemiological investigation where the results of a study tend to generate further questions. Here one would wonder whether individuals in these groups are vulnerable, in general, to other disorders as well, and to what extent their vulnerabilities are a reflection of their particular circumstances in Israeli society.

Another function of the epidemiologist is to investigate the etiology of psychiatric disorders. This can be done in a number of ways. One way might be to experimentally alter the independent variable presumed to be the significant etiological factor to see if there is a change in mental health. One can do this by changing certain features of a particular environment, then comparing the mental health outcome to that in a similar situation where no changes have been introduced. Another means of investigation might be to follow groups exposed to similar stresses over a period of time to determine the incidence of specific conditions which develop. In all such efforts, the epidemiologist faces the task of measuring the social or environmental variables presumed to have etiological significance. This is not a simple task.

The Rutter and Brown article which follows points to some of the major methodological obstacles likely to be encountered in such etiological studies; specifically it points to problems in the area of family life. They report on six different types of scales used to measure family life within the framework of four questions related to reliability and validity. "Can trained investigators agree about the emotions expressed and rated by a family member?" According to Rutter and Brown the simplicity and clarity of definition is important. Planned training with master tapes, group discussion, and the like are particularly important in insuring that investigators agree upon emotions expressed and related.

The second question is, "How far do the emotions expressed by the individual agree in different situations?" In their own investigations, the authors found that emotions expressed were highly consistent from one situation to another but, conversely, they found that the subject's report of someone else's emotions did not correlate well with other means of emotional measures. They felt that during the interview a high degree of involvement by the informant might influence the reliability. Therefore it was not good to rely on a single direct attitudinal questionnaire.

The third question they concerned themselves with was whether husbands or wives gave equivalent account of the family activities. There was a high correlation on concrete items and lower correlation on less concrete variables, such as parental interaction. The importance of distinguishing between objective and subjective variables was stressed.

Finally, Rutter and Brown considered factors influencing reliability and validity. Interviewer variables were not found to produce any differences in their study. Respondent bias was examined in relationship to sex differences and differences between patients and nonpatients. In this regard, differences were found only in the overall ratings of marriages.

Chapter 4

Epidemiology and Mental Disorder: A Review

MICHAEL SHEPHERD AND BRIAN COOPER

THOUGH IT IS NOW FASHIONABLE TO SPEAK OF THE EPIDEMIOLOGY of mental illness, this conjunction of terms appeared in the literature only rarely before 1949, when it was chosen as the title of a conference organized by the Milbank Memorial Fund to explore common ground betwen psychiatrists and public health workers.[1] Since then a spate of publications, especially in North America, the Scandinavian countries, and the United Kingdom, has signalized the confluence of two medical disciplines. The number of these investigations is now so large, and their nature so varied, that it is advisable to demarcate the boundaries of psychiatric epidemiology. In Britain this task has been made easier by the cataloging of current research projects by the M.R.C. Committee on the Epidemiology of Mental Disorder,[2] itself only some 4 years old. Just over 100 projects are listed, of which approximately one-third are focused on the psychological and social aspects of mental illness, either causal or concomitant; about one-quarter, which includes genetic studies, are concerned with the incidence or prevalence of different forms of psychiatric morbidity; one-

The authors would like to acknowledge the sources of several tables and figures in the text. They are: Professor K. Rawnsley (Table 1), *Pediatrics* (Table 2), the Editor and publishers of the *Journal of Psychosomatic Research* (Tables 3, 4 and 5), of the *Journal of Mental Science* (Fig. 2), and of *Annals of Eugenics* (Fig. 3, K. Pearson and G. A. Jaedevholm, on the inheritance of mental disease, *Ann. Eugen.* (Lond.), 4, 362, 1931).

sixth concentrate on prognostic or follow-up studies, and almost as many on primarily administrative issues; the remaining small miscellany comprises studies of diagnosis, vital statistics, and the evaluation of therapeutic procedures.

These topics can be taken as representative of the modern view of the scope of the epidemiological method in psychiatry; they fit well, for example, into the outline sketched by Lin in his recent W.H.O. monograph.[3] At the same time, it is apparent that to call the majority of such studies "epidemiological" is, in one sense, to do little more than attach new labels to old bottles: their objectives have been among the legitimate goals of psychiatric research for over a century. Clearly, some understanding of the evolution of psychiatric epidemiology is necessary if its present status and, still more important, its future prospects are to be assessed.

Historical Development

Many of our current notions on psychiatric epidemiology were in circulation before 1914, the year in which Goldberger published the first of a series of papers that were to demonstrate beyond argument the professional epidemiologist's contribution to the study of mental illness. There were several well-documented accounts of the so-called psychic epidemics. The development of intelligence testing and the early studies of suicide had established the value of the ecologist's method; and the older psychiatrists, as Lewis has pointed out, were familiar with such basic epidemiological themes as the relationship between mental disorder and migration, isolation, occupation, and socio-economic change.[4]

In view of these promising trends, it is of more than historical interest to examine the reasons for the relative neglect of the mass aspects of mental disorder in the earlier part of this century. How well the concepts of epidemiology had been established is clear from Frost's masterly review, published in 1927, which summed up the thinking of his day. Epidemiology, he wrote, being

> . . . essentially a collective science, its progress is largely dependent upon that which has been made in other fields. Since the description of the distribution of any disease in a population obviously requires that the disease must be recognized when it occurs, the development of epidemiology must follow and be limited by clinical diagnosis, and by the rather complex machinery required for the systematic collection of morbidity and mortality statistics. Epidemiology must also draw upon statistical methods and theory, because even the simplest quantitative descriptions must be stated statistically; and more minute descriptions, involving perhaps the demonstration of complex associations, may require the application of quite elaborate statistical technique. Moreover, quantitative epidemiological descriptions, in terms of frequencies of disease in different population groups, require, as part of their data, more or less detailed statistics of population, implying the prior development of demography.[5]

Unfortunately, Frost's vision was partially blinkered by the conventions of his day, for he goes on:

> . . . usage has extended the meaning of epidemiology beyond its original limits, to denote not merely the doctrine of epidemics, but a science of broader scope in relation to the mass phenomena of diseases in their usual or endemic as well as their epidemic occurrences. Although it is clear from current usage that the definition of epidemiology has been extended beyond its original sense, it is not clear just how far it has been extended. It is certain that its scope is not usually limited to the diseases in which epidemics are characteristic, since it is entirely in conformity with good usage to speak of the epidemiology of tuberculosis; and it seems customary also to apply the term to the mass phenomena of such non-

> infectious diseases as scurvy, but not to the so-called constitutional diseases, such as arteriosclerosis and nephritis. . . .
>
> In this sense epidemiology may be defined as the science of the mass phenomena of infectious diseases, or as the natural history of the infectious diseases.[6]

Inasmuch as this definition would exclude most mental illness from the purview of the epidemiologists, their disregard of psychiatry—with some rare and distinguished exceptions—could be attributed to the state of development of their subject. The failure of their leading psychiatric contemporaries to interest themselves in the mass phenomena of mental illness, on the other hand, can be more readily explained in terms of professional priorities. Many psychiatrists were preoccupied with a set of biological and phenomenological concepts, hoping to establish a scientific nosology with, in Adolf Meyer's words, "the psychological facts in their patients as mere symptoms of more or less hypothetical diseases back of them."[7] Yet to the more discerning epidemiologists these "psychological facts" were inseparably part of the mass phenomena of mental disorder; to Greenwood, for example, they figured prominently among his procatarctic factors of disease, and he wrote of them with characteristic hard-headedness:

> It is my business to point out that while a fairly consistent description of the aetiology of such crowd-diseases . . . can be provided by means of the hypothesis that the psychological element in the mixture of interactions expressed in bodily illness is the determinant, methods which have ignored that element have led to no consistent account of the facts at all. For this severely practical reason I hold that practical epidemiologists cannot afford to neglect psychology. *What* psychology they should study is not for me to say.[8]

Thirty years later, it is easier to appreciate that for the epidemiologist, concerned primarily with the study of populations, a meaningful psychology must extend beyond the individual organism. Unfortunately such a psychology was lacking a generation ago. Meyerian commonsense psychology, shaped by its originator's interest in the social sciences and construing mental illness as "the reaction of a personality (conceived as made up of constitutional endowment plus experience) to a situation in the social environment,"[9] might have provided an acceptable theoretical system had it not been for the clumsiness of most psychobiological formulations. At the same time, attempts to frame a theory of group behaviour based on instinctual propensities[10] became submerged by the growing influence of Freudian psychology, and were to remain neglected until the contemporary renewal of interest arising from comparative ethology. In his discussion of group psychology Freud gave lucid expression to the latent antithesis between his own outlook and that of the social psychologist:

> Group psychology is . . . concerned with the individual man as a member of a race, of a nation, or as a component part of a crowd of people who have been organized into a group at some particular time for some particular purpose. When once natural continuity has been severed in this way, if a breach is thus made between things which are by nature interconnected, it is easy to regard the phenomena which appear under these special conditions as being expressions of a special instinct ("herd instinct," "group mind"), which does not come to light in any other situations. But we may perhaps venture to object that it seems difficult to attribute to the factor of number a significance so great as to make it capable by itself of arousing in our mental life a new instinct that is otherwise not brought into play. Our expectation is therefore directed towards two other possibilities, that the social instinct may not be a primitive one and insusceptible of dissection, and that it may be possible to discover the beginnings of its development in a narrower circle, such as that of the family.[11]

While this point of view does not preclude an interest in the mass phenomena of disease, the emphasis of so authoritative a theorist tended to produce a concentration on individual psychopathology at the expense of a psychology of social involvement. Indeed, as one sympathetic critic has observed: "With certain exceptions, social psychology and psychoanalysis do not contradict each other—they no longer speak the same language."[12] Linguistic difficulties can be expected to impair communication. It is therefore not surprising that misunderstandings arose between epidemiologists and depth psychologists over questions of mutual interest. Psychodynamic embellishments, for example, lent a baroque façade to the severe outlines of the notion of accident proneness; and psychoanalysts have tended to show so little regard for the ecological approach to suicide that as late as the mid-1930's one of their most prominent representatives could claim that "... statistical data on suicide as they are compiled today deserve little if any credence."[13]

But if the growth of epidemiological psychiatry between the wars was retarded by these circumstances, a few investigators were able to anticipate the subsequent renaissance. Farsighted workers in the public health field, like Greenwood and Wilson, initiated collaborative studies with psychiatrists. Some psychiatrists—E. O. Lewis in Britain, Brugger in Germany, Rosanoff in the United States—affirmed their concern with public health aspects of their work by conducting large-scale community surveys;[14] while others were led to the same field of study by an interest in genetics.[15] In America statisticians like Malzberg and Pollock made use of data compiled in mental hospitals,[16] and sociologists of the Chicago school began to study the urban ecology of mental illness.[17] Scattered, uncoordinated, and deriving inspiration from several disciplines, these studies paved the way for the rapid expansion that was to follow the Second World War.

The rapidity of this expansion owed something to the unprecedented interest taken in the mental health of both the military and civil populations during the conflict. Its chief impulse, however, came from the postwar renewal of interest in the psychosocial components of morbidity and the emergence as a separate discipline of social, or "comprehensive," medicine. Epidemiological methods are fundamental to the aims of social medicine, which stands or falls by the ecological approach to illness—and especially to noninfectious, chronic illness where mental diseases take their natural place among Ryle's "diseases of prevalence, which also have their epidemiologies and their correlations with social and occupational conditions, and must eventually be considered to be in greater or less degree preventable."[18] Already in 1944 the Goodenough Report had underlined the importance of social medicine for British psychiatry; and what we now term social psychiatry has flourished to the point of preeminence in this country. The working assumption of the social psychiatrist is contained in Morris Ginsberg's statement that: "Though the individual consists largely of his social relations, there is a core of individuality in each person which is uniquely his own and which is in the last resort unshareable and uncommunicable."[19] It is an assumption that harmonizes not only with the undogmatic eclecticism of British psychiatry but also with the philosophy of the National Health Service in a welfare state where the conflicting claims of the citizen and his society constitute a basic political issue.

Problems of Method

An historical perspective, then, however limited in scope, can elucidate some of the reasons for the recent upsurge of interest in epidemiological psychiatry. It also helps to account for the comparatively meagre success so far attained. But this relative failure cannot be fully understood without reference to the factors which limit the application of epidemiological methods to mental disease. The limitations spring partly from a lack of basic information which time and effort can be expected to supply; but over and above these remediable deficiencies are more intractable problems; for convenience these may be subsumed under two main headings, the causation of mental illness, and the classification and measurement of psychiatric disorders.

THE CAUSATION OF MENTAL ILLNESS

To some modern epidemiologists, there are no *a priori* grounds for regarding mental illness as qualitatively different from other types of morbidity, so that the same tools that have proved so efficacious in the study of organic disease can be readily adapted to that of psychiatric disorder. Thus Reid comments that ". . . many mental illnesses are as much 'crowd diseases' as is typhoid fever," and again: "Although these (epidemiological) models were designed to fit the behaviour of infectious disease, there is no reason why some appropriate forms should not apply to the aspects of crowd behaviour, such as the dissemination of psychological disorders in human populations."[20]

This viewpoint overlooks some important aspects of psychiatric disorder, which are discussed in a report of the W.H.O. Expert Committee on Mental Health,[21] and can be summarized as follows: first, there are individual factors in the causes and manifestations of many psychiatric diseases that, because they belong to the sphere of values, cannot be fully quantified. Second, the aetiology of mental disorder is essentially multifactorial in nature. Third, there are considerable social and cultural differences in what is considered psychically abnormal in different surroundings, and in the way such abnormality is treated. Finally, human character and behaviour deviations show infinite variation, ranging from severe psychosis to mild personality disorders that many would regard as outside the boundaries of psychiatry.

In practice, mental illness is rarely infective, but it is often communicable. The extensive literature on mass outbreaks of irrational behaviour, extending from the so-called psychic epidemics to the more sophisticated modern studies of "socially shared psychopathology,"[22] testifies to the interest taken by many workers in the nature of this communication. Penrose has made a spirited attempt to retain the classical triad of host, environment, and agent in his mathematical model of crowd behaviour, with the morbid or exaggerated idea in the role of noxious agent.[23] For most workers, however, the causes of abnormal group behaviour are to be sought in the reactions of more or less predisposed individuals to particular sets of physical, psychological, or social circumstances. On this point there is agreement between attempted explanations otherwise as far apart in time and spirit as Hecker's "sympathy" or "imitation,"[24] Durkheim's "collective disposition"[25] and Kräupl and Taylor's "pluralistic emotions."[26]

This emphasis on host-environment interaction is carried over in the epidemiological approach to the large mass of non-infectious and noncommunicable psychiatric illness even when a physical agent like alcohol can be identified. Traditionally the study of factors pertaining to the host has been the domain of genetics, with a large contribution from epidemiology. Recent developments in genetics, to which reference is made later in this chapter, have brought the two disciplines still closer and if, as Böök has recently asserted, the geneticist must now ". . . ask the question 'what does the gene do to this individual' in the same sense as the virologist inquires about the effect of a specific virus,"[27] then the prospects of collaboration are closer still.

For the moment the epidemiologist's primary concern is with the influence brought to bear on the phenotype at different epochs of the life span. In the earliest paranatal phases of development the influences are dominantly physical; as the organism undergoes "psychosocial evolution," to borrow Medawar's phrase, so the social environment becomes increasingly important and the epidemiologist turns naturally to his colleagues in the social sciences for help. From them he has already received, and made good use of, such conceptual tools as class, mobility, isolation, and kinship; and when the delineation of social systems assumes primary importance, as with some forms of delinquent behaviour, the contribution of the social scientist becomes crucial. Unfortunately, however, the social sciences are still handicapped by what T. H. Marshall terms "a relative shortage of apparatus," which makes it difficult to ". . . provide schemes of analysis by which complicated problems are reduced to simple formulae."[28] Until these formulae become available the epidemiological study of social and interpersonal events, and the subject's perception of them, will remain gravely handicapped.

Classification of Psychiatric Disorders

The epidemiologist must identify his cases before he can count them, and he should be able to define and classify what he identifies. The nature of most psychiatric disorders, however, is so ill-defined as to preclude an aetiological classification. Within the major functional psychoses diagnostic practices have been shown to differ widely.[29] Variation is even more pronounced among the minor disorders, where the inadequacy of current systems of classification is most exposed. Estimates of the amount of neurotic illness dealt with by general practitioners, for example, have varied widely[30] and Crombie has pointed out that the International Classification of Disease does scant justice to the psychiatric case load in general practice, whose importance he has indicated by proposing a fivefold subdivision of total morbidity into (i) an illness, all or nearly all organic; (ii) an illness, mainly organic, but with some emotional content; (iii) an illness with emotional and organic components in equal proportion; (iv) a mainly emotional illness but with some organic content; and (v) an illness all or nearly all emotional.[31]

Along with the task of classifying declared morbidity goes that of identifying and classifying mentally ill persons who do not seek medical or social care. This ill-defined zone of disability is populated not only by individuals who exhibit psychological symptoms, anomalies of behaviour, and deviant personality traits, but also by those who fail to meet the "social-cultural expectations"[32] of their social group, and so demand assessment within a particular social context. The principal case-finding instruments available today are psychiatric and structured interviews, psychological screening tests and scales, and ratings of social adjustment to family, peers, work, and community.[33] For none of these methods is there at present adequate information as to reliability, validity, stability over time, or the importance of cultural factors in determining the accepted norm.

Uncertainties of diagnosis are closely linked to the problem of measurement. Mortality rates cannot often be applied usefully to psychiatric disorders, though when they are relevant, as in the case of suicide and of general paresis, they have been employed to good effect. Traditionally, the morbidity statistics for mental illness have been derived from mental hospital records, and first admission rates have provided a valuable guide to the incidence of major psychotic illness. Outside hospital practice, the records of industrial sickness absence and of general practice consultations have made it possible to use spells of sickness and doctor-patient contacts as indices of morbidity. By and large, however, the chronic, fluctuating course of much minor psychiatric disability places a heavy strain on the customary units of measurement. Duration may be difficult to determine, and operational measures such as "episodes" of illness are not easily defined. The definition of illness proposed by Hinkle and Wolff, for example, as "any symptom or syndrome that the American medical profession at the present time generally accept as evidence of ill-health,"[34] can be commended more on patriotic than on scientific grounds. More complex indices such as the "lifetime prevalence rate" are correspondingly less precise. The epidemiologist is thus seriously handicapped in his efforts to measure the rates of specific disease groups or reactions, and in the past he has tended to use global estimates of mental disorder, often lumped together with the rates for suicide, juvenile delinquency, crime and divorce, as catch-all indices of mental ill health. The case remains unproven for bringing together such disparate items on a linear scale to estimate the sickness of a society.

Applications of the Epidemiological Method to Psychiatry

This chequered background helps to explain why it is more informative to dwell on the uses rather than the achievements of the epidemiological method in psychiatry. Morris has suggested that there are seven uses for epidemiology, namely, for historical study, for community diagnosis, for study of the working of health services, for estimating the individual risks of acquiring disease, for completing the clinical picture, for identifying syndromes, and for establishing the causes of illness.[35] These several uses are, as he admits, no more than variations on a single theme, the "study of the health and disease of populations and groups in relation to their environment and ways of living." The spectrum of these seven variations passes from scientific analysis to public health action; each in turn can now be considered in relation to mental illness, the conncctions being illustrated with relevant examples.

Aetiological Studies

The primary scientific business of epidemiology is to do with the aetiology of disease, and its techniques are especially useful in assessing the relative importance of multiple causes. After nearly 50 years the studies of pellagra by Goldberger and his associates remain the most convincing demonstration of the value of this method applied to a neuro-psychiatric condition; or, to be more precise, of the method in the right hands, for it is not always recalled that the Thompson Commission, working at the same time on the same problem with the same methods, reached radically different conclusions.[36] Goldberger himself summed up the essence of his work as follows when he pointed out that to suggest a faulty diet as the root cause of pellagra was also to draw four inferences. "These are," he wrote, "first that a difference in diet as between pellagrins and non-pellagrins be demonstrable; second, that the disease must be curable by a proper diet; third, that it must be preventable by such a diet, and, fourth, that it may be experimentally produced by diet."[37] The establishment of these four postulates, and the coincident eradication of a major scourge, constitute one of the most remarkable achievements in modern medicine, whose details unfortunately still lie buried in the archives of the U.S. Public Health Reports, and merit much wider publicity. From the original accounts it is clear that although he was dealing with a condition in which the deficiency of a physical factor was both a necessary and sufficient cause, Goldberger was also alert to not only the massive socio-economic role of poverty in pellagra but also to the more subtle part played by psychological factors. Thus, in his first paper he suggested that, contrary to popular belief, pellagra was unlikely to be a communicable disease because of the exemption of nurses and attendants in mental hospitals where the disease was rife among the inmates. He commented drily: "The writer from personal observation has found that although the nurses and attendants may apparently receive the same food, there is nevertheless a difference in that the nurses have the privilege, which they exercise, of selecting the best and greatest variety for themselves. Moreover, it must not be overlooked that nurses and attendants have opportunities for supplementing their institutional dietary that inmates as a rule have not."[38] Again, on the appearance of deficiency symptoms among some residents of South Carolinian villages with adequate food supply, Goldberger wrote as follows: "A great variety of causes may operate to bring about individual peculiarities of taste with respect to food. They may have their origin in the seemingly inherent human prejudice against the new untried food or dish; they may date from some disagreeable experience associated with a particular food; they may arise as the result of ill-advised, self-imposed or professionally directed dietary restrictions in the treatment of digestive disturbances, kidney disease, etc.; they may originate as a fad; and in the insane they may arise because of some delusion such as the fear of poisoning, etc."[39]

All subsequent experimental studies, including the recent work on the inborn metabolic error of Hartnup's disease,[40] have served to confirm and elaborate on the broad picture of pellagra as defined epidemiologically. To be sure, the disease lent itself to this approach: it was well described clinically; the proximate causes were concurrent; and individual variation was relatively small. Goldberger himself was aware of these advantages and correspondingly cautious about the prospects of epidemiological research in other, more obscure, mental illnesses. Declining an offer to undertake research into schizophrenia, for example, he wrote: ". . . in five or more years I could probably find out nothing. Much work will be needed on the physiology of the central nervous system and on many collateral problems before dementia praecox can be understood."[41] Time has proved him right. A recent review of the epidemiological contributions to our knowledge of psychiatric aetiology suggests that the volume of work is more impressive than its results.[42]

The quest for causes has, in general, been directed towards the establishment of associations betwen significant events in the life history and the subsequent appearance of mental illness. These events can be subdivided chronologically into those with effects which are delayed in time, and those which are close enough to the outbreak of illness to be regarded as proximate or precipitant. The latter group has lent itself to population studies most conveniently in times of upheaval. Rawnsley, for example, has assessed the mental health of the Tristan da Cunha community evacuated to this country after the volcanic eruption in 1961 and has been able to compare his findings with those of a Norwegian expedition which visited Tristan in 1937–8.[43] The outstanding feature described by the Norwegians had been an outbreak of hysterical spells among the women of the island; the 19 survivors with a history of these "spells" were shown 25 years later to exhibit higher recent medical consultation rates and, in particular, to suffer from a form of psychogenic headache, which, in turn, proved to be significantly more often present among the wives of the island's leaders. Rawnsley's attempt to relate the two indices of morbidity, i.e., an earlier hysterical "spell" and a psychogenic headache, to the social factor of status suggests strongly that the paired associations are independent of the remaining variable.

For the study of proximal precipitants under more normal conditions Gordon has emphasized the value of analysing infrequently occurring, single events, by analogy with point epidemics, and has exemplified his argument with the psychoses after childbirth.[44] His suggestion has been followed up by Paffenbarger, who, by examining area hospital records over an 18-year period, identified a group of women whose first mental illness had occurred in relation to childbearing; 125 postpartum psychoses were detected, comprising a first-attack rate of 0.7 per 1000 live births.[45] A control group was derived from women of the same race whose deliveries immediately preceded or followed those of the index subjects. The two groups were compared in respect of age, parity, age at marriage, social class, period of gestation, birth weights, and the somatic complications of pregnancy and parturition. The small numbers involved limited detailed comparison, but there was a definite tendency for the frequency of recorded somatic complications to differentiate between the two groups. To test the specificity of these findings, Paffenbarger went on to make identical comparisons with two other index groups, namely, mothers who had developed late postpartum haemorrhage, and mothers whose infants had developed hypertrophic pyloric stenosis. In neither were the differences of the same order as those found with the psychotic mothers.

Essentially the same method of retrospective analysis of hospital records has been employed by Pasamanick and his co-workers to examine the significance of much earlier events in the individual life history. They collected information about the complications of labor recorded on birth certificates or hospital records, and compared the data obtained with those relating to infants selected from the same batch of birth certificates and matched for a number of relevant variables. The logic of this procedure, in the authors' own words, runs as follows:

> (1) Since prematurity and complications of pregnancy are associated with foeta and neonatal death, usually on the basis of injury to the brain, there must remain a fraction so injured who do not die. (2) Depending upon the degree and location of the damage, the survivors may develop a series of disorders. These extend from cerebral palsy, epilepsy, and mental deficiency through all types of lesser degrees of damage sufficient to disorganize behavioural development and lower thresholds to stress. (3) Further, these abnormal-

> ities of pregnancy are associated with certain life experiences, usually socioeconomically determined, and consequently (4) they themselves and their resulting neuro-psychiatric disorders are found in greater aggregation in the lower strata of our society.[46]

The use made of this method is illustrated most clearly by reference to mental subnormality, one stage along their "continuum of reproductive casualty." Their retrospective studies had suggested a significant association between subnormality and not only such physical features as prematurity, maternal complications of pregnancy and neonatal-abnormalities, but also socioeconomic status, race, and season of birth. To assess the individual importance of these several factors the authors then resorted to a prospective study, following up 500 premature babies and a control group of full-term infants matched for hospital of birth as well as for socioeconomic circumstances.[47] At 40 weeks the premature infants exhibited a higher incidence of neurological abnormalities and a lower development quotient on the Gesell development examination. These findings were confirmed when 300 of the children were reexamined more than 2 years later, but in addition it was then noted that whereas at 40 weeks the development quotients of white and colored control children were virtually identical the groups had diverged by the age of 3 years. Whereas the white children then exhibited an improvement of their adaptive and language skills, the opposite was true of the Negroes. The sharpest decline was recorded for the children whose mothers had received the poorest education. These differences, which were not evident in other fields of behaviour, are attributed by the authors to sociocultural factors.

Longitudinal studies of this kind, in which a cohort of normal subjects is followed up in order to define variations of development, and so to assess the significance of deviant behaviour, represent an epidemiological technique of increasing importance. Other examples include the study by Douglas of a national sample of British children born during 1 week in

1946,[48] and Mangus and Dager's survey of factors related to personality change in the second decade of life.[49] The information provided is especially valuable for child psychiatry which has long suffered from the lack of normative data against which to evaluate supposed disorders of behaviour. These studies, however, are slow to mature and can be usefully supplemented by cross-sectional surveys. In the Buckinghamshire Child Health Survey, for example, data have been collected about a 10 percent sample of all school-children between the ages of 5 and 15 in an English county.[50] There stands out a small but persistent group of daily bedwetters up to the age of 10–11, most of whom were receiving no medical attention, and were not regarded as presenting psychiatric problems.

As an aid to the study of human development, epidemiology helps to assess the impact of life experiences on innate characteristics. The newer technical advances have now made possible the extension of epidemiological research into the field of genetics proper. In mongolism, for example, Cohen, Lilienfeld, and Sigler have pointed out that the newly discovered chromosomal abnormalities have already made it necessary to estimate (1) the chromosomal constitution of a representative sample of phenotypically normal subjects; (2) the comparative incidence of mongolism, to examine the effect on nondisjunction of external events like ionizing radiation; (3) the possible association between trisomy and translocation and maternal age; and (4) the relationship between mongolism, leukaemia, and ionizing radiation.[51] All these questions are open to a form of epidemiological study that can be expected to proliferate in the wake of other cytogenetic discoveries.

Illness-expectancy Studies

Estimating the individual expectation of psychiatric illness has also been a joint concern of genetics and epidemiology. Some of the outstanding early investigations of mental disorder in communities were inspired by a primary interest in genetics, and indeed Fremming, whose longitudinal study of mental illness on the island of Bornholm is a model of its kind, wrote of survey methods that "the most important purpose of such research is to provide reliable figures for the expectation of hereditary mental diseases in the general population."[52]

The classical contribution of epidemiology in this sphere, however, has been the concept of accident proneness. The origin of this term can be traced back to 1919 when Greenwood and Woods, in their report to the Industrial Fatigue Research Board, suggested that the observed frequency distributions of accidents in a group of factories fitted best mathematically with the hypothesis of initially unequal liabilities to accidents rather than to pure chance or to a bias in the direction of individuals who had already sustained at least one accident.[53] Further work tended to substantiate this notion of "accident liability," but in 1926 Farmer and Chambers transmuted a statistical into a psychological concept, defining "accident proneness" as "a personal idiosyncrasy predisposing the individual who possesses it in a marked degree to a relatively high accident rate."[54] Though the evidence has never established a dichotomy between individuals who are and are not accident-prone, nonetheless, as Adelstein has commented, the concept "was seized upon as the open sesame to all accident problems" by many subsequent workers who were impressed by the more speculative assumptions of psychosomatic medicine.[55] That a more rigorous application of the concept may still prove rewarding has been demonstrated recently by Smart and Schmidt.[56] Basing their work on the suggestion that patients with psychosomatic illnesses tend to experience morbid tension, and seek release by physical action that is often ill-considered, they argued that such patients would therefore tend to be involved comparatively frequently in all forms of accidents, including traffic accidents. From a group of 271 male hospital patients in Ontario with an unequivocal diagnosis of peptic ulcer, they ascertained that 135 possessed driving licences, and that this subgroup did not differ in social or demographic essentials from either the remaining ulcer patients or from the male population of the province. They then compared the age-adjusted traffic-accident rates for the 135 index cases with those of male car drivers in the general population. This group experienced a significantly higher rate of accidents than average, and so constituted a high-risk group.

Completing the Clinical Picture

In the use of epidemiological techniques as aids to the completion, or extension, of the clinical picture of mental disease, perhaps the most interesting development in this country has been the new look taken at the general practitioner under the National Health Service. The crude statistics of the age-sex distribution of neurotic illness as obtained from hospital data and from general practice (Fig. 1) indicate the dimensions of the problem of neuroses in the community.[57]

Study of the nature of the clinical and social phenomena exhibited by these patients (only a small minority of whom are ever referred to a psychiatrist) constitutes a major task for the future. So does their outcome, for whereas prognostic studies of the major forms of psychiatric illness are well-established, our knowledge of the natural history of the minor disorders is still in its infancy. Meanwhile evidence is accumulating to suggest that psychological and social factors can affect the outcome of some established physical disease whose course is known to differ widely from case to case.[58] Recently, for example, Rutter has conducted an anterospective study of a sample comprising 80 cases of established peptic ulceration followed up for 6 months after their discharge from hospital in-patient care.[59] During their stay in hospital observations were made on the patients' physical condition and radiological

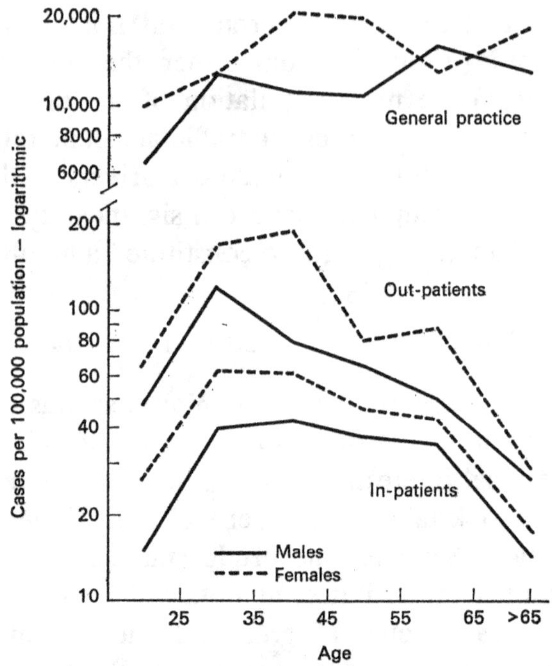

FIGURE I. Age prevalence of neurosis studied during I year.

status by a physician; at the same time the psychosocial variables were assessed independently by the psychiatrist and psychiatric social worker. After 6 months the patients were re-examined by all three observers independently. Surprisingly, outcome could not be correlated with any of the somatic or social factors but affective features present at the initial psychiatric examination were significantly related to the patient's state after 6 months, whether this was assessed either by the presence of ulcer pain or by incapacity for work.

Extending the clinical picture to include the subclinical or "incipient" cases with declared illness raises particular difficulties in psychiatry. How important this problem can be is well shown in the sphere of mental subnormality when intelligence test results are compared with clinical findings. In the study of Stockholm children cited by Penrose, for example, a group of 300 children, excluded from ordinary schools on the ground of feeble-mindedness, was examined with a modified version of the Binet-Simon test.[60] A sample of the normal school population was similarly examined. It was shown that the distribution of intelligence scores was quite continuous, with no indication of a natural boundary between the normal and the defective children. There was a close correlation (about + 0·8) between the test scores and the clinical diagnosis of feeble-mindedness, but the correspondence was by no means perfect; had the ascertainment of mental deficiency been made on test scores rather than on clinical examination, a somewhat different group would have been selected as abnormal.

The clinical picture can also be extended by comparisons between mental illness in different environments as by the description of the so-called exotic psychiatric disorders.[61] The possibilities of this approach have been explored by Murphy in his careful study of the urban distribution of mental illness in Singapore.[62] By relating the rates of mental hospital admission to areas of residence in terms of defined census tracts, he was able to show, in accordance with expectation, that positive relationships existed, some tracts being associated with much higher rates than others. Unlike his predecessors working in the Occident, however, Murphy did not find the highest rates of illness in the densely populated lower class slum districts. Again, when the residential areas were classified by cultural and ethnic characteristics, it emerged that, contrary to findings elsewhere, geographic mobility correlated positively with manic-depressive disorder, and negatively with schizophrenia. The key to these discrepancies, Murphy suggested, lay in the special sociocultural features of Singapore that dis-

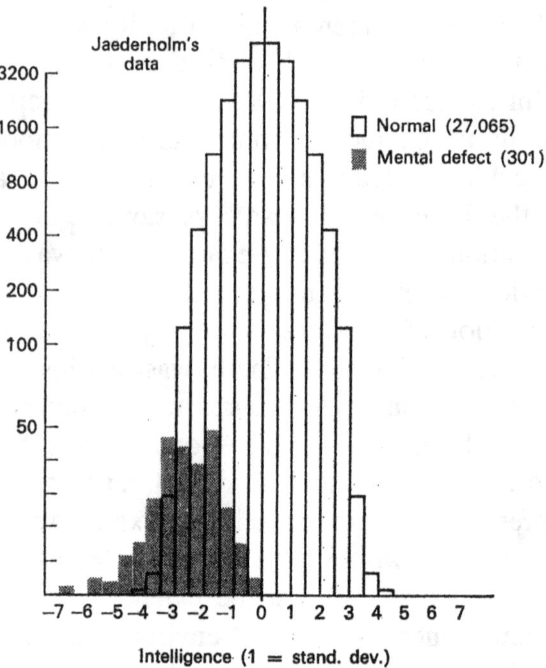

FIGURE 2. Distribution of intelligence.

tinguish it from the pattern of most Western cities. Emphasizing the importance of the supportive culture that exists in the Singapore slum areas, he commented: "There is a tendency in the West to think of the slums as being populated by people who have no ambition and have made no effort to get out of them; in Singapore one might say that a considerable proportion of the slum dwellers are there precisely because they have ambition—at least the ambition to leave their native land in search of something better." With regard to the unexpected distribution of the functional psychoses, he suggested that the association found in other societies between high rates of schizophrenia and lack of cultural support is understandably absent in Singapore, because "what causes or at least is linked to the rise in the schizophrenia rate is not the absence of cultural support but the efforts of both society and the individual to regain or retain such support." In Singapore, where the stranger must contend with an attitude of *laissez-faire* indifference, "the evidence," says Murphy, "suggests that an affective type of breakdown may be encouraged when the individual lacks the support of a surrounding culture and is not led to make an effort to assimilate."

Delineation of Syndromes

A W.H.O. expert committee[63] has recommended that this method be employed in all prevalence surveys on the grounds that symptoms constitute the most easily standardized and measurable units of observation, and that knowledge of their distribution in populations, independent of the charting of formal illness, leaves the way open for new discoveries. There is, however, an understandable reluctance on the part of clinically trained psychiatrists to revert to purely symptomatic levels of description perhaps for the reason that Lewis has advanced: "It is humiliating because it throws us back to the infancy of medicine."[64]

The recording of enumerated symptoms has proved most valuable so far in screening techniques, employed mainly where large numbers have to be examined rapidly, as in induction procedures.[65] The use of a similar technique in an area prevalence survey has been described by MacMillan.[66] A more promising field for mapping new syndromes, however, is that of child psychiatry, where an established nosology is still lacking and the clinician relies less on symptoms than on signs of morbidity, particularly on disturbances of behaviour. Case identification is here more difficult in that it may depend, not so much on the observation of intrinsically abnormal behaviour, as on exaggeration of normal traits or the persistence of certain kinds of behaviour beyond the appropriate stage of development. To this extent, pathological disturbance may be equated with deviation from the norm, and the significance of any observed item of behaviour cannot be assessed without some knowledge of its frequency by individual age groups. Thus in a current British research project, the Buckinghamshire Child Health Survey, information has been gathered on a sample of 6000 normal school-children, and also on child guidance clinic attenders with known psychiatric disturbance.[67] The data, collected from questionnaires completed by parents and teachers, cover the occurrence and frequency of most commonly recognized symptoms, and also provide for rating various characteristics on a simple three-point scale. In this way, a picture is being built up of behavioural norms for this population, and the significance of the least common characteristics tested by comparison with the child guidance sample. Observed clustering of symptoms or uncommon characteristics can then provide a basis for the delineation of syndromes or abnormal patterns of behaviour.

Community Diagnosis

With this type of study epidemiology enters the realm of public health and medical administration. Though its more immediate concern is likely to be with the planning of health services, the diagnosis of health and disease in whole communities has prevention as its ultimate goal. In this context, the survey of mental deficiency carried out over thirty years ago by E. O. Lewis can still be regarded as a model.[68] He took six geographical areas of England and Wales, each with a population of about 100,000, and of widely differing type; three were urban and three rural, and they included a metropolitan suburb, a mining area, and a northern cotton town.

Lewis was able to show that they were representative of the country as a whole in respect of such characteristics as social class and occupation, incidence of treated mental disorder, and ascertained mental deficiency. He then carried out in each area a survey of adult mental deficiency based on the reports of all available medical and social agencies, together with a screening of all school children. This latter, the most important part of the investigation, was carried out in three stages. First, the teachers in each school were asked to pick out the children of each age whose school work and general performance were poorest; about 15 percent of the whole school population was sorted out on this basis, so that there was no possibility of any significant number of retarded children being missed. Secondly, all these children were then submitted to group intelligence tests, which were supervised and scored by Lewis's assistants. Thirdly, all children whose scores on the group tests suggested a degree of mental retardation were examined individually by Lewis, using both intelligence tests and medical inspection. In the infants' departments, where group tests were inapplicable, 6 percent of the most backward children were examined individually. By these methods Lewis obtained a total prevalence rate for the six areas surveyed of 8·57 per 1000, a figure that still commands substantial agreement.

Where sufficient knowledge has been established a psychiatric condition, like any other, can be identified by screening procedures, and prophylactic measures can be introduced by the public health authorities. In the case of phenylketonuria, for example, it has already proved possible for 124 British local health authorities at the request of the Ministry of Health to undertake the routine screening of infants aged 4–6 weeks and so to identify 39 cases from more than 650,000 tests; the possibility of treating these early cases with low phenylalanine diets then opens the way to preventive action.[69] Unfortunately few psychiatric disorders are sufficiently well defined for large-scale, rational prophylactic or therapeutic measures to be feasible and most community studies have been concerned chiefly with the prevalence of mental ill health. The results of these surveys are least equivocal when the patient's condition is clearly identified by contact with a medical or social agency.

In Britain the National Health Service has led to so wide a coverage of the population by general practitioners that the extent of such conspicuous morbidity can be estimated from their returns. The amount of illness is not inconsiderable. A study of our own, for example, has recently shown that the reported one-year period prevalence rate for adult psychiatric illness reported by some eighty practitioners in the London area was as high as 140 per 1000.[70] These estimates, however, represent only a fraction of the reported rates of medically inconspicuous morbidity. Here the investigator is compelled to employ an operational definition of mental ill health and to examine whole populations or samples of them by questionnaire or interviews: often he undertakes a large, extensive survey supplemented by a smaller intensive study. For the purpose some workers adopt a pragmatic approach with reliance on the subjects' reports, supplemented by direct questioning. In a study of a new housing estate, for example, Martin *et al.* interviewed a sample of 750 families at home, using a check-list of symptoms: 22 percent of the adults admitted to "nerves," 17 percent to "depression," 12 percent to sleeplessness, and almost as many to undue irritability.[71] Other workers assume that there is a scale along which mental health or personality can be placed and measured; the authors of the midtown Manhattan project,[72] for example, quote with approval the view . . . "that an emotional adjustment exists on a quantitative continuum and that trained psychiatrists or psychologists are able to place an individual in his position on this continuum . . ."[73] On either assumption the results are disconcerting. The families on the housing estate exhibited at least one symptom in 35 percent of cases; of the midtown residents only 18.5 percent were deemed mentally "well." It must be concluded either that mental ill health approaches the rule or that the criteria by which it is assessed are inadequate. As present the operational criteria of individual investigators differ so widely as to render comparative studies in place or time more useful than attempts to chase the chimera of "true" prevalence.

Comparison between the prevalence rates of mental ill health in more than one area usually goes with a search for ecological correlates, ranging from relatively simple factors like overcrowding to complex indices of social structure like those used by Leighton in North America[74] and Loudon in southern Wales. Comparisons over time are harder to come by, but the results of Essen-Möller's forthcoming second survey of the overt and latent mental disability in south Sweden should be of particular interest.[75] Mention must also be made of the large anterospective study of Wilner and his colleagues who examined the effect of the quality of housing on mental and physical health by a three-year follow-up of 300 families moved from slum to superior accommodation with a control group of 300 slum families; they succeeded in demonstrating that determination and half a million dollars can prove the obvious, but their work stands as a monument to the practical use of epidemiology in social research.[76]

Historical Studies

As a means of demonstrating changes in the character or distribution of illness the use of the historical method in psychiatry has been limited until recent years. With the help of this method it is possible to analyse time trends to determine, above all, whether the amount of mental illness has altered and whether it has been affected by therapeutic or other measures. Anecdotal studies like those of Haeser (1882) and Hecker (1859) on the dancing manias of the Middle Ages are descriptively important, but their value is much enhanced when reliable statistics are also available. Hare, for example, from a study of contemporary records and clinical descriptions, was able to plot the spread of general paresis across Europe, and to adduce a certain amount of evidence supporting the hypothesis of a neurotropic strain of spirochaete originating in northern France at the end of the fifteenth century.[77] He was able also to make use of statistical data to examine more recent trends, thereby demonstrating a steady decline in the prevalence of general paresis which has long antedated modern methods of treatment.

To the long-standing controversy on the putative increase of mental disorder, Goldhamer and Marshall made a useful contribution by comparing mental hospital admission rates in Massachusetts over an interval of 100 years.[78] They found that the nineteenth and twentieth century age-specific rates were radically different; in the earlier period there was a relatively high concentration in the 20–50 age group, whereas in the more recent period the majority of patients admitted were in their fifties and sixties. On the evidence, they suggest that while a large part of the seeming increase was due to a growing tendency to admit to hospital patients with mental disorders associated with the senium, some of the increment might be attributed to a true rise in the incidence of these conditions, especially cerebral arteriosclerosis.

In a different field, Halliday has studied the patterns in the incidence and distribution of certain "psychosomatic" disorders over the first half of this century.[79] He found evidence of a marked increase in the incidence of peptic ulcer among males, but not among females, so that the sex ratio for this group of disorders had changed considerably during the period under review. Conversely, for diabetes there had been a marked increase among females, but not among males. Over a period of 50 years the male/female ratio for deaths ascribed to this disease had fallen from 2 to 0·5. Halliday postulated that such striking changes in the sex distribution of disease must be associated with some corresponding changes of male and female psychosocial roles in our society.

Studies of Health Services in Action

The perspective obtained from historical studies can be of service in the assessment of current health services and the prediction of future needs. The present debate on the future of British mental hospitals, for example, has been largely inspired by the recorded fall in mental hospital residents over the past decade. According to one prediction the need for beds will have fallen about 40 percent by 1975, largely because of an anticipated rundown of the population of chronic hospital inmates.[80] As this decline has coincided approximately with the introduction of tranquillizing drugs, some workers have claimed a causal association between the two events. That this is not necessarily so has been shown by the static picture obtained from individual institutions that had enjoyed the benefits of a major program of administrative reform, with favourable consequences for the bed state, before the advent of tranquillizers.[81] Such figures suggest that the social concomitants of drug therapy play an important part in affecting the flow of patients from hospital.

Attempts to examine directly the workings of the mental health services in action have been surprisingly few. Recently, however, Lawrence has made an operational study of the emergency procedures in London by concentrating on the social determinants of admission to a metropolitan observation ward.[82] She was able to obtain relevant information about not only a group of patients but also a sample of the 20 percent of people who were referred to the mental welfare department without further action being taken. Her findings indicate that however important the medical aspects of the case both the breakdown in tolerance that initiated referral and the decision of the D.A.O. to take action were also affected strongly by social and administrative pressures and by the attitudes and beliefs of contiguous figures in the immediate environment.

Future Prospects

No survey, however brief, of the past and present status of psychiatric epidemiology can be complete without some reference to its future. At a recent American conference devoted to the future of psychiatry hopes were pinned to the development of giant electronic digital computers "permitting the posing of questions and obtaining of answers which were never dreamed of in the past."[83] It would seem to be more realistic to recognize that the questions are already with us and that most of the answers are more likely to come from human than from mechanical brains. Nor is it necessary to accept the complementary American prophecy of "the continued application of human ignorance and error to research method and analysis and interpretation of data," provided the clinical and the social investigator can be imbued with a viewpoint which was clearly outlined by Sir James Spence:

> His main task is to place the phenomena (of disease) in temporal and in quantitative relationships with each other. This leads him to know the course of a disease as it may be expected commonly to occur. His next task is to determine the variation from that course, and to find correlations between these variations and aetiological factors or alternative treatments. When possible he uses statistics to express these variations. He uses statistical estimates of variations also in designing the extent of his study. If the disease under study is one which varies little in its course he limits his number of examples. . . . He thus comes to know disease as a predictable sequence of events, and the knowledge gained becomes the basis,

> the only basis, by which the underlying process of disease in the living patient can be rationally interpreted.[84]

Spence was talking here about clinical science but his summary of its logic might be transposed verbatim to what is now being called clinical epidemiology. This discipline can and should supplement and expand the psychiatrist's traditional concern with the individual patient. "Psychiatry," as Odegaard has insisted, "is forced to study groups and populations because it deals with individuals, not in spite of that fact."[85]

Chapter 5

On the Social Epidemiology of Schizophrenia

MELVIN L. KOHN

MY INTENT IN THIS PAPER IS TO REVIEW A RATHER LARGE and all-too-inexact body of research on the epidemiology of mental illness, to see what it adds up to and what problems it poses for further research. I shall be highly selective, and I shall be highly summary. Instead of reviewing the studies one by one, I shall talk of general issues and bring in whatever studies are most relevant. It hardly need be stressed that my way of selecting these issues and my evaluation of the studies represent only one person's view of the field and would not necessarily be agreed to by others.

Before I get to the main issues, I should like to make four general comments, by way of introduction:

1. Much of what I shall discuss will concern not mental illness in general, but schizophrenia in particular. The emphasis on schizophrenia is because of its singular importance as a public health problem, because so much of the relevant research has been focused on schizophrenia, and perhaps most of all because I happen to think of schizophrenia as the most theoretically challenging of the mental disorders.

When I speak of schizophrenia, I shall generally be using that term in its American, not its Scandinavian, sense—that is to say, I shall mean roughly what is meant by the *two* Scandinavian diagnostic entities, schizophrenia plus reactive psychosis. I use the term in its American sense not because that usage is superior, but because it is the usage that has been employed in much of the relevant research, and because any comparative discussion must necessarily employ the more inclusive, even if the cruder, term.

2. I want to mention only in passing the broadly comparative studies designed to examine the idea that mental disorder in general and schizophrenia in particular are products of civilization, or of urban life, or of highly complex social structure. There have been a number of important studies of presumably less complex predominantly rural societies that all seem to indicate that the magnitude of mental disorder in these societies is of roughly the same order as that in highly urbanized, Western societies. I refer, for example, to Lin's study of Taiwan,[1] the Leightons' in Nova Scotia,[2] Leighton and Lambo's in Nigeria,[3] and Eaton and Weil's of the Hutterites.[4] For a historical perspective within urban, Western society Goldhamer's and Marshall's study in Massachusetts[5] is the most relevant; it indicates that the increasing urbanization of Massachusetts over a period of 100 years did *not* result in any increase in rates of disorder, except possibly for disorders of old age. The data are hardly precise enough to be definitive, but they lead one to turn his attention away from the general hypothesis that there are sizable differences in rates of mental disorder between simpler and more complex social structures, and to look instead at differences *within* particular social structures, where the evidence is far more intriguing.

3. I shall not attempt here to review the data on possible genetic factors in schizophrenia, although these are certainly relevant to any discussion of the epidemiology of mental disorder. That field, as you may know, is in quite a ferment at the moment. A reanalysis of the data from twin studies by David Rosenthal[6] has strongly suggested that past studies, particularly because of the methods used for the selection of

cases for study, have greatly exaggerated the concordance figures for identical twins. (By concordance is meant the probability that if one twin becomes schizophrenic his co-twin will too.) Preliminary studies by Tienari[7] in Finland and Kringlen[8] in Norway have substantiated Rosenthal's conclusion to a startling degree. Since Kringlen is now conducting what promises to be the definitive study, it might be best to reserve final conclusions for awhile. But one conclusion has long been clear: whatever the degree to which genetic factors predispose to schizophrenia, they do not provide a *sufficient* explanation of that disorder, and one must look elsewhere too.

4. Finally, much of what I shall do in this paper will be to raise doubts and come to terribly tentative conclusions from inadequate evidence. If you wonder why this is worth doing, the reason is that we know so little and the problem is so pressing. Genetics does not provide a sufficient explanation, and, I take it from Kety's critical review,[9] all biochemical and physiological hypotheses that have been advanced to date have failed to stand the test of careful experimentation. And so, inadequate as the following data are, they are the best that are available to us.

I.

It seems to me that most of the important epidemiological studies of schizophrenia can be viewed as attempts to resolve problems of interpretation posed by the pioneer studies, Faris & Dunham's ecological study of Chicago[10] and Clark's analysis of occupational rates.[11] Their findings were essentially as follows:

Faris & Dunham: The highest rates of first hospital admission for schizophrenia are in the central area of the city, with diminishing rates as you move toward the periphery.

Clark: The highest rates are for the lowest status occupations, with diminishing rates as you go to higher status occupations.

Let us consider the issues that arise in trying to interpret these findings.

1. The first issue, the simplest but nevertheless a strangely perplexing issue, is whether or not the findings are somehow peculiar to Chicago. This much we can say with certainty: the findings are not unique to Chicago. The essential finding of the Faris and Dunham investigation, on the ecological distribution, has been replicated or partially replicated in a number of American cities—Providence, Rhode Island; Peoria, Illinois; Kansas City; St. Louis; Milwaukee; Omaha, Nebraska[12]—and in Oslo, Norway.[13] The essential finding of the Clark investigation, on the occupational distribution, has been confirmed again and again, in these same investigations, in Hollingshead and Redlich's study of New Haven,[14] in the research by Srole and his associates in midtown, New York City,[15] and in several other investigations.[16] Svalastoga's reanalysis of Strömgren's data for northern Denmark is consistent,[17] as is Leighton's for "Stirling County," Nova Scotia. Ødegaard has presented some partial data for Norway that seem to lead to the same conclusion.[18]

But there are some exceptions. Clausen and I[19] happened across the first, when we discovered that for Hagerstown, Maryland, there was no discernible relationship between either ecological area or occupation and rates of schizophrenia. On a reexamination of past studies, we discovered a curious thing: the larger the city, the stronger the correlation between rates of schizophrenia and these indices of social structure. In the metropolis of Chicago, the correlation is large, and the relationship is linear: the lower the social status, the higher the rates. In cities of 100,000 to half a million (including Oslo, as Sundby and Nyhus showed), the correlation is smaller and not so linear: it is more a matter of a pile-up of cases in the lowest socio-economic strata, with not so much variation among higher strata. When you get down to a city as small as Hagerstown—36,000—the correlation disappears. This proved to be the case not only for Hagerstown, but for the tiny city of "Bristol," Nova Scotia, in the Leighton's investigation,[20] and for the rural area of Scania, in Sweden, that Hagnell and Essen-Möller have been investigating.[21] So one must conclude that although there is overwhelming evidence for a correlation of both ecological area and occupation to rates of schizophrenia, it has been demonstrated only for larger cities. We are dealing then with the social structure of the larger urban environment.

2. The second issue is, depending on how you look at it, either a trivial technical issue or a substantive issue of great importance. As a technical issue, it is generally referred to as the "drift hypothesis"; as a substantive issue, it is the issue of mobility.

The drift hypothesis was first raised as an attempt to explain away the Faris and Dunham findings. The argument is that in the course of their developing illness, schizophrenics tend to drift down into lower status occupations and lower status areas of the city. It is not that more cases of schizophrenia are produced in these strata of society, but that schizophrenics who are "produced" elsewhere end up at the bottom of the heap by the time they are hospitalized, and thus are counted as having come from the bottom of the heap.

There have been odds and ends of evidence for and against the drift hypothesis,[22] none of it definitive, but the best-designed studies seem to indicate that schizophrenics have been no more downwardly mobile than other people coming from the same social backgrounds. The really critical evidence in the controversy, it seems to me, are the recent findings of Srole and associates that rates of mental disorder correlated nearly as well with their *parents'* socioeconomic status as with patients' own socioeconomic status. Certainly the parents didn't drift downward because of the patients' disease, and so the simple drift hypothesis does not hold. (More complicated formulations, that include genetic factors, may still have some merit.)

The mobility issue as a substantive issue is another thing again. Ever since Ødegaard's classic study of rates of mental disorder among Norwegian migrants to the United States,[23] we have known that mobility is a matter of considerable consequence for mental illness. We have not known *how* and *why* it is a matter of consequence—whether it is a question of who migrates or of the stresses of migration—and unfortunately subsequent research has failed to clarify this issue. This question is one of considerable importance, but since it takes me afield from the main theme of my discussion I shall not pursue it here. My concern for the moment is not with mobility but with social structure.

3. The third issue in interpreting the Faris and Dunham and the Clark investigations is the most serious of all: the question of the adequacy of hospital admission rates as a measure of the incidence of mental disorder. Faris and Dunham tried to solve the problem by including patients admitted to private as well as to public mental hospitals. This was insufficient because, as several subsequent studies have shown, many people who become seriously mentally ill never enter a mental hospital. Subsequent studies have attempted to do better than Faris and Dunham by including more and more social agencies in their search for cases; Hollingshead and Redlich in New Haven, and Jaco in Texas,[24] for example, have extended their coverage to include everyone who falls into any sort of treatment facility—Jaco going so far as to question all the physicians in the state of Texas. This is better, but clearly the same objections hold in principle. And Srole has demonstrated that there are considerable social differences between people who have been treated, somewhere, for mental illness, and severely impaired people, some large proportion of them schizophrenic, who have never been to any sort of treatment facility. So we must conclude that using

treatment—*any* sort of treatment—as an index of mental disorder is suspect.

The alternative is to go out into the community and diagnose everyone—or a representative sample of everyone—yourself. This has been done by a number of investigators, for example Essen-Möller in Sweden, Srole and his associates in New York, Leighton in Nova Scotia. They have solved one problem, but they have run into two others, perhaps equally serious.

One problem is finding a reliable and valid criterion of mental illness.[25] For all its inadequacies, hospitalization is at least a reliable index, and you can be fairly certain that the people who are hospitalized are really ill. But can one really be certain that the Leighton's estimate that approximately 48 percent of their population suffer at least 10 percent impairment,[26] or Srole's that 23.4 percent of his are impaired are meaningful? Psychiatric diagnoses, even of hospitalized patients, are notoriously unreliable. Psychiatric diagnoses of people in the community, usually based on second-hand reports, are likely to be even more unreliable.

Personal examination by a single psychiatrist using presumably consistent standards is one potential solution, but applicable only to relatively small populations. Another is the further development of objective rating scales, such as the Neuropsychiatric Screening Adjunct first developed by social scientists in the Research Branch of the U.S. Army in World War II[27] and later used in both the Leighton's and Srole's investigations, but not developed to anything like its full potential in either study. Meantime, we have to recognize that the community studies done so far have been based on indices whose reliability and validity are at any rate suspect.

The other problem with community studies is even more serious. In most of these studies we are no longer dealing with the *incidence* of mental disturbance, but with its prevalence.[28] That is, we are no longer measuring the number of new cases arising in various population groups during some period of time, but the number of people currently ill at the time of the survey. This reflects not only incidence but duration of illness. And, as Hollingshead and Redlich have convincingly shown, duration of illness is highly correlated with social class. Various approximations to incidence have been tried, and various new—and often fantastic—statistical devices invented, to get around this problem, but without any real success. Clearly, what is needed is *repeated* studies of the population, to pick up new cases as they arise and thus to establish true incidence figures. (This is what Hagnell and Essen-Möller are attempting in Scania, and it is a very brave effort indeed.) The crucial problem, of course, is to develop a reliable measure of mental disorder, for without that our repeated surveys will measure nothing but the errors of our instruments. Meantime, we have to recognize that the many prevalence studies of communities—including all the recent large studies in the United States—are using an inappropriate measure that exaggerates the relationship of socioeconomic status to mental disorder.

So the results are hardly definitive. It may even all wash out —one more example of inadequate methods leading to premature, false conclusions. I cannot prove otherwise. Yet I think the most parsimonious interpretation of all these findings is that they point to something real. Granted that there is not a single definitive study in the lot, the weaknesses of one are compensated for by the strengths of some other, and the total edifice is probably much stronger than you would conclude from knowing only how frail are its component parts. A large number of complementary studies all seem to point to the same conclusion: that rates of mental disorder, particularly of schizophrenia, are correlated with various measures of socioeconomic status, at least in large cities, and this probably is not just a matter of drift or duration of illness or who gets hospitalized or some other artifact of the methods we use. In all probability, more schizophrenia is actually produced at lower socioeconomic levels. At any rate, let us take that as a working hypothesis and explore the question further. Assuming that more schizophrenia occurs at lower socioeconomic levels, Why?

II

Is it really socioeconomic status, or it is some correlated variable that is operative here? Faris and Dunham did not take socioeconomic status very seriously in their interpretation of their data. From among the host of variables characteristic of the high-rate areas of Chicago, they focused on such things as high rates of population turnover and ethnic mixtures and hypothesized that the really critical thing about the high-rate areas was the degree of social isolation they engendered. John Clausen and I later produced more direct evidence that seems to refute the social isolation hypothesis.[29] But there are any number of other possibilities. Ethnic composition is a possibility, and one recent study in Boston suggests that the reason large cities show strong correlations of social class to rates of mental disorder, and small cities do not, is that the small cities do not have the right mixtures of lower-class ethnic groups.[30] Perhaps. Or perhaps genetics provides an explanation. If there is a moderately strong genetic linkage in schizophrenia, then one would expect a higher than usual rate of schizophrenia among the fathers and grandfathers of schizophrenics. Since schizophrenia is a debilitating disease, this would be deflected in grandparents' and parents' occupations and places of residence. In other words—it could be the drift hypothesis after all, in a rather complex version.

There are several other possibilities, but in the absence of any compelling evidence it hardly seems worthwhile reviewing them. All we can say for now is that some correlated variable might prove critical for explaining the findings; it might not be social class, after all, that is the truly operative variable. But until that is demonstrated, the wisest course would seem to be to take the findings at face value and see what there might be about social class that would help us to understand schizophrenia.

III

What is there about the dynamics of social class position that might affect the probability of people becoming schizophrenic? How does social class operate here, what are the intervening processes? Is it stress, or childhood experience, or something else about the conditions of life in different social classes that really matters for the differential likelihood of developing schizophrenia?

The stress hypothesis is in some respects the most appealing, in part because it is the most direct. We have not only our own observations as human beings with some compassion for less fortunate people, but an increasingly impressive body of scientific evidence, to show that life is rougher and rougher the lower one's social status. The stress explanation seems especially plausible for the very lowest socioeconomic strata, where the rates of schizophrenia are the very highest.

There has to my knowledge been only one empirical investigation of the relationship of social class to stress to mental disorder, that by Langner & Michael in New York.[31] This study, as all the others we have been considering, has its methodological defects—it is a prevalence study, and many of the indices it uses are at best questionable—but it tackles the major issues head-on, and with very impressive and very intriguing results. It finds a strong, linear correlation between stress and mental disturbance, specifically, the more sources of stress, the higher the probability of mental disturbance. It also finds the expected relationship between social class and stress. So the stress hypothesis has merit. But stress is not all that is involved in the relationship of social class to mental disorder. No matter how high the level of stress, social class continues to be correlated with the probability of mental disturbance; in fact, the more stress, the higher the correlation.* Thus, it seems that the effect of social class on the rate of mental disorder is not only, or even principally, a function of different amounts of stress at different class levels, but of something else again. What else? Langner and Michael have no direct evidence, but they make a suggestion that has long been popular with psychiatrists and clinical psychologists: that their childhood experiences, perhaps especially their relationships with their parents, have somehow better prepared middle- and upper-class than lower- and working-class people for dealing with the hazards of life.

And now we enter what is perhaps the most complicated area of research we have touched on so far, and certainly the least adequately studied field of all.

Allow me to speak for a moment about studies of family relationships and schizophrenia, leaving social class out of the picture for a brief while. There has been a huge research literature, most of it inadequately designed. One has to dismiss the majority of studies, because of one or another incapacitating deficiency.[33] In many, the patients selected for study were a group from which you could not possibly generalize to schizophrenics at large: either because the samples were comprised of chronic patients, where one would expect the longest and most difficult onset of illness with the greatest strain in family relationships, or because the samples were peculiarly selected not to test a hypothesis but to load the dice in favor of a hypothesis. In other studies there have been

* The latter finding is in part an artifact of the peculiar indices used in this study, and reflects differences not in the incidence of illness but in type and severity of illness in different social classes at various levels of stress. At higher stress levels, lower-class people tend to develop incapacitating psychoses and middle-class people less incapacitating neuroses.

inadequate control groups, or no control group at all. One of the most serious defects of method, to which we shall return, has been the comparison of patterns of family relationship of lower- and working-class patients to middle- and upper-middle-class normal controls—which completely confounds the complex picture we wish to disentangle. In still other studies, even where the methods of sample and control selection have been adequate, the method of data collection has seriously biased the results. This is true, for example, in those studies that have placed patients and their families in stressful situations that are bound to exaggerate any flaws in their interpersonal processes, especially for people of lesser education and verbal skill who would be least equipped to deal with the new and perplexing situation in which they found themselves.

Still, some of the studies have suggested respects in which the family relationships of schizophrenics seem unusual, and unusual in theoretically interesting ways—that is, in ways that might conceivably be important in the dynamics of schizophrenic personality development. Some of the recent investigations by Bateson and Jackson, on communication processes in families of schizophrenics,[34] for example, and by Wynne and his associates on emotional processes in such families,[35] are altogether intriguing.

But—and here we must once again bring social class into the picture—there has not been a single well-controlled study that demonstrates any substantial difference between the family relationships of schizophrenics and those of normal persons *from the same social class backgrounds.*[36] Now, it may be that the well-controlled studies simply have not dealt with the particular variables that do differentiate the families of schizophrenics from those of normal lower- and working-class families. My study with John Clausen,[37] for example, deals with only a few grossly-measured aspects of family relationships, and does not take up the very processes that more recent psychiatric case studies have emphasized as perhaps the most important of all. It may be that investigations yet to come will show clear and convincing evidence of aspects of family relationships definitely different for schizophrenic-producing families and normal families of the same social background.

But if they do not, that still does not mean that family relationships are not important for schizophrenia, or that it is not through the family that social class exerts one of its principal effects. I have said that there is no evidence of any difference between the family relationships of schizophrenics and those of normal families of the lower and working classes. Another way of putting the same facts is to say that there is increasing evidence of remarkable parallels between the dynamics of families that produce schizophrenics and family dynamics in the lower classes generally,[38] which *may* indicate that the family patterns of the lower classes are in some way broadly conducive to schizophrenic personality development. Clearly these patterns do not provide a sufficient explanation of schizophrenia. We still need a missing *x*, or set of *x*'s, to tell us the necessary and sufficient conditions for schizophrenia to occur. Perhaps that *x* is some other aspect of family relationships. Perhaps the lower-class pattern of family relationships is conducive to schizophrenia for persons genetically predisposed, but not for others. Or perhaps it is generally conducive to schizophrenia, but schizophrenia will not actually occur unless you are subjected to certain types or amounts of stress. We do not know. But these speculative considerations do suggest that it may be about time to bring all these variables—social class, early family relationships, genetics, stress—into the same investigations, so that we can examine their interactive effects. Meantime, we must sadly conclude that we have not yet unravelled the relationship of social class and schizophrenia, nor learned what it might tell us about the etiology of the disorder.

IV

Throughout this discussion, I have emphasized the methodological deficiencies of past studies, for that is essential to any proper evaluation of their substantive results. I should hate to conclude this paper, however, with the implication that improvement in method is what is principally needed to advance this field. Important as that is, it is not nearly so important as a new stance toward ideas. The epidemiology of mental illness has been a dreadfully dull field of study: again and again, investigators have done little more than see whether or not the same stereotyped set of demographic characteristics correlate with some index of mental disorder. Rarely have investigators designed their studies to pursue some definite idea—the stress hypothesis, for example—or to choose definitively between two alternative interpreations of past results. There has, in fact, been a fear of theory in this field of investigation, with the predictable result that the most preposterous *ad hoc* theories have been dragged in to explain or explain away ambiguous findings. Perhaps the most important thing to be learned from an examination of past research is the desperate need for bringing theory in, in time, when we are designing our investigations.

Chapter 6

The Reliability and Validity of Measures of Family Life and Relationships in Families Containing a Psychiatric Patient

MICHAEL RUTTER AND GEORGE W. BROWN

THE IMPORTANCE TO THE PSYCHIATRIST OF INVESTIGATIONS of family life and relationships no longer needs arguing. Much of psychiatric theory is concerned with the role of abnormal family structure or deviant parental attitudes and behaviour in the genesis of psychiatric disorder. Stemming from observations that mental illness often affects several people in the same family at about the same time,[1] psychiatrists have become increasingly concerned with the diagnosis and alleviation of *family* psychopathology in contrast to the previous more exclusive concern with the individual patient.[2] Brown[3] has shown that family attitudes and relationships may influence the course of schizophrenia, and recently too, evidence has accumulated which points to the adverse effects of long-standing illness in a parent on the health of the rest of the family.[4] Investigations by Clausen and Yarrow, Grad and Sainsbury, and Brown and Wing[5] have all emphasized the extent of the burden on the families of mentally ill patients.

Mental illness may have deleterious effects on the rest of the family through the direct social effects of certain symptoms, by alterations in the balance of family activities and structure and through adverse effects on interpersonal relationships.[6] If these effects are to be investigated effectively, it is essential to have reliable and valid tools for the measurement of different aspects of family life and relationships, and it is with this problem that the present paper is concerned.

Review of Literature

The volume of research on the family over the last 40 years has been considerable,[7] but other writers have pointed to the methodological weaknesses of much of the work.[8] Consequently in this brief review of the literature we shall comment only on a few investigations that have been concerned with methodological issues and in which the findings illustrate some of the major problems.

Issues involved in the assessment of the reliability and validity of measures of family life have been considered by a number of writers;[9] others have compared the value of interview, observational, and questionnaire techniques,[10] and the relative merits of retrospective and longitudinal approaches have also been discussed.[11] A basic distinction must be made between concrete happenings or activities in the family on the one hand and on the other, feelings, emotions, or attitudes concerning these events or the individuals participating in them.[12] Dean and Whyte, Garrett, and Hoffman and Lippitt[13] made a similar distinction between objective and subjective items, and Yaukey and his colleagues[14] between facts and feelings. Approaches to the assessment of validity are necessarily quite different for these two types of measure.

With events and activities there is an objective reality to be measured. Regardless of people's feelings about it there are *factual* aspects to the number of contacts the family have had with kin or with friends, the amount the husband helps with the housework, the frequency of quarrelling, etc. With such items the concern is to eliminate any distortions and biases involved in the reporting of the informant in order to get as close as possible to the objective reality. It is, of course, necessary that the report be reliably scored or rated but the main issue is the *accuracy* of the report and the major way this may be tested is the comparison of the informant's account with the accounts given by others.[15]

With feelings and attitudes the situation is quite different. Comparison of different accounts is unhelpful. The wife's account of her husband's attitudes in no way validates his own account. Here the problem is to get the informant to express his attitudes in a way that does not distort his inner feelings and then to get investigators to agree on their ratings. Similarly the main problem in the assessment of emotional states such as warmth or hostility is the interjudge agreement on what is observed. In contrast to the situation with objective happenings, ambiguities and ambivalence are frequent with feelings. Someone may feel both warmth and resentment about another person. Nevertheless, if measures are valid, it may be expected that somewhat similar emotions should be manifest in similar situations on different occasions, so that repeated observations offer some test of validity if the observations are carried out independently by different observers. A further important distinction should be made between observed emotions, self-reported emotions, and an informant's report of someone else's emotions. Unfortunately, very few studies have made these distinctions between happenings and feelings about happenings, and between observed and reported emotions, and frequently the data relevant to the assessment of reliability and validity have not been reported. Nevertheless, as far as possible these distinctions will be made in reviewing previous studies.

I. Attitudes and Emotions

Attitudes to child rearing, for example, have been assessed from a number of different approaches including questionnaires, self-ratings and interviews. Many questionnaires, of which Schaefer and Bell's parent attitude research instrument (PARI) is perhaps the most used,[16] have involved the parents' agreement or disagreement with general statements such as "children should realise how much parents have to give up for them." A fundamental problem with this approach is that it does no allow the measurement of attitudes to *individual* children or the comparison of attitudes to different children in the same family. Becker[17] and others have produced evidence suggesting the importance, for predictive purposes, of focussing on specific parental behaviour with the child in question rather than on general parental personality or attitudinal variables. Furthermore, such scales are so seriously influenced by an acquiescence-response set and by the educational level of the respondent that it is to be doubted whether it is worthwhile persisting with this approach.[18]

Interview measures of attitudes and emotions have often had only a moderate level of reliability. For example, Peterson[19] on measures of parental warmth, strictness, etc., obtained correlations of .45 to .81 and McCord[20] correlations of .52 to .76. Sears' figures[21] on parental variables, some of which were attitudinal and some behavioural, were also mainly in the .50 to .70 range. The validity of such measures has also often been less than satisfactory. Many studies have used self-reports of emotions and reports of someone else's emotions as if they were directly comparable. However, Becker[22] showed that there were often serious disagreements between a mother's evaluation of the emotions of the father, and ratings based on interviews with the father, or father's self-ratings. Similarly, the correlations between interview methods and self-rating methods were usually only fair (.41 to .51) and were sometimes poor.

Validity may also be assessed indirectly by retest reliability, that is whether the person expresses the same attitudes when he is re-examined after an interval of time. Baldwin, Kalhorn, and Breese's study[23] (1949) utilizing the Fels Parent Behaviour Scales was one of the most thorough to examine this question. They used the Fels scales to measure some 30 variables, many of which were attitudinal, on the basis of a combination of interview and observations. Interrater agreement on the same observations was genuinely quite high (correlations were in the range .50 to .90 with most .60 to .70) and agreement between two ratings of the *same* observer with a 6-month interval between the ratings was of the same order. However, the agreement between ratings of *different* observers separated by a 1 year interval was less good; correlations were mostly about .40 to .50 but some were as low as .10 to .20. Tizard and Grad[24] in a family study of mentally handicapped children and adults also interviewed the same informants twice to obtain information on family relationships, attitudes, and mental health. They reported rather low agreement between the ratings of the two interviews, but no actual figures were quoted.

There are many studies of the reliability of judgements about simulated emotions (using actors) but few on the reliability of judgements about natural emotional states. Hamburg's study of the reliability of ratings of expressed anxiety, anger, and depression is a key study of the latter type.[25] Comparisons between the ratings of different judges produced correlations of .78 to .87 and it was found that over 70 per cent of the ratings of one observer fell within 1 point of the rating of the other observer (unfortunately the distribution and range of ratings was not given). Bandura and Walter[26] obtained equally reliable ratings of emotions such as hostility and warmth, but it was noteworthy that ratings based on interviews with fathers were somewhat less reliable than those based on interviews with mothers. It is difficult to evaluate the validity of their ratings. Retest reliability was not assessed and ratings of observed emotions were treated as comparable with ratings based on the informant's report of someone else's emotions. Brown *et al.*[27] also achieved high interrater agreement on expressed emotions but reliability of ratings of emotions in other studies has usually been appreciably lower. The methods used may be important but Harris and Metcalf's[28] findings suggest that the training and experience of raters also greatly influences the level of reliability achieved.

Several studies have shown that different emotional components (for example the content of what is said, the vocal characteristics of speech and facial expression) can be used as reliable indicators when taken independently or in combination. Ekman[29] showed that whole person photographs could be matched with speech typescripts at a better than chance level, Alpert and his colleagues[30] demonstrated that the intensity of speech varied with the accompanying emotions, while Starkweather and Waskow[31] found that both speech transcripts and content-free (filtered) speech could be rated for emotions with moderate reliability. These and other studies suggest that in rating emotions it is important to consider both the content of what is said and the tone of voice used. Facial expression and other bodily characteristics are also useful, probably to a lesser extent.

II. Events and Happenings

"Objective" items such as disciplinary techniques, amount of interaction with the children, husband's participation in household tasks and child care, frequency of contact with kin and with friends, leisure activities, etc., involve different methodological problems. The validity of measures (whether based on questionnaire, observation or interview) has usually been more in question than the reliability.

Of questionnaires, that developed by Herbst[32] is a good example of one that aims to measure family relationships and activities. Answers to such questions as "Who mows the lawn?" "Who does the ironing?" or "Who decides whose job it is to do the dishes?" are used to determine participation in family activities, decision-making, and tension in the home. The validity of some of the measures derived from the questionnaire has been questioned by Yamamura and Zald.[33] Most of their criticisms can be met by modifications of the scale and rather more serious is Hoffman and Lippitt's finding[34] that each family member tends to exaggerate his relative participation in tasks. They did not report the extent of the differences found.

Questionnaires, such as that used by Tharp,[35] which require answers of "much," "some," "a little," etc. to items on activities like the amount of housework usually done by the husband have similar methodological problems. Husband-wife agreement on the scale has not been reported but obviously the level of the agreement obtained will depend in part on both having a similar reference or comparison group from which to judge how much is "much."[36] It is also likely that attitudes towards the spouse may influence judgements as to whether his participation can be considered "much" or only "some."

One of the very few studies to examine the agreement between fathers and mothers on questionnaire measures of family life was that by Radke.[37] Each parent filled in a questionnaire requiring answers of the "usually"—"sometimes" variety on parental discipline and relationships to the child. Agreement between parents was only moderate and the agreement between parents and their children was worse. As already suggested, the use of responses like "usually" or "sometimes" may be particularly open to the biases introduced by different attitudes and different parental concepts.

Observation of family interaction in the home has not been much used, perhaps largely due to practical difficulties, but observations of experimental situations have been increasingly employed.[38] Most approaches of this kind have been concerned with family communication and decision-making, variables particularly difficult to assess by other techniques. Goodrich and Mishler[39] have shown that these variables can be rated with high reliability in experimental situations but their validity is less certain. Interaction patterns usually remain stable in the experimental situation,[40] but O'Rourke[41] found differences between patterns shown in the home and in more formal settings. The question of validity needs further examination, but it may be that this kind of approach will prove to be the most useful for the assessment of communication and decision-making.

Interview methods have also been widely used to measure family activities and, when assessed, the inter-rater reliability of scores of ratings has usually been quite high. For example, Marshall[42] reliably measured children's interaction with their parents and with other children, and Bandura and Walters[43] achieved correlations of about .70 to .90 on such items as parental restrictions of the child's activities and the amount of time parent and child spent in affectionate interaction. The validity of interview measures has been less often considered. In spite of Blood and Wolfe's claim[44] that "many previous studies have shown a close correlation between what husbands and wives say about their marriages," we have been able to find few studies which have examined the problem and most do not support Blood and Wolfe's statement.

Perhaps the highest level of husband-wife agreement has been on the frequency of coitus, where correlations have ranged from .54 to .72.[45] However, these correlations are sufficiently low for there to be major differences in conclusions according to which informant's account was taken. Furthermore, Clark and Wallin[46] produced some evidence to suggest that the extent of the informant's dissatisfaction with sexual relationships influenced the level of agreement.

Kohn and Carroll[47] interviewed mothers, fathers and children to find out which parent was more encouraging to the child and to which parent the child turned for advice and reassurance. Mothers and fathers agreed in 77 percent of cases but there was agreement between mother, father and child in less than half the cases. Andry[48] also interviewed both parents and the children on the adequacy of parent-child communication, which was the most affectionate parent and similar variables. There was about 70 percent agreement between the parents and the delinquent children and a higher agreement between the parents and nondelinquent children. However, some of the scales were bipolar and extremely skewed, thus artifically inflating the level of agreement, and there was possible contamination of data in that all interviews were conducted by the same person.

Eron[49] found that mother-father agreement, on child-rearing practices and related variables was quite poor; correlations ranged from—.04 to .64 (excluding a correlation of .91 on residential mobility) and only 10 of 22 correlations were significantly better than zero. Many of the items were a mixture of the subjective and objective or referred only to the informant (rather than to both parents) so that interparent agreement on events and happenings cannot be readily assessed from their data.

Three rather more peripheral studies also report low levels of agreement between different informants. Young and Young[50] found that for many items the reliability of "key informants" as used in anthropological work was poor. High disagreement between husbands and wives on the contraceptive methods they used is reported by Yaukey and his colleagues, and Kenkel and Hoffman[51] found that people were rather inaccurate both in their forecast of which marriage partner would do the most talking in an experimental decision-making situation and also in their report afterwards of who did the most talking.

Haggerty[52] examined father-mother agreement on both interview ratings and questionnaire responses concerned with a wide range of family, social and medicosocial variables. Agreement on items such as medicines kept in the home, type of recreation, children's discipline, etc. (interview ratings) and social mobility, stress in job, etc. (questionnaire responses) varied from 21 percent to 93 percent or 50 percent to 100 percent if moderate agreement was accepted. Thus, although a moderate level of husband-wife agreement has sometimes been found, in many studies the agreement has been poor. Unfortunately a number of other major studies which gathered information separately from both husbands and wives did not report the level of agreement between the two accounts.[53]

III. Summary Measures

Summary measures of overall marital adjustment, tension or family functioning have been obtained from interviews and questionnaires. On the whole, questionnaires have been shown to have a satisfactory reliability and there is fair agreement between scales,[54] but it is not always clear what is being measured. The only study to assess husband-wife agreement on such measures is Geismar and Ayres' investigation of changes in family functioning following social casework. A detailed manual[55] gives instructions on the rating of eight areas of marriage according to seven point scales (with about 71 percent of ratings on the middle three points). Interrater reliability was quite high; in only 19.4 percent of cases were there disagreements of two points or more on family relationships and family unity, and on social activities. The overall husband-wife agreement for the eight areas in a small sample of ten couples was, surprisingly, reported to be even better than the interrater agreement based on the *same* interview.[56] The husband-wife agreement on individual scales was not reported.

In view of the contradictions in methods and findings only limited general conclusions can be drawn from this selective review of the literature. The reliability of ratings, especially on emotions, has often been only moderate but the validity of all kinds of measures has been more in question. It seems that poor results have often stemmed from a conceptual confusion between "objective" events and "subjective" feelings about events. Questionnaires involving agreement or disagreement with general statements are seriously biased by the educational background and social attitudes of the respondent. For related reasons specific and detailed answers are usually to be preferred to choices between such general phrases as "often" or "sometimes." For most purposes information from *both* parents and about *both* parents will be required. Retrospective accounts will rarely be satisfactory as they have been shown to be both unreliable and subject to important biases.[57] Questionnaires are of value as screening instruments but probably they have only a limited place in intensive studies. For certain variables direct observation of natural or experimental situations may be the preferred approach but in spite of trenchant criticisms[58] the interview offers the greatest chance of measuring a wide range of variables and if it can be shown to be reliable and valid it may be the most useful tool for many purposes. The present study was planned to test some of these conclusions and to examine other outstanding questions on reliability and validity.

Research Design

The measures of family life and relationships which we have developed over the last three years have been primarily designed to study the interaction between illness and family variables. Thus an important aspect of this reliability and validity study has been an examination of the effects on reporting of the informant's status of psychiatric patient. After interviewing some 80 families during the period when measures were being developed, there was a systematic study of 30 families, in all of which there were children of school age or younger and in which one parent had newly attended a psychiatric facility.* Consecutive cases of newly referred patients

* Findings were reviewed after the first 20 cases and it was decided to omit the joint interview and retrospective measures for the last 10 cases. Consequently the results for measures referring to a period one year ago are based on 20 cases only and those for the joint interview on 18 cases only (two families refused a joint interview).

living in one London borough were used. Three patients were too ill to be interviewed and there were 9 partial refusals. All but 3 of the refusals were willing to participate in part but for the purposes of this part of the study, agreement to interviews with the patient, with the spouse, and with both together was demanded. Of the 18 female patients, 11 were diagnosed as having a neurotic depressive disorder, 3 other neurotic conditions, 3 manic-depressive psychosis, and 1 schizophrenia. Of the 12 male patients, 5 were diagnosed as having a personality disorder (usually associated with some neurotic symptoms), 3 an anxiety state, 2 manic-depressive psychosis, 1 neurotic depression, and 1 drug addiction.

For each family there was a 2–3 hour interview with the patient, a 3–4 hour interview with the spouse (usually in two sessions) and a third interview of about an hour with the two of them together. All interviews were recorded on tape. The two interviews with the informants singly covered the same ground (illness, social impact of illness, and various aspects of family activities and relationships) and ratings were made on identical variables. The joint interview was on a different topic (family utilisation of medical and social services) and was used to observe the interaction of the married couple. At each interview there were two investigators who made independent ratings, and there were different investigators for each of the three interviews so that there were six investigators and six sets of independent ratings for each family.

The study was designed to make two basic kinds of comparison. The first was between ratings made by the two investigators present at the same interview, thus constituting a *within*-interview comparison to test whether different investigators can agree on ratings based on the *same* material. The second comparison was *across* different interviews, that is between ratings based on *different* material; between the spouse interview and the patient interview, or between either of these and the joint interview.

In this report we shall concentrate on giving an account of

our methods and some detailed findings on the reliability and validity of six representative scales in three areas: 1. family events and activities; 2. emotions and feelings of individual members of the family; and 3. summary scales. A companion paper[59] gives comparative material on a greater number of scales. Methods and findings on measures concerning clinical material, the social context and impact of symptoms, and the characteristics of the children will be reported elsewhere.

Method

I. Events and Activities

Since we are concerned in these scales with concrete events and the frequency with which they occur during a specified period of time, we assume that there is a true answer and it is the interviewer's job to get as close as possible to it by skilled questioning—to get beyond the informant's attitude to what actually happened. With respect to participation in household tasks, for example, an informant's attitude may influence how she feels about her husband's involvement in housework, but in measuring participation we are concerned only with how much the husband actually *did* participate in the last three months. People's feelings about activities are equally important but are evaluated by a different group of scales.

To keep the measurement of events, and what people feel about events, as independent as possible we rely on a detailed and flexible cross-examination about recent events, using what Richardson and his colleagues have termed a "nonschedule standardised interview."[60] The codings are firmly structured and quantitative and most consist of some form of frequency count. There are detailed instructions on the information to be obtained, the interviewer must confine himself to specified events or activities in the schedule, he must cover *all* the happenings which are listed and he must question about a specified period of time. Although the information to be obtained is structured, the way in which it is obtained is, within certain specified limits, left to the interviewer's judgement. We do not feel that complex information about the distribution of household tasks or the impact of symptoms on family life can be obtained by sticking rigidly to a limited number of structured questions. This is particularly the case where some of the informants are mentally ill and the families come from differing social backgrounds. Questions using the same words may mean different things to different informants. An unvarying order of questions is also undesirable for many things. To aid memory the subject is encouraged to build up a train of associations about the event in question. Cooperation is generally better if emotionally important items spontaneously raised by the informant are covered first. To reduce forgetting of items or conscious distortion, the interviewer is expected to get the informant involved in the interview so that there is good rapport or participation.[61] The interviewer should continue questioning until he is satisfied that he has obtained a full and consistent account or until it is clear that further questioning—at least at that stage of the interview—is not going to elicit further useful information.

We aim to get accurate accounts of events by insisting on reports of actual happenings, not generalisations and by focussing on a defined, recent and usually short period of time. With most measures we question in detail about the week preceding the interview and then go on to find out about rarer events in the last three months and also to determine in what ways the last week differed from other weeks during the same period.

We have completely rejected such questions as: "How much does your husband help in the house?" as we believe that the answers to questions of this type may be greatly influenced by the attitudes of the informant. Instead, detailed questioning on actual recent events may make it possible to get nearer the truth. Hoffman[62] has described the technique in detail and has suggested that the set to recall specific details rather than meaningful wholes may result in a fragmentation of the event described. By weakening many of its gestalt qualities the event is divested of much of its emotional meaning so minimising unconsciously motivated omissions and distortions. Thomas and his colleagues[63] have used a somewhat similar technique to measure the behavioural characteristics of children.

Another issue in the questioning on which we have laid emphasis is the use of a number of different approaches to the same activity. For example, in asking about leisure activities we first ask about the number and type of contact with kin and with friends. Later in the interview we ask how many evenings a week they have gone out and what they did when they went out. Finally we go through a check list of specified activities asking if the informant or his spouse went to the cinema, swimming etc., in the last three months. The interviewer is expected to be constantly on the alert for contradictions and inconsistencies and to question further on the topic when necessary. We have found that the ordering and lay-out of the interview schedule makes a lot of difference to how well this cross-checking is carried out.

On the content of the various activities measured we have often followed outlines described by other workers. For example, the section on household tasks has much in common with Herbst's questions,[64] that on prohibitions is similar to Bandura and Walters' questioning on restrictions[65] and that on parental expectations similar to (although fuller than) those used by Hoffman and her colleagues[66] to measure parental granting of autonomy to the child. The three main differences from other scales are: 1. concentration on a defined recent period of time (rather than asking about the usual pattern);

2. questioning about actual frequencies (rather than relying on answers of "often" or "sometimes"); and 3. use of scores based on frequencies (rather than general ratings).

II. Emotions and Attitudes

Our approach to the measurement of emotions and attitudes is rather different in that we are no longer dealing with "objective" events and in that inconsistencies and ambivalence are an intrinsic part of emotional states and not merely methodological difficulties to be eliminated. Under no circumstances is the interviewer allowed to point out inconsistencies in attitudes or feelings. It is common, for example, for someone to deny dissatisfaction with something at one stage in the interview in response to a direct question but then later to go on to grumble about it. Similarly, it is not infrequent for people to express both strongly negative and strongly positive feelings about their marriage partner or their children.

Because ambivalence of feelings is common we have made nearly all scales unipolar. For example, warmth is rated quite independently of the amount of criticism expressed. For the same reason and to avoid halo effects we have largely relied on unidimensional scales, although there are also a small number of summary scales.

Our attempt to use the interview as a standard stimulus for eliciting emotions and attitudes has much in common with the principles outlined by Chapple[67] in describing his standard experimental interview. As much of our interview is concerned with eliciting precise factual material it is particularly important to establish early on that we are interested in feelings as well as events. Warm expressive movements[68] and verbal and vocal encouragements[69] have been shown to influence the quantity of responses of the type that have been reinforced and we use these techniques to encourage the production of spontaneous emotional and attitudinal material. Care is taken to encourage positive and negative attitudes to an equal extent. Where the informant's feelings are in doubt questions such as "how do you feel about (it)?" are also used. More direct probes (e.g., "Does this kind of thing ever cause an atmosphere in the home," or "Does that ever make you feel on edge?" are also used sparingly but to ensure comparability between interviews the occasions and frequency with which such direct probes may be used are specified in the interview instructions.

As with events and activities we lay little emphasis on answers to such general questions as "How do you get on with your husband?" Rather we have found that emotions and feelings about the spouse, for example, are usually best elicited by getting the informant to talk about him in connection with questions about actual everyday activities. Informants who don't criticise their spouse when asked directly will often do so spontaneously when talking about leisure activities or his participation in the care of the children.

Our recognition of emotions and feelings was not mechanical. The content of what was said was taken into account but more emphasis was laid on the *way* things were said. Interviewers were expected to recognise emotions by observing differences in the speed, pitch, and intensity of speech. To a lesser extent facial expression and gesture were taken into account. During the training of interviewers, efforts were made to develop these observer skills and to achieve uniform thresholds in the recognition of emotions. As suggested by Johnson,[70] we tried to facilitate this process by having interviewers meet together regularly to listen to tape recordings, make independent ratings and then discuss their interpretations of the same material and attempt to describe the features they used in coming to their decisions. Special tape recordings were produced which included excerpts of several interviews to illustrate different levels of criticism, warmth, hostility, etc. Interview techniques were developed by having interviewers go out in pairs and discuss afterwards the style of questioning and the informant's responses.

Tone of voice was particularly important in the recognition of emotions expressed during the account of symptoms. Informants who are highly critical and scathing and ones who are sympathetic and understanding may sometimes use much the same words to describe the illness and its effects. The difference lies in the way things are said and in the tone of voice used.

In judging tone of voice it was important to recognise not only absolute tonal qualities but also differences in tone within the range of emotional expression of that informant. Interviewers were instructed to be on the alert for the vocal qualities evident when the informants said things obviously positive and approving and things obviously critical and hostile as judged by the content of the words used. Having established levels in this way, the recognition of emotions was easier when the content of speech was neutral or ambiguous. Occasionally personal idiosyncrasies were helpful. An unusually striking example was provided in one interview where it soon became obvious that the informant gave a brief "nervous" laugh every time she made a pejorative remark about her husband and that she rarely gave this laugh other than at times when she was being critical. Of course the laugh was not in itself enough to label a remark "critical" but thereafter in the interview the presence of the laugh served to alert the interviewer to the possibility of a critical remark.

A somewhat intuitive approach of this kind seemed necessary if we were to be able to rate the kind of emotions and feelings in which we were interested, but clearly there was the risk that unreliable and unrepeatable ratings might result. We attempted to deal with this in six ways:

1. At all times we were concerned with specific not general attributes. The question was not whether the informant was a very warm person but rather did he show warmth in the way

he talked about the person specified (in the single interview) or in his behaviour at interview towards the person specified (in the joint interview).

2. As far as possible we aimed to be noninterpretative. Interviewers were instructed to deal only with feelings *demonstrated* by verbal or nonverbal behaviour and at no time to attempt to infer what were the "real" feelings.

3. Although emotions were recognised intuitively in the first instance, we attempted to improve reliability and validity by (a) specification of the main cues to be used in the recognition of emotions and (b) exclusion of cues which proved unreliable or of dubious validity. For example, a remark might be regarded as critical on the content of the words alone (that is without consideration of tone) only if there was an explicit statement that the informant resented, disliked or disapproved of the specified person or his behaviour.

4. Common thresholds for deciding that an emotion was present and common scales for the degree to which it was shown were established by master tape recordings for which there were detailed annotations pointing out which remarks were critical, warm, hostile, etc., and why. Group discussions of tape recordings and of disagreements over ratings were also important.

5. We attempted to provide reasonably uniform stimuli by regulating the form of the interview and the style of questioning.

6. "Halo" effects have been reduced by having independent unipolar, unidimensional scales with detailed rules for rating each.

As with the scales on events and activities, the types of scales on emotions for the most part follow those used by other workers, at least in general outline. For example, the rating of warmth is somewhat similar to that used by Bandura and Walters[71] and the scale on dissatisfaction has something in common with Baruch's[72] measures of tension. In contrast to some investigators, however, we have not used bipolar scales and some of the scales are more narrowly defined in an attempt to avoid halo effects and to increase validity.

III. Summary Scales

Finally there were a few summary scales that were not closely related to any single portion of the interview and most of which relied on the subjective judgement of the interviewer. One such scale (concerning the marital relationship) is described in the results section.

Results

I. Scales on Emotions

There were two types of scales concerned with emotions, and results will be given for one example of each: 1. ratings on observed emotions (example: warmth); 2. frequency counts of the number of emotive remarks (example: critical comments).

(a) Warmth toward the other marriage partner

In the single interview (with either the patient or the spouse) this rating was based on the amount of warmth *demonstrated* by the informant when talking about the other marriage partner, and in the joint interview with the husband and wife together on the amount of warmth directed by the one towards other marriage partner. In general, stereotyped endearments were regarded as irrelevant for this rating, but positive comments about the spouse, especially if made spontaneously, were important. Sympathy and concern, interest in the spouse as a person, interest in what he did and expressed enjoyment in mutual activities were all relevant. Particular note was taken of warmth and enthusiasm in the tone of voice. Whereas the presence or absence of criticism, or even hostility, was deliberately disregarded, the failure to express warmth in relevant situations was taken into account. For example, an unsympathetic detached "clinical" account of the illness or a flat unenthusiastic account of the spouse's characteristics would suggest a low rating on warmth. Warmth was most readily noted in the sections dealing with illness, leisure, household tasks, marriage, and communication, but could be observed in any portion of the interview.

Interrater reliability was high, showing that trained investigators could agree well in their judgements about warmth. Reliability was as good on judgements which concerned the patient's warmth (r=.79) as on the warmth of the non-patient (r=.75). However there was a slight tendency for agreement to be less good when the subject was male (r=.60) rather than when female (r=.88). It is doubtful whether this sex difference is of general importance in that it appeared to be due solely to large inter-rater differences on three men of abnormal personality and it was not found for other measures of emotions. Inter-rater reliability for ratings based on observed warmth in the joint interview was as high (r=.85) as for ratings based on the single interview.

Considerations of validity raise the important question as to how far feelings expressed about the spouse when he is absent agree with the feelings shown towards him when the husband and wife are together. This was assessed by comparing the *across*-interview correlation between ratings based on the single interview and ratings based on the joint interview. This provides a measure of the degree to which feelings are persistent across different situations. It is not strictly speaking a measure of validity in that somewhat different feelings may well be expressed in the two situations.* Nevertheless a low association between the two sets of ratings would suggest that

* Tables of results may be obtained from authors.

expressed feelings are highly situation specific and so throw considerable doubt on the usefulness of the measure. In fact, the level of agreement between ratings made in the single and joint interviews was moderately high (r=.68) indicating the validity of the ratings of warmth.

The findings so far all apply to *observed* warmth and it remains to consider *reported* warmth. The reliability of ratings about the amount of warmth is just as reliable when based on the respondent's account of the other person's emotions (r=.80) as for observed emotions, but the *across*-interview agreement is poor. The product moment correlation between reported emotions in one single interview and the observed emotions of the same person in the other single interview was only .35 and with the observed emotions in the joint interview it was only .42. This suggests that the validity of reported emotions may be low although the reliability is high. As observed with other scales the level of reliability is a very poor guide to the level of validity.

Observed warmth of one marriage partner toward the other has been shown to have good reliability and good validity. Findings on other comparable emotional variables such as warmth shown to the child and hostility to the other marriage partner were very similar.

(b) Number of critical comments made about or to the other person

Critical comments were judged either on tone or on content. For a remark to be judged critical in content there had to be clear and unambiguous statement of resentment, disapproval or dislike. Any remark could be critical on tone alone and great emphasis was laid on the interviewers' judgements of tone of voice. The unit for a remark was a statement terminated either by a change of topic or by a question from the interviewers. A generally critical remark followed by a specific criticism in the form of an example (e.g., "He's so lazy about the house . . . . why yesterday he even refused to bring in the fuel") was not counted as a change in topic.

Realiability and validity was judged in the same manner as for warmth. Inter-rater reliability was equally high on critical remarks made by patients (r=.88), by nonpatients (r=.92), by men (r=.87) and by women (r=.93). Agreement across interview was also high. Criticisms were made much less frequently in the joint interview but when there were *any* criticisms in the joint interview there were nearly always (11 out of 13 cases) ten or more criticisms in the single interview. Similarly, if there were *no* criticisms in the joint interview it was quite rare (2 cases out of 23) for there to be as many as ten criticisms in the single interview. Because of the high number of cases with no criticisms in the joint interview (due to this difference in threshold) the correlation is lower (r=.51) than for warmth, but it is still substantial.

Thus a count of the number of critical comments has been shown to be a reliable and valid measure. The count of the number of positive remarks showed similar findings.

II. Scales Measuring Events and Activities

These scales concern actual happenings that are observable by anyone present at the time. However, the happenings may reflect emotions and attitudes in a fairly direct way, as with "irritability" the first example taken. The second, "participation in household tasks" was chosen as an example of one rather more neutral in tone.

(a) Irritability

The amount of "negative" behaviour in the home was assessed on several specific scales (for example, frequency of quarrelling, scapegoating, etc.) but it was also assessed on an overall scale of irritability. Irritability was taken to include quarrelling, bickering and tiffs, "flying off the handle," active and specific scapegoating or picking on someone, and *severe* snapping and shouting. It was a five point frequency scale that was rated on the basis of the informant's account (once per month or less=0, more than once a month to once a week=1, more than once a week to four times a week=2, 5–7 times a week=3, and more than daily=4). In the same way as for all other emotional measures ratings were made of irritability shown to a specific person, not irritability in general.

No respondent bias in reporting could be found. The mean irritability score for men was similar when based on the man's own report (1.14) as when based on the woman's report (1.14). Similarly, the mean irritability score for women was of the same order when based on the woman's own report (1.50) as when based on the man's report (1.46). Neither could any differences be found between patients and non-patients in the reporting of irritability. The mean irritability score for patients based on the patient's report was 1.64 and on the nonpatient's report it was 1.39.

Interrater reliability was high and was equally high for irritability shown by the patient when the informant was a patient (r=.79) as when the informant was a non-patient (r=.85). Interrater reliability was equally good for irritability shown by the non-patient (r=.80 on the spouse's report and .91 on the patient's report).

Although attitudes may influence the informant's judgement as to what is or is not irritability, there is a certain objective reality as to how often irritability is shown by someone. Thus, more important than reliability is the question as to whether husbands and wives, when interviewed separately, give comparable accounts of irritability. The issue here is one of validity —unless the account given by the husband agrees fairly well with that given by the wife there can be little confidence in the measure. The agreement between ratings of the irritability shown by the patient to his spouse, as judged on the patient's account and on the spouse's account, was moderately high (r=.67) suggesting that the measure is valid as well as reliable.

Two further questions arise. One of the difficulties involved in making ratings over a three month period is that the patient's clinical state may vary and so some form of averaging must be done in order to make a single rating. Clearly this might add a source of error to the ratings so that a further "peak" rating of irritability was also made for the one week in which there was the most irritability. The *across*-interview agreement (reflecting the validity of the measure) was slightly higher (r=.78) for this worst week than for the rating on the whole three month period (r=0.67) suggesting that a rating concerning a shorter period of time may reduce averaging errors.

It also seemed desirable to obtain a measure of the irritability shown by the patient before he became ill. Often patients had been ill for several years and in view of previous reports of the lack of validity of retrospective accounts it was decided, during this pilot study, to make ratings for a three month period a year ago (i.e., between 15 months and 12 months before the interview) in order to test the value of such retrospective accounts. Inter-rater reliability was as good for ratings based on this period but the *across*-interview agreement was only slight (r=.26) suggesting that a rating of irritability based on retrospective accounts had poor validity and was therefore of little use.

b) Husband or wife's participation in household tasks

The aim of this scale was to compare the *relative* participation in household tasks of husbands and wives in different families, rather than to measure the actual physical work done or hours spent on household tasks. Informants were systematically questioned on who performed ten tasks (shopping for food, cleaning the house, washing up, shopping for children's clothes, cleaning windows, bringing in fuel, household repairs, washing clothes, preparing meals, and looking after the garden or yard) so that details were obtained on the frequency with which each member of the household undertook these activities during the three months preceding the interview. Trivial participation (e.g. buying an occasional loaf of bread) was not counted and when the major part of the week's activity in a certain area was carried out on one occasion (e.g. a main shopping expedition on Saturday) this was given a score of 3.5. The total score for each item was seven and for daily activities this was subdivided as one point for each day of the week. The score for each day was subdivided equally among the number of people participating in the task that day, irrespective of the actual amount of work done.

On an "objective" scorable item like this, interrater reliability was scarcely in question. For the husband's participation the inter-rater reliability was .91 and for the wife's participation it was .87. As with "irritability" the important question was the degree to which husbands and wives, when interviewed separately, gave equivalent accounts. For the husband's participation the correlation expressing *across*-interview agreement between the husband's account and the wife's account was .75 and for the wife's participation it was .67. Thus the measure appeared to have satisfactory validity.

Although the *across*-interview correlation was moderately high, it was still important to consider why agreement was not better than it was. Hoffman and Lippitt[73] reported that, using a questionnaire approach to participation in household tasks, respondents tended to overestimate their own participation. This did not occur in the present study in which intensive interviewing was used to obtain the measure. There were no differences between the scores based on reports of men and of women, nor were there any differences between the reports of patients and nonpatients. Thus, there was no evidence of respondent bias related to sex or to patient status.

As noted above, the form of the questioning and the construction of the scale was designed to eliminate attitudinal biases as far as possible. The extent to which this was successful was assessed by examining the effect on husband-wife agreement of the respondent's dissatisfaction with that area of the marriage (separate ratings for dissatisfaction in each area were obtained and these have been shown to be reliable).[74]

It was found that, compared with the account of the other marriage partner, dissatisfied wives tended to slightly underestimate* the participation of their husbands (on average, by 15.7 percent) and satisfied wives to overestimate his participation (on average, by 11.4 percent). Put another way, 8 of 12 dissatisfied wives underestimated their husband's performance but only 5 of 16 satisfied wives did so. Similarly, dissatisfied husbands tended to slightly underestimate the participation of their wives (8 of 9 cases) and satisfied husbands to overestimate (12 of 19 cases). None of the differences mentioned above was large and none was statistically significant. It may be concluded, therefore, that the emphasis on facts rather than feelings, largely eliminated attitudinal biases. Nevertheless, a slight effect remained and occasionally this might be enough to influence conclusions. The wives who were dissatisfied with their husband's participation in household tasks reported that their husbands participated significantly less than the husbands of satisfied wives but this difference was not found when the husband's account was taken. Similarly, different conclusions would also be drawn about the participation of wives when the husband was dissatisfied with her performance according to whose account was taken.

As with irritability, the participation during a three month period a year ago was also measured. Again, although the inter-rater reliability was high, the *across*-interview agreement was less good suggesting that restrospective accounts, although reliable, were less valid.

The inter-rater reliability and the *across*-interview agree-

* "Underestimate" only in relation to the account of the other marriage partner. There is no satisfactory means of determining which is the true figure.

ment were as good or better for nearly all other "objective" measures (e.g. positive interaction with the children, frequency and range of contact with kin, joint leisure activities, etc.) but it was somewhat lower in a few, for example, frequency of coitus.[75] Respondent biases related to sex or patient status were not found in any other scales of this kind and the only other scale to show any significant bias related to dissatisfaction was participation in child care. However, although not reaching the 5 percent level of significance, slight biases associated with dissatisfaction were found in a few other scales.[76]

III. Summary Scales

Overall rating of the marital relationship

This is a summary rating by the interviewer of the husband-wife relationship (it is *not* the perception of the informant). The rating was not mechanical but involved the interviewer's judgement, which took into account the amount of expressed affection and concern, the degree of dissatisfaction in each area of marriage, communication between husband and wife, joint activities, the frequency and severity of quarrelling and bickering, etc. The rating was on a four point scale with a mean of 2.57 and a standard deviation of 0.78 (two points were subdivided to make a six point scale for the last ten cases but reliabilities are based on the four point scale) and there was a good distribution across all points (13.8 percent on 1, 34.6 percent on 2, 39.3 percent on 3, and 12.3 percent on 4). Inter-rater reliability was high (r=.82) and the *across*-interview agreement was equally high (r=.82) indicating the validity of the measure. As with most other scales the *across*-interview agreement on the rating for the relationship a year ago was less good (r=.49) and thus less valid.

Possible respondent biases were examined in the same way

as for other scales. The mean scores on the scales were exactly the same (2.57) when based on interviews with husbands as when based on interviews with wives so that there was no sex bias. However there was a slight and just significant tendency ($t=2.14$, $p<.05$) for the marriage to be rated worse (2.79) on the basis of patient's information than of nonpatients (2.36). There was complete agreement between ratings in 50 percent of cases but where there were differences, ratings based on patient's account tended to be one point worse. The difference was not large enough to greatly influence any conclusions based on this rating but it should be noted that systematic differences in rating were found in spite of a high correlation between the ratings based on different interviews.

IV. Other Scales

There are also one or two scales which do not fit easily into the above classification; one example is given.

"Parent preferred by child" is a scale involving a combination of the child's behaviour and his attitudes as perceived by the parent. It aims to assess which parent the specified child tended to prefer, that is which parent he went to when upset or for comfort or advice.

A rating was made of mother preferred, father preferred or no consistent preference. There was high interrater reliability; in 98.2 percent of cases there was complete agreement between raters. Furthermore, there was good agreement between the two parents as to which parent was preferred. In about half the cases there was no definite preference and in the remainder about an equal number of fathers and of mothers were preferred. There was complete agreement between the accounts of the two parents in 69.2 percent and in only 1 case (3.8 percent) was there a complete contradiction between the two accounts so that the perceptions of fathers and mothers as to which parent was preferred were highly consistent.

Discussion

Data concerning six scales, which were representative of the different types of scale used to measure family life and relationships, have been presented in the context of the four major questions concerning reliability and validity which we set out to answer.

1. Can trained investigators agree in their judgements about the emotions expressed by an informant in relation to his spouse or his children? Ratings of emotional states and counts of emotive remarks have both been shown to have high levels of interrater reliability. Comparisons with other studies, many of which reported lower interrater agreement are difficult in that most provided insufficient data on method and findings to allow considerations of factors influencing reliability. Our experience during the development of the measures suggested that simplicity and clarity of definition of scales together with carefully planned training are the most important elements leading to increased reliability. "Master" tapes providing examples of emotions expressed in different interviews together with group discussions of rating have proved particularly useful.

2. How far do emotions expressed by someone in one situation agree with the emotions expressed by him in another situation? It was found that emotions showed moderately high consistency in different situations, that is to say, they were not situation-specific and were valid in the sense that they could successfully predict responses in other situations. On the other hand, a subject's report of someone else's emotions, which in many studies has been taken as directly comparable to observed emotions, proved to correlate quite poorly with other emotional measures. Observed emotions and reported emotions cannot be equated, as also shown by Becker.[77] Again there are no adequate data which can indicate which features of our

approach were most important in increasing the validity of measures. In addition to the aspects noted as possibly influencing reliability, a high degree of involvement or participation in the interview by the informant, standard measures taken to increase emotional expression in the interview, and a lack of reliance on single direct attitudinal questions (of the "how do you feel about your husband?" variety) were probably important. We also regard the use of unipolar, unidimensional scales of emotions that are directed towards a single specified person as likely to be of greater predictive value than general ratings of emotive characteristics (for example we believe a rating of expressed warmth by the father towards his eldest son to be more useful than a rating of parental warmth or even paternal warmth towards children).

3. Do husbands and wives, when interviewed separately give equivalent accounts of family activities? In contrast to many other studies, we found a moderately high level of agreement between husbands and wives on most (but not all) scales. This was so on such highly concrete items as the frequency of kin contacts and less concrete variables as the amount of parental interaction with the children. By comparison with methods in the different studies which have examined husband-wife agreement it appears that the most important feature leading to good *across*-interview agreement is a careful distinction between events and feelings about events, that is between "objective" and "subjective" variables. Detailed and intensive questioning involving systematic cross-checking appears more likely to lead to accurate measures than questionnaire or interview approaches requiring answers of the "often" "sometimes" variety. Attitudes are much more likely to influence an informant's judgement of whether the spouse "often" did something than they are to distort his account of who did something on each day during the last week.

Summary measures of the overall marriage relationship and

of the amount of tension in the home also gave very similar ratings whether based on the husband's account or the wife's account.

4. What are the features which influence reliability and validity? The answers to this question are perhaps more important than the actual levels of agreement achieved in that they may offer leads to ways in which reliability and validity can be increased and also they may offer insights into some of the dynamics of family interaction. Some of the issues have already been mentioned and others are covered in a very useful review by Hoffman and Lippitt and in Richardson's thoughtful discussion of interviewing techniques.[78] The main issues may be summarised under the following headings:

a) *Interviewer variables.* That these may be very important in some kinds of interviewing has been clearly shown in other studies,[79] but they did not appear so in the present study. The study was not specifically designed to test interviewer variability, but no consistent differences between the interviews or the ratings of male and female interviewers were found nor were there any differences in the ratings of medical and nonmedical investigators. In large part, patients were interviewed by medically qualified people and nonpatients were interviewed by nonmedically qualified people, and it is conceivable that this might account for the very occasional differences found between patients and non-patients. On the other hand, that this is unlikely is suggested by the finding that where differences did occur these were equally prominent in the few interviews of patients done by non-medical investigators.

b) *Respondent bias* was examined in relation to sex differences and to the differences between patients and nonpatients. No sex differences were found and patient differences were small and affected only a very few scales. There were slight but not significant differences on most scales of "negative" behaviour (e.g. irritability) but the only scale in which the difference reached significance was the overall rating of marriage by the interviewer.*

It might be argued that as the only significant difference was on a scale involving attitudes and judgements (marriage) and as there were no significant differences in the reporting of actual irritable behaviour or events there is likely to have been no distortion or concealment in the accounts of either the patient or the nonpatient. Rather, the slight differences found related to the more gloomy view of the marriage conveyed by the patients (most of whom were depressed) to the interviewer who rated the marriage. This seems to be the most likely explanation for the main effect (which was slight) but, in that there were also occasional differences in the reporting of behaviour, there may also have been some distortion in the accounts of one or other marriage partner. In a very few cases there was evidence from other sources (including incidental observations during interviews) that the non-patient sometimes concealed or "played down" certain negative features of their family life. However, in general there were very few patient-non-patient differences and the fact that one informant was a patient seems to have had remarkably little influence on the validity of findings. Perhaps most important, the fact that they had come for psychiatric help may have increased their cooperation in the interviews. On the other hand, it might be expected that mental disorder would sometimes distort or impair memory, and it should be noted that 10 percent of patients were too ill to have an intensive interview of the kind we used.

c) *Attitudinal biases* were shown to have a slight distorting effect on the reporting of participation in household tasks.

* The scale measuring the amount of quarrelling also showed a marked patient/non-patient difference on the first 20 cases. The scale at that time showed poor *across*-interview agreement but following measures to improve the scale, *across*-interview agreement on the last 10 cases was much better. This was also accompanied by a striking reduction in the patient/non-patient difference which was quite slight on the last 10 cases.

They were also found with the scale for participation in child care but not to a significant extent on other scales such as positive interaction with the children, leisure activities, etc. Anecdotal evidence from interviews where there were large husband-wife differences suggested that dissatisfaction is most likely to influence the reporting of frequencies of events or activities when the dissatisfaction is specifically with the *quantity* of the spouse's participation in the activity rather than the *quality* of participation but this hypothesis can only be tested by a further investigation. We believe that our efforts to keep separate the measurement of events and feelings about events have been largely responsible for our relative success in eliminating attitudinal biases. This may be illustrated by one interview in which, in answer to the introductory remark, "We would like to ask now who does the various jobs in the family?" the informant immediately intervened with, "Well, I can tell you straight away my husband does nothing!" On questioning about specific tasks individually (shopping for groceries, cleaning the house, etc.) she reported several activities in which her husband took an active part. At the end of the section she said spontaneously in a surprised tone of voice, "He really does quite a lot doesn't he?" The general question elicited a quite misleading answer greatly influenced by her critical attitude to her husband. Detailed questioning on actual recent events made it possible to get nearer the truth.

d) *Variability and averaging*. Where there is a variable pattern of behaviour during the period of time to which the measure refers difficulties in "averaging" may lead to error. To test this the *across*-interview agreement was compared for ratings based on a 3 month period and those based on the week showing the most of whatever was being measured. In general, agreement was equally good in both but in a few scales the ratings based on the worst week showed appreciably better husband-wife agreement suggesting that "averaging" errors may occasionally be important.

e) *Forgetting.* Hoffman's discussion of techniques to reduce consciously and unconsciously motivated forgetting has already been mentioned. In addition the effect of duration of time on memory for events needs to be considered. Other workers have shown the biases involved in retrospective accounts[80] and we also find that husband-wife agreement was usually appreciably worse for events a year ago than for events in the immediately previous three months. Retrospective accounts, however reliable in their ratings, appear to have very dubious validity.

We have shown that it is possible to achieve satisfactory levels of reliability and validity for interview measures of many aspects of family activities and relationships. The results were obtained by fairly intensive interviewing in families where one member was a psychiatric patient and it cannot be assumed without further investigation that similar results could be obtained for families not under medical care, nor can the findings be applied to studies using questionnaire or structured interview techniques. Further study of the factors which may influence reliability and validity are particularly needed.*

* This study would not have been possible without the co-operation of many other people. In particular we are much in debt to Mrs. Sandra George, Dr. P. Graham, Mr. D. Quinton, Miss Rita Lang, Mrs. Margaret Rayfield, and Mr. P. Ziffo, who have been jointly responsible for the development of the measures and the interviewing in the study described. We are also grateful for the helpful advice of Dr. J. K. Wing, and to Mrs. Bridget Bryant, Mrs. Margaret Bone, Mrs. Judy Gerhold and Miss Anne Hurley who took part in the early stages of the project.

We also thank the consultant psychiatrists who allowed us access to the families of their patients. The study was supported in part from a grant from the Association for the Aid of Crippled Children.

Chapter 7

Emotional Disorders in an Israeli Immigrant Community

A Comparison of Prevalence Among Different Ethnic Groups

ASHER HOEK, RAFAEL MOSES, AND LESLIE TERRESPOLSKY

PRESENT PREVALENCE STUDIES IN ISRAEL ARE LIMITED TO mental hospitals Halevi[1] and to a psychiatric out-patient clinic.[2] However many persons with emotional disorders do not come to the attention of psychiatric services at all. Hence, to establish a rate which reflects the true prevalence of emotional disorders, study of a community is essential.

Prevalence studies of emotional disorders in communities outside Israel have been carried out by Rennie and Srole,[3] Leighton,[4] Pasamanick,[5] Kessel,[6] Primrose,[7] and others. As reported[8] the rates arrived at range between 2 percent and 70 percent.

Due to the organization and use of health services in Israel, especially in smaller communities, the general practitioner or family doctor of the local health clinic is usually the first person to whom the population turns when medical attention is desired. Thus he is by training and circumstances in a unique position to recognize emotional disorders, while at the same time being a key figure in the administration of care. The present study was undertaken in one such general practice area and determined the prevalence of emotional disorders, as recognized by the family doctors (RED–Recognized Emotional Disorders).

In Israel, with its large immigrant population, persons of divergent cultural origins are exposed to a process of rapid economic development and social change, a way of life often different from that known and established in their country of birth. Several investigators, among them Weinberg[9] in Israel and Opler,[10] Malzberg,[11] Murphy,[12] Leighton and Hughes[13] abroad show that the emotional health of diverse culture groups is differently affected by migration and social change. Ruesch[14] stated: "The difficulties encountered in the process of acculturation are largely reflected in the statistics of mental disease."

On the basis of this postulate, a community study of RED prevalence amongst different ethnic groups of the Israeli population should also throw light upon the absorption difficulties and may be regarded as instrumental in the allocation of mental health programs to the various sectors of the community. Hence, the present investigation selected an immigrant community as its study population.

Since the results of prevalence studies are comparable only if the same methodology is used, attention has been paid to the development and use of a replicable method.[15]

Objectives

The objectives of this study were formulated as follows:

I. To determine the prevalence of emotional disorders as recognized by the family doctors (RED), among adults in a defined general practice population.

II. To compare the prevalence of RED among persons of different ethnic groups.

III. To develop a method of investigation, which can be

used in other community studies, so that comparable data on RED prevalence may be obtained.

Materials and Methods

The Study Population

The population selected for study are adults, aged 20 and above,* residing in a Jerusalem housing estate, who are registered for medical care with the local "Kiryat Hayovel Family and Community Health Center." On June 30th, 1963, this population comprised 963 adults in 441 family units.† This population is composed mainly of persons who immigrated into Israel after its independence was established: 255 or 26.5 percent originated from European countries; 634 (65.8 percent) were born in North-African and Asian countries, while 62 (7.7 percent) were Israel born. At least 72 percent of the immigrant population arrived during the years 1948–1951. Of the population studied 446 (46.3 percent) were men and 517 (53.7 percent) women.

The total immigrant population from Europe was found to be much older than the African-Asian population: 60 percent male and 67 percent female from Europe being over 50 years old, while only 27 percent of the African-Asian males and females had reached this age. (The median age for males is: Europe 57, Africa-Asia 38; the median age for females is: Europe 56, Africa-Asia 38.)

The range of social class, based on the occupation of the head of the household, was chiefly between 3–5.‡

The Health Center is located on the fringe of the residential

* Included in the study are persons born before January 1, 1944. This was done to exclude the age of obligatory army service—during which draftees are not expected to make use of the Health Center.

† 5 of these families had not attended the health center during the preceding 12 month period.

‡ On the basis of a rating system adopted from and similar to that of the British Registrar General for the determination of social class in Britain.

area. It is family oriented, rendering both curative and preventive care, and each family is in principle—though not always in practice—attended by one doctor and one nurse.

Definitions

Recognized Emotional Disorder. A person has been included in the RED population when the family doctor considered him or her to fit the following operational definition: *"Bodily, psychological or social manifestations, recognized by the doctor as symptoms of emotional disorder."**

As has been shown by Redlich,[16] the boundaries of emotional health and disease are not always clearly defined and are at times an issue of difference of opinion between leading authorities. Ryle[17] showed that this was one factor in the different prevalence rates arrived at in the various studies he examined. The definition used in this study attempts to avoid this issue.

Major Manifestation. For every person listed as RED, the physician was required to designate the major manifestation [MM] of the disorder as follows:

Bodily (B)—when the major form in which the doctor recognized the emotional disorder is through complaints of pain or bodily tensions.

Psychological (Ps)—when the major form is through psychopathological phenomena.

Social (S)—when the major form is through the patient's interaction with other people or by social maladjustment.

Diagnostic Category of RED. For every person listed with RED the physician was required to determine the diagnostic category according to the Classification of Mental and Emo-

* The definition of RED was pretested by asking six physicians in health centers all over town how they recognized a person with emotional disorder. It became evident that alert physicians base their decision not on the presenting complaint of the patient but on their own observations as to organic findings, affective and/or thought processes, or interaction with surroundings.

tional Diseases of American Psychiatric Association, 1952. The RED were divided accordingly into five categories: Psychotic Disorders (P); Psychoneurotic Disorders (N); Psychophysiologic, Autonomic and Visceral Disorders (Psph); Personality Disorders together with Sociopathic Personality Disturbances (D); Disorders caused by or associated with impairment of brain tissue functioning (O). Persons who were considered to be mentally deficient were excluded from the study in view of the special acculturation difficulties of this group.

Chronic Organic Disease (COD). A person has been listed as RED with COD if an organic disease caused moderate or severe impairment of the major daily activity (whether employment, study or housekeeping). A person with slight impairment of major daily activity was not classified as having COD.

Methods of Collecting Data

1. *Universal data.* The denominator data for year of birth, sex, and country of birth were abstracted from the Kiryat Hayovel population census which had been carried out in June 1963. The universal data of the RED population were abstracted from the face sheet of the medical record.

2. *Prevalence.* To determine which patient was recognized as having an emotional disorder several methods were utilized. About half (210) of the 441 families were surveyed in staff meetings of the health center team (three physicians and four nurses participating). The list of persons with RED, type of disorder and major manifestation was then handed to the investigator who was present at some of these staff meetings to observe how decisions were arrived at. His impressions were (a) the staff "know their patients" and would not label a person as RED on the basis of a one-time impression; (b) careful consideration was given to each adult and the staff used the occasion to review the population; (c) if there was

any disagreement about diagnosis, the patient was excluded or was regraded. The conclusion reached was that this method was reliable and that the rate of prevalence obtained is a minimal rate.

As a cross check to the listing of names in this way, the investigator perused the case-file of all members of 30 consecutive families that had been surveyed by the team in his absence. The independent listing on the basis of file notes correlated highly with the names listed by the team. Four persons of a total of 65 adults in these families, who were listed as RED by the investigator and not by the team, were ruled out by the team because there was disagreement about the presence of emotional disorder.

The 230 families not surveyed in staff meetings were reviewed by the senior family doctor. When he did not feel sufficiently acquainted with the case another physician or nurse or both were called upon. Of these families, 50 were also independently reviewed by another physician who had been working in the unit for two years. A comparison of the lists of RED made by the two doctors showed agreement in all but three cases: The junior physician had left out three persons. Two of those had not made use of the service lately. The third person responded to the senior family doctor in a "withdrawn way, hardly answering my questions," while the younger physician "had not noticed any peculiar behaviour." A further check of this group of families was carried out by asking nurses to review some of the families to which they were assigned. Here again the concurrence of opinion was confirmed.

Major Manifestation, Type of RED and COD

These items were listed at the same time as RED. The pretest showed that doctors had sometimes a difficult time in making an unequivocal decision on type of RED and MM. Especially in regard to the manifestation it was found sometimes that two or three forms were more or less equally present. On the cases reviewed in staff meeting, further discussion led usually to a consensus. In cross-checking the case records, the investigator almost always found notes about recurrent manifestations that correlated well with staff decisions. When the staff did not reach agreement, the case-notes in the file were used as the basis for the final decision.

The same block of 50 families, which were listed independently by two doctors, was used for a reliability test. Of the 21 persons listed as RED, the diagnosis was dissimilar in two (between Neurosis and Personality disorder). Major manifestation showed three differences (between Bodily and Social manifestation). On the strength of this finding the error is probably less than 15–20 percent.

The methods used for gathering data (objective II) have been described in detail, for they are the basic material in this study.

The use of checks and cross-checks has reduced the effects of subjective bias, a phenomenon described by Kessel.[18] He showed the importance of "the doctor's attitude towards psychiatry, psychiatrists, neurotic patients, and the so-called psychosomatic group of illnesses" in establishing prevalence "if his clinical judgment is to play a part in case identification." Balint[19] demonstrated this clinically. It is thought that the operational definition used in this study, and especially the method used in identification of RED, has reduced the effect of this phenomenon as much as possible.

Analysis of data

In the comparison of E-born and AA born the following points should be noted:

I. Persons with organic mental disease were not included since the RED was not thought to be brought about as a result of psychogenic factors.

II. Persons born in Israel were excluded as their emotional disorder cannot be related to immigration.

III. Comparisons were made twice, first including and then excluding persons with COD. It was thought that the bodily manifestation in this group might unduly influence the findings.

IV. To ensure equitable distribution by age between the two ethnic groups, a dichotomy was set up, attempting to divide the population approximately into two halves. Since the AA population was found to be younger, the dividing age was set at age 40, while for the European group the age of 50 was decided upon.

Four cell Chi-square tests were used for measuring significance. The level of significance used was 5 percent.

Major Findings

A. Total Prevalence

Of 963 adults studied, emotional disorder was recognized in 200 (20.8 percent), i.e., in more than one of five persons. In more than one of three households (37.2 percent) at least one person has RED.

The prevalence of RED in Europe and among Afro-Asian immigrants is similar.

Neither are there differences among males and females, when not controlling for age.

Emotional disorder is not equally recognized at all ages.

In the group of 35–49 years 33 percent or one-third of all persons are RED ($p < 0.001$) while only 13 percent of persons aged 65 + are included ($p < 0.05$). Women aged 20–34 from Asia-Africa have a much higher prevalence than their counterparts from Europe ($p < 0.001$), while at age 50–64 women from Europe are preponderant ($p < 0.01$). Men from Europe and Asia-Africa show similar rates of RED when controlling for age.

Old women from Europe have more RED than those from Asia-Africa ($p < 0.01$).

When comparing the "young" against the "old", the Asia-Africa group shows significant difference on a 5 percent level: old men and young women are preponderant. The European born group shows no differences.

A further interesting finding was an outstanding peak for Asia-Africa men in the 40–44 year age group: 16 of 28 men in this group are RED as compared with 8 of 44 in the 35–39 years old and 6 of 21 in the 45–49 years old. ($x^2 = 5.330$ $0.05 < p < 0.02$)

B. Prevalence by Type of RED

Ten and a half percent of the RED population is diagnosed as psychotic (only of the 21 cases was not confirmed by a psychiatrist), 81 cases (40.5 percent) as neurotic; 51 (25.5 percent) as personality disorders and 43 (21.5 percent) as psychophysiological disorders.

More than half of the women are diagnosed as neurotic and about half of the men as personality disorders ($p < 0.001$). The comparison of Europeans and Afro-Asian immigrants showed no significant difference in the distribution. Neither were the diagnostic categories affected by age.

C. Prevalence by Type of RED and Major Manifestations

To study the distribution of MM and type of RED, patients with Chronic Organic Diseases were excluded so that this group should not unduly influence the results.

Patients *without COD*. A striking finding is the distribution of P—80 percent show psychological manifestations and none show bodily manifestations. Neurotics have mainly B or Ps, and no male neurotic has social manifestations. The Psph group is scattered among the three manifestations but men have more S ($P < 0.05$). Sixty-seven percent of D have social manifestations but this relates mainly to women, since 9 of 10 women who are diagnosed as D are in the S group, while 35 percent of the men with this diagnosis are in the B group (not significant).

Discussion

Whether the emotional ill health in every fifth adult in this community is to be attributed more to individual psychopathology or to factors inherent in the acculturation process is a moot question. On the one hand Weinberg concludes that

> a mentally healthy person himself will create conditions to keep up his inner security by satisfying his need for belonging, not only by trying to remain with his fellow immigrants and seeking the proximity of fellow countrymen . . . but also and above all, by active adjustment through choosing and creating conditions which may make it easier for him to take up his institutional roles in the new environment and acquire the esteem of his new co-citizens.[20]

On the other hand, at least one of the findings—the high prevalence among Afro-Asian born men aged 40–44, would lead one to assume that without emotionally satisfying substitutes the breakdown of traditional institutions causes excessively severe stress situations even for the mentally healthy person. The lower (14.5 percent) rate of RED among Israel born, especially among men, would tend to corroborate this interpretation. If additional investigation confirms this finding, modification in the absorption methods should contribute to a reduction of the prevalence of emotional disorders among future newcomers.

Though the definition of RED is unequivocal, the doctor does not necessarily have equal opportunity to make use of it with every patient. Diagnosis of emotional disorder requires, in addition to observation, also the existence of communication, i.e., a common language. In one specific case of lack of common language the doctor stated: "It would not be fair to put him in the RED group, since I can't talk with him." It is also well known that many persons tend to hide their emotional difficulties because they are shameful in our civilisation. Thus, even if we assume keen observation and alertness in diagnosing RED on the part of the doctor, it is probable that the overall rate of 20.8 per hundred is below the true prevalence, which will remain unknown until a community study[21] is carried out.

Yet it may be stated safely that the organization of the community health center—with its family orientation, the relative stability of its personnel, the combination of preventive and curative care, the fairly comprehensive medical records as well as an awareness of the social and emotional needs of the population—ensured a reasonably high level of case finding. This may not be the case in a differently organized health service.

Prevalence rates among European born (23.1 percent) and Afro-Asian immigrants (20.8 percent) may in addition be influenced by language differences. The staff of the Center is mainly of European or Anglo-Saxon origin. They are able to talk with Europeans in a tongue other than Hebrew, but they do not know Arabic, the most frequent other tongue among the Afro-Asian group. Communication with Afro-Asians is thus considerably more difficult for them. In addition, the cultural distance between the staff and European born is less than with Afro-Asian born. It is interesting that, notwithstanding these factors, no appreciable difference in the prevalence was found.

When we turn to the significant age/sex specific differences of RED, three groups emerge with conspicuously high rates among women—(a) those aged 20–34 from Afro-Asia, and

(b) those aged 50–65 from Europe; among men—(c) those aged 40–44 from Afro-Asia.

The strikingly high rate among the 20–34 year old women from Afro-Asia may be because they are better known to the health center staff than the European women in that age group. They tend to marry young, bear a larger number of children, and, consequently, frequent the pregnancy and well-baby clinic, where they are attended by the same doctor as in the curative service. A study carried out in a health center that uses different personnel in preventive and curative care will be needed to test whether the high prevalence rate is due to the intensive use of services or is caused by psychosocial factors.

The higher prevalence among older women from Europe can be explained on a psychological and cultural basis. In line with the considerations of Lilli Stein,[22] it is suggested that elder women from Afro-Asia continue to have a clear function in their large families: taking care of children who have not yet married, and helping the married children with their little ones. The European women, on the other hand, with their small families, have a much more limited function and become unoccupied and lonely. A related aspect, hinted at here and requiring further study, is the difference in the psychological meaning of the menopause and the mechanisms for adjustment to biological change in European as opposed to Afro-Asian born women.

The peak among the AA born men, aged 40–44, may reflect the common difficulties encountered by the Afro-Asians, which can be summed up as a break in continuity occurring in middle life. The characteristics of the Afro-Asian men who immigrated soon after the establishment of the state of Israel were: little or no schooling; transition from small commerce to physical labor; transit camp living conditions; separation from relatives and little or none of the security provided by the continuation of the traditional extended family system in which they had grown up.

A survey of all 71 Afro-Asian men aged 35–49 who had immigrated between 1948–1951, revealed that of the 13 men who at the time of immigration had a child age 7 or older, none belonged to the RED group. But 22 men with RED are among those whose eldest child was younger than 7 years ($x^2=7.11$ $p<0.01$). This finding may be fortuitous, yet one is tempted to speculate that children of school age were of considerable help to their fathers in the process of acculturation. This point requires further study—especially in view of the implication for absorption services; it might present an important clue as to the particular nature of services to be focused on specific family groups.

The overall rate of 2.2 percent of psychosis (or 2.6 percent when organic psychosis is included) is probably not far below the true prevalence. It is unlikely that the health center staff, acquainted as it is with the local population, would not know about an overtly psychotic person. Three factors may raise the actual figure: (1) the five families not attending the health center; (2) persons who are psychotic, but not severely enough to be recognized as such—and consequently have not been referred to a psychiatrist; and (3) psychotics among the mentally deficient. According to Srole et al.[23] 6.1 percent of the Midtown Manhattan population are in the "probable psychotic type." However our rate of psychosis is considerably higher than the rates established elsewhere—as summarized by Plunkett and Gordon,[24] and by Primrose[25]—except for Bremer, who in a Northcoast village in Norway arrived at a rate of 28.7 per thousand.

The highly significant preponderance of neurotics in women and of personality disorders in men corroborates findings by previous investigators.[26] The meaning is clear neither to them nor to us.

Conclusions

By a conservative estimate at least one out of every five adult immigrants of the lower income class has an emotional disorder, amongst the European born as well as amongst the Afro-Asian born. Yet, as shown by the age/sex specific distribution neither the stress situations nor the manifestations of the emotional disorders appear to be the same in the two groups. This indicates the need for specific understanding of differences in psychological make-up and in modes of acculturation. There is evidence that young women and middle-aged men who immigrated from Afro-Asian countries and 50–65 year old women from Europe are the most vulnerable groups, and services should consequently be geared to these groups.

The established rates of RED cannot be simply extrapolated to other communities. This is so, for in addition to the chief variable selected—ethnic groups as measured by continent of birth—other factors such as socioeconomic status, education, age and family status at time of immigration to Israel, as well as care provided by community services will have influenced the process of acculturation as it is reflected in the prevalence of RED. To confirm or correct the RED rate so that it will reflect the true prevalence for Israel, similar studies should be carried out in a number of carefully selected localities. The results are comparable only if the same methodology is used.

PART III

Community Psychiatry

Introduction

NEW DEVELOPMENTS IN COMMUNITY PSYCHIATRY, ESPECIALLY the reorganization of mental health facilities and programs have special virtue in bringing psychiatry closer to the patient, family, and community. The first article in this section surveys the professional services and preventive educational programs developed by the Mental Health Association of the 13th Arrondissement in Paris, and underscores many of the advantages to be gained by coordinating all relevant activities for a circumscribed geographic area.

Recent developments such as the above have generated a great range of questions about the changing role of the psychiatrist, the use of hospitalization as a treatment technique, the problems associated with the acceptance by the population, of new programs, and the long term effects of community care. These and other issues must be faced if we are to avoid the kind of apathy that, as Kathleen Jones notes, has been shown in the past regularly to follow waves of reform.

In the next article, Dunham critically examines what he considers to be the difficulties or weaknesses inherent in recent developments in community psychiatry. He notes that as the concerns of psychiatry have moved beyond the treatment of the severely disturbed, there has been, in some quarters, a tendency to neglect their needs and to take on other responsibilities for which psychiatrists are inadequately equipped. He questions the possibility of present day psychiatry to effectively develop techniques to treat the mentally ill on a community level. Whether or not psychiatrists will be truly more effective as they become involved in the community power structure must also be considered; in particular, one must consider whether or not this is a proper role for psychiatrists in view of the natural obligations imposed by others in the power structure.

Plaut's comprehensive discussion of the psychosocial aspects of public health provides additional perspective on community psychiatry. He notes that while the task of health education is important in influencing individual action, more emphasis should be placed on the reorganization of institutions. Changes in administrative policies which pertain to such things as visiting hours, admission application, and the like, often have significant effects on mental health. The fact that lower class groups are more accustomed to authoritative than democratic methods, adds to the difficulty of involving these particular groups in effective community action.

That the advent of powerful psychopharmaceutical agents has altered the natural history of the severe psychiatric disorders can be seen in changing patterns of admission, duration, discharge, and readmission to state and private hospitals. Many have avoided hospitalization and have been able to adjust to community and family life. The report of Englehardt and Freeman is therefore of particular interest, for it points to the importance of the limited effect of the drugs on the more formal aspects of psychopathology and social participation and to the possibility that in certain patient groups the effect of the drugs may be only to delay ultimate hospitalization. Their report underlines the importance of assessing in addition to psychology the personality and the family resources of patients for determining those who will and those who will not need hospitalization.

Jones' article reminds us further that there is still at present, in many quarters, a controversy concerning institutional or community care. Some see the institution as being appropriate only when other facilities are unavailable. Others view the institution as one of several means of care, especially for those in need of a controlled environment.

Chapter 8

An Experience with Sectorization in Paris

PHILIPPE PAUMELLE AND SERGE LEBOVICI

It is the purpose of the authors to report on the professional services of the Mental Health Association of the Thirteenth Arrondissement, an administrative section of Paris with a population of 165,000. Privately operated, it is supported by public funds and philanthropic gifts in its endeavor to provide for the inhabitants of the arrondissement an integrated mental health service, including neuropsychiatric facilities for children and adults, a program for the prevention and treatment of alcoholism, and a coordinated effort in mental health education. Because of its emphasis on serving a specific geographic area or sector, the work of the Mental Health Association of the Thirteenth Arrondissement has become known as a sectorization project.

While the residents of the arrondissement have always had public mental health services available to them, these were seldom sufficient to meet the need and were rarely coordinated to provide optimal results. Specialized residential or outpatient facilities were frequently located at a geographic distance, had limited communication with referring clinics, and had little contact with rehabilitation centers. Hospital stays were unduly prolonged by the difficulty of coordinating social readaptation. All too often, essential family ties were loosened or broken, thus retarding the reintegration of the patient in the community.

It is the aim of the Thirteenth Arrondissement Plan to create a whole range of extramural facilities with clearly organized and defined roles, all centering around the community Mental Health Center and each entrusted to a specialized team. In this way, patients can be served in the reality of their home environment, and professional workers motivated toward the goal of prevention. Toward these ends the Association de Santé Mentale et de Lutte contre l'Alcoolisme dans le XIIIe Arrondissement worked in close partnership with authorities, practitioners, and the general public.

With the program outlined in the Ministry of Public Health memorandum of March 15, 1960, it became possible to coordinate mental health services provided by hospital, day hospital, aftercare centers, and workshops. The way in which this was developed in the Thirteenth Arrondissement, as well as plans for the future, will be delineated in the following sections. Throughout the emphasis is on a coordinated and continuing mental health approach, with the same team assuming and retaining responsibility for a patient once an initial contact has been made. The team is part of a multiple-service organization, recommending whatever treatment may be most appropriate and available at a specific moment, given the patient's particular problems and circumstances. The dangers of passing a patient from one isolated agency to another, without adequate consultation or follow-up, are avoided. By further focusing on key organizations and contacts, an extensive mental health education effort is mobilized, facilitating the concepts of prevention and early diagnosis and treatment.

The Thirteenth Arrondissement

Situated on the river Seine, the Thirteenth Arrondissement is the equivalent of a large French town with a population of about 165,000. It may be considered a complete urban unit, taking the Place d'Italie as its geographic and spiritual center.

Like all Paris arrondissements, the section is subdivided into four administrative districts. Of these, the two to the south are economically less well endowed. The two northern ones, comprising the big railway network of the Gare d'Austerlitz and the large hospitals of la Salpétrière and La Pitié are less densely populated, their inhabitants enjoying a higher socio-economic standard.

The two southern districts differ slightly from each other. The southwest area, that of Maison Blanche, has a standard of living that is slightly superior to that of the southeast, known as the station quarter, where the automobile plants of Panhard and the aviation works of Snecma are surrounded by the homes of workers and their families, including a large number of North Africans. There are also small precision industries with workmen who still take pride in their traditional skills.

On the whole, the arrondissement is a reflection of the poorest parts of Paris with a sufficiently typical population composition, e.g., workers and minor employees, foremen, a few executives, some professional people, and comfortable shopkeepers. Because of lack of services and overcrowding, housing conditions have been, and often still are, very poor.

The 1954 Paris census reflects the unfavorable ecological factors in the Thirteenth Arrondissement; conditions of life might be termed "pathogenic." Sociological reports on the arrondissement record a greater number of deaths due to tuberculosis, more frequent behavioral disturbances in children, and the highest figures for juvenile delinquency. These conditions may change, for the arrondissement is due for reconstruction. Important industries will move elsewhere, and the resident population is likely to increase by 10,000 to 15,000 within the next few years. This will probably effect changes in the social character of the population, and the newcomers are likely to introduce fresh aspects for future ecological studies.

The Alfred Binet Center

The Alfred Binet Center for Child Guidance is organized into four teams under the expert guidance of a director and a social assistant director. Each team is responsible for a geographic area of the arrondissement and is composed of a number of psychiatrists, psychologists, and social workers, together with secretaries and various professional assistants (psychoanalytic psychotherapists, psychomotor therapists, remedial teachers, etc.). Teamwork among the psychiatrists has produced highly dynamic aspects: theory as well as practical treatment is applied to every case. All the professionals work constantly at every level in the field of psychotherapeutic action from the moment of undertaking responsibility for a patient. Specialized psychotherapeutic treatment includes psychoanalysis, individual and group therapy, and psychodrama.

Every team directs its clinical and intermediary action as seems most appropriate, but for both theoretical and practical reasons it speedily became evident that the leader of each team could undertake an additional form of service. Thus, one of our number has organized an extensive facility for the study and treatment of speech difficulties, while another is the professional adviser to the Day Hospital for Children (described below).

Placement of a center for child psychiatry in a clearly defined geographical sector has immense advantages. Disturbances treated are so closely involved with reaction toward home surroundings and family circumstances that realization of the ecological dimension is important, particularly in an area like the Thirteenth Arrondissement. The children we examine and treat are preselected by means of constantly improving cooperation between, for example, school social workers and the center's social psychiatric assistants. By coordinating our plans, the waiting list can be shortened to reasonable proportions.

Similarly, time spent on patients who suddenly arrive or are brought for consultation can be reduced if it is realized that today's noisiest cases will not necessarily be tomorrow's gravest problems and that the "best-behaved" children may be harboring serious inhibitions of a neurotic or psychotic nature.

Continuity of treatment, vital in mental health work, is assured at the Alfred Binet Center, since the team responsible for a case keeps that responsibility throughout the period of treatment and aftercare. The role of the social worker who follows the family's progress is particularly important; the "key contacts" at her disposal in the arrondissement facilitate follow-up at critical moments in the near or distant future. This continuity adds a longitudinal dimension to the center's services, as noted by the return of families at times of crisis.

The whole staff of the Alfred Binet Center is engaged in a series of research endeavors, with current emphasis on epidemiologic studies, involving the detailed recording of cases, including psychosocial, diagnostic, prognostic, and therapeutic indications noted in the course of treatment, all under the expert guidance of a member of the French National Institute of Health. Extensive reports are made on each patient at intervals of one, three, and five years after admission to the center or earlier in the case of discharge or discontinuation of treatment for other reasons. It is, of course, impossible in this brief space to give details on the appproximately five hundred new cases treated every year. The majority are children aged from six to fifteen. The fact that preschool children and adolescents are rarely brought for treatment indicates the importance of cooperating with the school services in the area. The referral of patients by family social workers, vocational guidance counselors, police, court authorities, and other key contact organizations provides practical proof of our success in integrating the center with the neighborhood. Research studies indicate that the great majority of children sent for examination come from reasonably secure social and economic backgrounds and are generally members of natural, adopted, or foster families; factors of apparent psychosocial etiologic importance may, however, be elicited. It is evident, for example, that among the lower social classes pathogenic tendencies are encouraged by overly large families and overcrowded housing conditions. We hope to utilize our research for effective preventive care in relevant areas and are particularly interested in studying the structural, plastic, and social aspects of what may be seen as a single unit from a dynamic point of view—structural diagnosis and prognosis.

Coordination between the Alfred Binet Center and the Mental Health Center for Adults is of additional assistance in certain difficult cases, as, for instance, when parents of a child are themselves known mental patients or psychopaths. In addition, we hope eventually to establish a well-equipped specialized facility for adolescents, to which patients may come of their own accord.

Perhaps the ultimate advantage of our community system is the emphasis placed on the utilization of intermediary bodies, whether in a technical or a theoretical sense. The inevitable discrepancy between the ever more urgent needs and the sadly slow and limited development of services makes it imperative to distribute the implementation of psychiatric action, thus creating the most hopeful conditions for the prevention of mental illness in the new generation. Use can and must be made of key contacts for the practical promotion of mental health in all phases of prevention, case finding, and early treatment. Frequently key contact persons possess knowledge of the circumstances which, with the aid of practical discussion or of informal but productive seminars, enable them to take charge of cases that are less complicated or in which their action is more acceptable than perceived interference by a psychiatrist. One example of an important key contact is a pediatrician who sees the parents of very young children. We are also endeavoring to extend counseling for social workers in pediatric, school, family, educational, and leisure-time fields and for educators interested in the prevention of delinquency.

Intermediary action demands new methods of approach. At the Alfred Binet Center, we have found particularly productive the utilization of group-dynamic techniques and, at times, psychodrama. Many other approaches may be pertinent. Over the last two years, under the auspices of the center's section on speech therapy, case-finding efforts have been conducted in some local schools. The ultimate goal is to provide remedial teaching for children unable to read, write, or draw without transferring them to a special school. This is intended particularly for children who come from families that are not oriented materially or culturally to the needs and difficulties of scholastic educational achievement and are unlikely to welcome special schooling for their children. The development of these services in the schools also provides further opportunities for the counseling of teachers.

Another helpful collaborator in problems of child development is the visiting psychiatrist, appointed by the Mental Health Center to the various welfare stations for mothers and children in the arrondissement. Would-be assistants in this field could tell a long story of their efforts to gain a local foothold. At first the consultant psychiatrist was overwhelmed by the task of treating obviously hopeless cases; valuable time was lost before a number of pediatricians and their colleagues realized the necessity for coordinated efforts and a team approach. Only now has an effective atmosphere been created for counseling with kindergarten and primary school teachers, as well as with psychologists.

The Alfred Binet Center welcomes trainees seeking experience in a variety of fields. Participation is provided in the daily program, plus supervised responsibility for individual cases. Trainees also assist in keeping up to date the coordination of our numerous personnel and the organization of the variety of services to be provided; these include not only case conferences but also staff meetings from all specialized facilities and interprofessional scientific and technical discussion groups.

Other Children's Services

The *Day Hospital for Children* was instituted as an extension of the Alfred Binet Center. Supported by the Rothschild Foundation, it provides services in temporary buildings, to which the children are transported by bus. It is intended for treatment of severely neurotic or psychotic children of school age and serves approximately twenty-five patients. They receive schooling adapted to their various capacities, as well as suitable remedial teaching, planned along carefully thought-out lines of progression. Briefly, it is our aim to develop a therapeutic atmosphere in the Day Hospital, both by treatment and by introducing the children to work adjusted to individual requirements (e.g., in educational workshops). Parents are constantly seen by the center's social workers and are required to participate in group psychotherapeutic sessions. After leaving the Day Hospital, a child may be sent, if necessary, to the Alfred Binet Center for follow-up treatment. Roughly speaking, we can say that the annual turnover of children is about 50 percent. The Day Hospital has now been in existence since 1960, and intensive follow-up studies are in progress.

We do not pretend that the Alfred Binet Center and its associated services can solve single-handed all the problems of child mental health in the Thirteenth Arrondissement. In our judgment, the most financially practicable plan is gradually to develop a variety of facilities, once the parent organism is fairly well established. By the time this is published we expect to open a *family placement service for children,* to be coordinated with that projected for adult mental patients, in the neighborhood of the psychiatric hospital at Soisy-sur-Seine.

The service would begin in a small way, dealing with temporary and urgent family placement cases. A few educators could take charge of a number of those children whose family conflicts would be assuaged by a separation of a few weeks; there would be no question of cutting a child off from his familiar surroundings, particularly important where school is concerned.

Establishment of a *day facility for severely oligophrenic children,* designed to combine various full-, half-, and part-time services, is in the planning stage. We also hope to initiate special classes, in cooperation with the consultations given by the Ligue Fraternelle des Enfants de France; these could constitute a particularly useful and necessary stepping-stone between the highly specialized pedagogic services of the Day Hospital and the ordinary schools attended by the children.

Finally, we have hopes of instituting, within the next few years, a *child neuropsychiatric center,* most probably located within the immediate neighborhood of the Soisy hospital for adult mental patients. This might be composed of a number of separate units, providing facilities for observation and hospital treatment along the lines of the medicopedagogic residential centers and psychotherapeutic clinics.

To complete the scope of these facilities, a *day hospital for adolescents* should be included among our projects, and also provisions for *specialized night services.* In our judgment, a careful review should be made of mental health resources for children, adults, and the aged, considering the future organization of the social centers that will inevitably follow in the wake of the large-scale building developments already under way in the Thirteenth Arrondissement.

The Mental Health Center for Adults

The child psychiatrist has come to realize the importance of the whole question of adaptation, its characteristics, and evolution in relation to family or school; similarly, yet with different aspects, the full importance of social rejection or alienation of the mental patient must be realized by the psychiatrist before he can hope positively to affect it. It should be remembered that the patient has often been excluded from the community of his fellowmen for years before he ever comes for treatment. His experiences probably range from isolation when he is quiet to police intervention and neighbors' fears if he becomes violent. He has met with more or less acute disappointment and degradation in his efforts to work and live and has finally been rejected. It becomes the task of specialized medical therapy to combat these disastrous social reactions, but it is no longer a question of the psychiatrist's working alone. Technically, the psychiatrist is the leader of a team composed of a variety of professional associates to facilitate the necessary approaches, including social workers, psychologists, psychotherapists, rehabilitation workers, and nurses. All join in diagnostic and therapeutic efforts which go beyond "treating" the patient in the strictest sense of the term. The team seeks to attain an understanding of the patient's surroundings, background, family, and work conditions, that is, the milieu in which he lives.

To facilitate adult psychiatric services, the Thirteenth Arrondissement has been subdivided into three administrative areas, each of 50,000 to 60,000 inhabitants and each initially equipped with a medicosocial unit. Another unit is to be provided for each area, and together the teams will be expected to offer all required services. The hub of organization has been located in the Centre de Santé Mentale, 76 Rue de la Colonie. Facilities are being developed for consultation and for ambulatory, domiciliary, and emergency care. Consultations are timed preferably for the evening, after working hours, and are arranged beforehand in an attempt to allot adequate time (generally three-quarters of an hour for first, and half an hour for subsequent, consultations). All team members are available, thus facilitating cooperation and precise diagnosis for treatment. Taking into consideration the full circumstances of the patient's condition and difficulties before he comes, a welcoming atmosphere is seen as essential; the receptionists and social workers focus on this aspect, and team members' timetables are programmed to ensure constant availability.

Ambulatory care of all types is being developed to maximum capacity. Pharmacological treatment is dispensed by nurses. Psychomotor and relaxation therapy are provided in individual or group sessions. Many forms of psychotherapy are available to meet individual requirements, from psychoanalysis to supporting therapy. Special mention may also be made of our efforts to assist schizophrenics to avoid apparently inevitable hospitalization through intensive psychotherapy. A regular, psychotherapeutically oriented consultation has been developed to select appropriate therapeutic action for individual cases.

An occupational counselor is always available to advise team members on problems of rehabilitation and readaptation. His task is primarily to find work for patients, which involves information and contacts with prospective employers. He must also discover the best ways of reinserting patients into the productive life of the community, which requires observation and participation in the activities of the rehabilitation workshop.

The facility for domiciliary and emergency care was initiated in 1963. From a preventive and therapeutic point of view, it is essential to have immediate access to patients' homes, to step in at the first suggestion of an appeal for help, or perhaps even to investigate an ominous lack of communication. While physicians and social workers play an important role, primary responsibility rests with the team for domiciliary care. As of 1964, there were four nurses, who arrange between themselves to be constantly on call at the center, providing assistance for cases not actually requiring hospitalization; for example, senile patients with somatic disturbances, depressive conditions, anxiety disorders, etc. The nurse on duty is available to calm a troubled situation when an appeal is received from the patient's family, to accompany a patient for treatment, and so on. In some cases, domiciliary care of the severely mentally ill amounts to hospitalization within the home. Here, too, the contacts made by the nursing assistant in visits with the family and neighborhood are of extreme importance in the patient's ultimate social reintegration.

It is, of course, impossible to treat all sick persons at the center; the teams have not yet at their disposal a sufficient array of extramural facilities. So far, including the newly established rehabilitation workshop, we have the Day Hospital, established in 1959. This is intended for all instances in which consultation and domiciliary care are insufficient and especially for those persons who would formerly have been hospitalized, probably under committal. A fully integrated therapeutic and occupational program is planned for each patient and regularly discussed at weekly reviews of treatment progress.

A more distant project is the Club des Peupliers for former mental patients, envisaged as a social rehabilitation service with planned leisure-time programs. In close collaboration with the Élan Aftercare Center, we provide lodging and upkeep for convalescent patients in a sort of hostel, operated under medical and social supervision. This home is particularly oriented toward rehabilitation, and patients are, as a rule, reintegrated into normal occupational work. Plans have been drawn for an extensive chain of sheltered workshops and rehabilitation services for those patients whose readaptation to normal working conditions is likely to take a longer time. In these specialized facilities, the type of work and its remuneration must be considered with careful attention to detail, taking individual requirements into account insofar as possible. Patients especially affected include the retarded and those who have experienced long treatment processes, that is, the group that usually constitutes the "dead weight" in psychiatric hospitals, where their problems are often merely aggravated and rendered chronic.

Coordination of Services

The general plan of action for the various links in the chain of community services involves an initial contact between the patient and a team from the Mental Health Center. This contact is maintained throughout, the team following each patient's progress through the various facilities. Practical experience has shown how difficult it is for this program to run smoothly; constant meetings, discussions, and correspondence are necessary. It is of primary importance to help the patient, from the very first, to realize that he has not been thrust into a clinic where he knows nobody and nobody knows him (the classic situation), but that he is secure—a feeling even more important for the mentally ill person than for the physically sick. To achieve this ideal, each psychiatrist responsible for the general mental health of an area must also understand his responsibility as a functional leader of a service. In this capacity he is no longer only a physician in charge of individual patients but the captain of a team, delegating the application of individual treatment to his colleagues. Considering the long-established, private, confidential nature of medical practice in France, leading only too often to successive treatments by isolated physicians, it becomes apparent that our team effort is breaking new and difficult ground in requiring everyone to coordinate his actions with all the others involved in the treatment process.

The physicians who administer the arrondissement's hospital as Soisy-sur-Seine (the Eau Vive) are also responsible for a medical sector team and are thus familiar with this type of cooperation. The Eau Vive operates on a small scale: 1 bed per 1,000 inhabitants, or a total of 175 beds when complete. These limitations of size impose conditions requiring intensive treatment over as brief a period of time as possible. To achieve maximum results we concentrate on continuity between services; the team continually surveys all patients. Since hospitalization is voluntary except in emergency or acute cases, we endeavor to stimulate active patient collaboration and adjust treatment to individual requirements. Patients progress positively, reaping the benefits of a varied daily timetable, adapted to their personal needs and leading away from completely isolated treatment to a social way of life opening onto the community.

Large-scale wards have been completely eliminated. Instead, the rooms vary in capacity from one to six beds. In addition, each section has its own functional aspects, ranging from facilities for patients in intensive treatment (where they may, if necessary, be completely cut off from noise, light, and normal social contacts) to the practically open areas, where men and women together may partake in a community life that, in its diversity, nearly resembles the outside world. After a conference with the architect, we also established for every section small units of a familial character, each containing seven beds, under the care of a nurse. These units facilitate temporary patient groupings of a therapeutic nature (as, for example, when their patterns of behavior are similar and they follow the same course of treatment). Feelings of human individuality and security are fostered, an important consideration usually impossible to attain when patients are crowded into vast wards.

It is hardly necessary to mention that the therapeutic goals of the hospital cannot be realized unless the number of qualified personnel is increased. We hope to achieve a ratio of one physician per twenty-eight patients and one nurse per seven patients, this being considered the absolute minimum requirement. Yearly we have to ask ourselves whether the per diem allowances should not also be raised.

Meanwhile, to the administrators and organizers of the responsible services, our projects and requirements are always new and often quite unprecedented. We must weigh in the balance human and financial responsibilities and the consequences of prolonged intramural care under conditions which, to say the least, often have little therapeutic effect. We are persuaded that our experience is well worthwhile on all counts if we can achieve the aims described: prevention of mental illness; treatment, primarily extramural, applied as early as possible; intramural treatment, continuously and intensively sustained; and, finally, social and professional rehabilitation of patients at appropriate levels of recovery.

Mental Health Education

In the centers for both child and adult mental health care, all workers hold to the principles previously described. As guardians of the mental health of the Thirteenth Arrondissement, we have come to realize the importance of screening candidates for treatment in the service facilities. It is our long-term aim gradually to orient key contact persons to an even greater awareness of mental hygiene and to bring them into ever-closer contact with the centers.

The various efforts to promote mental health in the sector's child and adult population come under the general supervision of the Mental Health Association of the Thirteenth Arrondissement. The association has organized a committee, under the direction of a social worker, which includes mental health advisers as well as representatives of the general public and individuals in useful positions and related professions.

The Club des Peupliers has among its members former patients from the Mental Health Center for Adults; it aims to provide assistance in leisure-time occupations and rehabilitation. Its executive committee is composed entirely of former patients, particularly those from the Day Hospital. The director of the Mental Health Service, a social worker, serves as professional adviser to the club and its sixty members. Twice a month, outings are arranged, including visits to theatres, day excursions, etc. For a number of former patients, the club provides their only link with the Mental Health Center, thus maintaining contact with the therapeutic community. Another useful function is that, by inviting individuals from the arrondissement to participate, we can gradually bring the general public to accept and understand behavioral symptoms of the mentally ill.

In the field of assistance to parents, the Mental Health Service has organized a film club. Meetings are held once a month in a community room in the arrondissement and are always attended by at least 150 parents. After the film presentation, difficulties of interpersonal relations within the family and educational problems are discussed.

The Mental Health Center also holds seminars for the educators of clubs for potential juvenile delinquents. At each meeting a specific problem of dynamic psychology is studied, information exchanged, and a case history reported by a staff member.

In considering the various mental health activities of the arrondissement, mention should be made of the educational coordinator, a psychologist who works on a half-time basis for the association, seeing both parents and schoolteachers. Using a schoolroom, she gives lectures for parents twice every term in each school in the arrondissement. Thus, a number of parents, unable or unwilling to discuss their problems at first, tend to do so more readily when the psychologist has become a familiar figure, either during the time for general discussion or at the close of the session. The psychologist tries to explain causes of children's behavioral problems (leading often to further discussion) and to help parents to adjust their attitudes.

More advanced educational activities are conducted by groups attached to various family associations. The same psychologist also directs group occupational facilities for young people. She is available for consultation as a staff member of the Alfred Binet Center and of the social assistance teams. A number of mothers ask for personal interviews to discuss their children's problems; for some, these individual consultations have become an excellent form of psychotherapeutic treatment.

Conclusions

In a practical sense, our endeavors to improve psychiatric assistance in the Thirteenth Arrondissement are still in their early stages, although we have followed the guiding lines of historic trends of development in France and, more specifically, in Paris. The Mental Health Association of the Thirteenth Arrondissement is a private organization, whose professional staff works in collaboration both with representatives of the population and with members of the administrative departments financing our efforts.

At this writing, a statistical research survey is in progress to determine results and direct future programs, with special emphasis on epidemiologic approaches. In addition, more specific research efforts have been initiated in an endeavor to understand the general characteristics of the arrondissement's "normal" population and plan for its future needs.

Because of its unique organization and services, the Mental Health Association frequently receives professional visitors from other parts of France or abroad. Some of these visitors, supported by grants from diverse agencies, stay with us for quite a long time, working or studying under our supervision. In the Mental Health Center for Adults, special provisions have been established for colleagues from abroad to learn about both hospital and community services.

Summary

A brief survey has been presented of the professional services and the preventive educational program for children and adults developed and implemented by the Mental Health Association of the Thirteenth Arrondissement of Paris, France, in collaboration with local administrative authorities and other public and private organizations. By coordinating facilities within a geographic area, serving 165,000 persons, and demonstrating the practical effectiveness of a community mental health team that retains responsibility for a patient from the moment of initial contact to social reintegration, it is hoped to learn more about the conditions favorable to mental health and the prevention of incapacitating mental illness.

Chapter 9

Community Psychiatry

The Newest Therapeutic Bandwagon

H. WARREN DUNHAM

THE PROPOSAL TO ADD COMMUNITY PSYCHIATRY TO THE ever-widening list of psychiatric specialties deserves a critical examination. Thus, my purpose in this paper is fourfold. First, I intend to examine the nature of community psychiatry as it is taking shape. Second, I want to consider our continuing uncertainty about mental illness which is manifested in a widening of its definition. Third, I discuss some of the historical landmarks and cultural forces that have brought about the proposal for this new subspecialty of psychiatry. Finally, I examine some of its hidden aspects with respect to the future role of psychiatry.

Community Psychiatry: The Newest Subspecialty

Let us begin by examining the nature of community psychiatry that is apparently emerging as judged by a mounting chorus of voices from those who jump on any bandwagon as long as it is moving. In doing this I will focus first on community psychiatry in relation to community mental health and the various programs, plans, and social actions that are currently getting under way, with emphases that are as varied as the cultural-regional contrasts of American society.

A pattern concerned with maximizing treatment potential for the mentally ill is gradually taking shape. This newest emphasis points to a declining role of the traditional state hospital and the rise of the community mental health center with all of the attendant auxiliary services essential for the treatment of the mentally ill. In its ideal form the community mental health center would provide psychiatric services, both diagnostic and treatment, for all age groups and for both inpatients and outpatients in a particular community. In addition, the center would have attached closely to it day and night hospitals, convalescent homes, rehabilitative programs or, for that matter, any service that helps toward the maximizing of treatment potential with respect to the characteristics of the population that it is designed to serve. Also attached to this center would be several kinds of research activities aimed at evaluating and experimenting with old and new therapeutic procedures. In the background would still be the state hospital that would, in all likelihood, become the recipient for those patients who seemingly defy all efforts with available therapeutic techniques to fit them back into family and community with an assurance of safety to themselves and others. This reorganization of psychiatric facilities as a community mental health program also implies an increased and workable coordination of the diverse social agencies in the community toward the end of detecting and referring those persons who need psychiatric help.

This ideal structure does appear to be oriented toward the urban community. Therefore, the need arises to clarify the size and type of the population that would be served. Further, a breakdown of the population into the several age and sex categories along with several projected estimates of the number of mentally ill persons that will occur in these population categories would be required. Estimates should be made for the psychoneuroses, the psychoses, the psychopathies, the mentally retarded, and the geriatrics cases that will be found in a community.

Indeed, we should attempt to mobilize and to organize our psychiatric resources in such a manner that they will maximize our existing therapeutic potential for any community. At all events, such a structure seems to suggest to certain professionals at the National Institute of Mental Health that if there comes into existence a realistic community mental health program, there must be a community psychiatry that knows how to use it. While the logic here escapes me, it seems to be quite clear to Viola Bernard who states that, "Recognition of the need to augment the conventional training for mental health personnel to equip them for the newer function of community mental health practice parallels wide-scale trends toward more effective treatment methods at the collective level to augment one-to-one clinical approaches."[1] Dr. Bernard goes on to say that community psychiatry can be regarded as a subspecialty of psychiatry and that it embraces three major subdivisions—social psychiatry, administrative psychiatry, and public health psychiatry.

While Dr. Bernard may see clearly the nature of a community psychiatry that transcends the traditional one-to-one clinical approach, this is not the case with departments of psychiatry in some medical schools as the recent National Institute of Mental Health survey attests.[2] In reviewing the limited literature it is all too clear that different conceptions abound as to what community psychiatry is and while these conceptions are not always inconsistent they nevertheless attest to the fact that the dimensions of the proposed new subspecialty are by no means clear-cut. These conceptions range all the way from the idea that community psychiatry means bringing psychiatric techniques and treatments to the indigent persons in the community to the notion that community psychiatry should involve the education of policemen, teachers, public health nurses, politicians, and junior executives in mental hygiene principles. A mere listing of some of the conceptions of what has been placed under the community psychiatry umbrella will give a further notion of this uncertainty. Community psychiatry has been regarded as encompassing (1) the community base mental hospital, (2) short-term mental hospitalization, (3) attempts to move the chronically hospitalized patient and return him to the community, (4) the integration of various community health services, (5) psychiatric counseling and services to nonpsychiatric institutions such as schools, police departments, industries, and the like, (6) the development of devices for maintaining mental patients in the community, (7) reorganization and administration of community mental health programs, and finally (8) the establishment of auxiliary services to community mental hospitals, such as outpatient clinics, day hospitals, night hospitals, home psychiatric visits, and the utilization of auxiliary psychiatric personnel in treatment programs.[3]

Perhaps we can come close to what someone visualizes as the content of community psychiatry by quoting an announcement of an opening for a fellowship in community psychiatry in Minnesota. In the announcement the program is described as follows: "One year of diversified training and experience, including all aspects of community organization, consultation, and training techniques, administration, research, and mass communication media." Such a psychiatric residency program certainly represents a great difference from the more traditional training program and points to a type of training that might be more fitting for a person who wants to specialize in community organization.

There is no clearer support for this conception than Leonard Duhl's paper[4] where he discusses the training problems for community psychiatry. In this paper he speaks of three contracts that the psychiatrist has, the traditional one with the patient, the more infrequent one with the family, and still more infrequent one with the community. In connection with his community contract, the psychiatrist states, according to Duhl, "I will try to lower the rate of illness and maximize the health of this population." Duhl continues, and I quote, because the direction is most significant.

> In preparing psychiatrists for these broadened contracts, a new set of skills must be communicated. For example, he must learn how to be consultant to a community, an institution, or a group without being patient-oriented. Rather, he must have the community's needs in central focus. He must be prepared for situations where he is expected to contribute to planning for services and programs, both in his field and in others, that are related: what information is needed; how it is gathered; what resources are available, and so forth. Epidemiology, survey research, and planning skills must be passed on to him. He must be prepared to find that people in other fields, such as the legislature, often affect a program more than his profession does. He must find himself at home in the world of economics, political science, politics, planning, and all forms of social action.[5]

While these remarks of Bernard and Duhl may not represent any final statement as to what community psychiatry will become, they point to a probable direction that this newest addition to psychiatric subspecialties may take. However, in this conception of the community psychiatrist as a person skilled in the techniques of social action there lie so many uncertainties, unresolved issues, and hidden assumptions that it is difficult to determine where it will be most effective to start the analysis, with the role of the psychiatrist or with the nature of the community.

Perhaps sociologists can garner some small satisfaction in the fact that the psychiatrist finally has discovered the community—something that the sociologist has been studying and reporting on for over half a century in the United States. However, once the psychiatrist makes this discovery he must ask himself what he can do with it in the light of his professional task, how the discovery will affect his traditional professional role, and how working on or in the community structure can improve the mental health level of its people. Now, it seems that those leaders of psychiatry who are proposing this new subspecialty imply several things at the same time and are vague about all of them. They seem to be saying, in one form or another, the following:

> 1. We, psychiatrists, must know the community and learn how to work with the various groups and social strata composing it so that we can help to secure and organize the necessary psychiatric facilities that will serve to maximize the treatment potential for the mentally ill.
>
> 2. We must know the community because the community is composed of families which, through the interaction of their members, evolve those events and processes that in a given context have a pathic effect upon some of the persons who compose them.
>
> 3. We must know the community in order to develop more effective methods of treatment at the "collective level," to eliminate mentally disorganizing social relationships, and to achieve a type of community organization that is most conducive to the preservation of mental health.
>
> 4. We must know the community if we are ever to make any headway in the prevention of mental illness. For we hold that in the multiple groups, families, and social institutions which compose the community, there are numerous unhealthy interpersonal relationships, pathological attitudes and beliefs, cultural conflicts and tensions, and unhealthy child training practices that make for the development of mental and emotional disturbances in the person.

An analysis of our first implication shows that no new burden is placed upon the psychiatrist but it merely emphasizes his role as a citizen—a role that, like any person in the society, he always has had. It merely emphasizes that the psychiatrist will take a more active part in working with other professionals in the community such as lawyers, teachers, social workers, ministers, labor leaders, and business men in achieving an organization of psychiatric facilities that will maximize the therapeutic potential in a given community. To be sure it means that in working with such persons and groups, he will contribute his own professional knowledge and insights in the attempt to obtain and to organize the psychiatric facilities in such a manner as to achieve a maximum therapeutic potential. Thus, this is hardly a new role for the psychiatrist. It only becomes sharper at this moment in history when a social change in the care and treatment of the mentally ill is impending, namely, a shift from a situation that emphasized the removal of the mental patient from the community to one that attempts to deal with him in the community and family setting and to keep active and intact his ties with these social structures.

The second implication is routine in the light of the orientation of much of contemporary psychiatry. Here, attention is merely called to the theory that stresses the atypical qualities of the family drama for providing an etiological push for the development of the several psychoneuroses, character disorders, adult behavior disturbances and, in certain instances, psychotic reactions. Thus, it follows that to change or correct the condition found in the person, some attention must be paid to the family as a collectivity, to grasp and then modify those attitudes, behavior patterns, identifications, and emotional attachments that supposedly have a pathogenic effect on the family members. From the focus on the family the concern then extends to the larger community in an attempt to discover the degree to which the family is integrated in or alienated from it.

However, it is in the third implication that many probing questions arise. For here the conception is implicit that the community is the patient and consequently, the necessity arises to develop techniques that can be used in treating the community toward the end of supplementing the traditional one-to-one psychiatric relationship. This position also implies a certain etiological view, namely, that within the texture of those institutional arrangements that make up the community there exists dysfunctional processes, subcultures with unhealthy value complexes, specific institutional tensions, various ideological conflicts along age, sex, ethnic, racial, and political axes, occasional cultural crises, and an increasing tempo of social change that in their functional interrelationships provide a pathogenic social environment. Thus, when these elements are incorporated into the experience of the persons, especially during their early and adolescent years, they emerge as abnormal forms of traits, attitudes, thought processes, and behavior patterns. In a theoretical vein, this is the Merton[6] paradigm wherein he attempts to show the diverse modes of adaptation that arise as a result of the various patterns of discrepancy between institutional means and cultural goals.

The influence of the social milieu in shaping, organizing, and integrating the personality structure, of course, has been recognized for a long time. What is not so clear, however, is the manner in which such knowledge can be utilized in working at the community level to treat the mental and emotional maladjustments that are continually appearing. In addition, the nature and function of those factors in the social milieu contributing to the production of the bona fide psychotics are by no means established.

These issues point to some very pressing queries. What are the possible techniques that can be developed to treat the "collectivity"? Why do psychiatrists think that it is possible to treat the "collectivity" when there still exists a marked uncertainty with respect to the treatment and cure of the individual case? What causes the psychiatrist to think that if he advances certain techniques for treating the "collectivity," they will have community acceptance? If he begins to "treat" a group through discussions to develop personal insights, what assurances does he have that the results will be psychologically beneficial to the persons? Does the psychiatrist know how to organize a community along mentally hygienic lines and if he does, what evidence does he have that such an organization will be an improvement over the existing organization? In what institutional setting or in what cultural milieu would the psychiatrist expect to begin in order to move toward more healthy social relationships in the community? These are serious questions and I raise them with reference to the notion that the community is the patient.

If a psychiatrist thinks that he can organize the community to move it toward a more healthy state I suggest that he run for some public office. This would certainly add to his experience and give him some conception as to whether or not the community is ready to be moved in the direction that he regards as mentally hygienic. If he should decide on such a step he will be successful to the extent that he jokingly refers to himself as a "head shrinker" and that he becomes acceptable as "one of the boys." But if he does, he functions as an independent citizen, in harmony with our democratic ethos, bringing his professional knowledge to bear on the goal he has set for himself and his constituents. However, successful or not, he will certainly achieve a new insight concerning the complexity involved in treating the community as the patient.

While I have poked at this proposition from the standpoint of politics, let me consider it with respect to education. If this becomes the medium by which the pathology of the community is to be arrested, one can assume that it means adding to and raising the quality of the educational system in the community. The dissemination of psychiatric information with respect to signs and symptoms, the desirability of early treatment, the natural character of mental illness, the therapeutic benefits of the new drugs, and the correct mental hygiene principles of child training have been going on not only through the usual community lectures and formal educational channels but also by means of the mass media—radio, television, the newspapers, and the slick magazines. I hasten to add, however, that this may not be to the advantage of the community, for it may do nothing else but raise the level of anxiety among certain middle-class persons, who, when they read an article on the correct procedure for bringing up children realize that they have done all the wrong things. Also, the media are frequently sources of misinformation and sometimes imply a promise that psychiatry cannot fulfill.

Further, I observe that in this proposal for a community psychiatry, the psychiatrist seems to be enmeshed in the same cultural vortex as is the professor. For it is becoming fashionable for a professor to measure his success in having hardly any contact with students—he is too busy on larger undertakings, research, consultations, conferences, and the like. Likewise, some psychiatrists think that they have arrived if they have no contact with patients. For example, I have heard of one psychiatrist who has not seen a patient for several years —he spends his time educating teachers, nurses, policemen, business men, and the laity in psychiatric principles.

The third and fourth implications of the new focus provided by community psychiatry are closely related because each position partially views the structures and processes of the community as containing certain etiological elements that make for the development of certain types of mental and emotional illness. However, the third implication, as we have shown, points to the development of treatment techniques on the collective level, while the fourth emphasizes that knowledge of the community is essential if mental illness is ever to be prevented.

There is do doubt that the word prevention falling on the ears of well-intentioned Americans, is just what the doctor ordered. It is so hopeful that no one, I am sure, will deny that if we can prevent our pathologies this is far better than sitting back and waiting for them to develop. But, of course, there is a catch. How are we going to take the first preventive actions if we are still uncertain about the causes of mental disorders? How do we know where to even cut into a community's round of life? And if we did cut in, what assurance do we have that the results might not be completely the opposite to those anticipated? Of course, there is always secondary prevention—that is, directing our efforts to preventing a recurrence of illness in persons who have once been sick. This is a laudable goal but in connection with mental and emotional disturbances we are still uncertain as to the success of our original treatment efforts.

Prevention of Behavioral Pathology—Some Previous Efforts

There is no doubt that the possibility of prevention is something that will continue to intrigue us for years to come. Therefore, it is not without point to take a look at several other programs that, while they have not all been exclusively oriented toward the treatment of the community, have been launched with the hope of preventing the occurrence of certain unacceptable behavior on the part of the members of a community. I cite two experiments which are widely known with respect to the prevention of delinquency.

The first is Kobrin's statement concerning the 25 year assessment of the Chicago Area Project.[7] Kobrin has presented us with a straightforward, modest, and sophisticated account of the accumulated experience provided by this project in the efforts to bring about a greater control of delinquency in certain areas of Chicago. This project has been significant on several counts, but in my judgment its greatest significance was that it helped to initiate various types of community organizational programs that logically proceeded from an empirically developed theory of delinquency. This theory, in general, viewed delinquency as primarily a "breakdown of the machinery of spontaneous social control." The theory stressed that delinquency was adaptive behavior on the part of adolescents in their peer groups in their efforts to achieve meaningful and respected adult roles, "unaided by the older generation and under the influence of criminal models for whom the intercity areas furnish a haven." This theory, in turn, rests upon certain postulates of sociological theory which emphasize that the development and control of conduct are determined by the network of primary relationships in which one's daily existence is embedded.

The significance of this experiment was that this theory of delinquency provided a rationalization for cutting into the community at certain points and seeking persons there who were ready to organize themselves to secure a higher level of welfare for themselves and their children. The results of this experiment are relevant to those advocators of the preventive function of a community psychiatry because there was not only the difficulty of determining what actually had been accomplished in the way of the prevention of delinquency but also a difficulty in assessing the experience in relation to community welfare.

Kobrin, in his opening sentence has stated this problem most cogently.

> The Chicago Area Project shares with other delinquency prevention programs the difficulty of measuring its success in a simple and direct manner. At bottom this difficulty rests on the fact that such programs, as efforts to intervene in the life of a person, a group, or a community, cannot by their very nature, constitute more than a subsidiary element in changing the fundamental and sweeping forces which create the problems of groups and of persons or which shape human personality. Decline in rates of delinquents—the only conclusive way to evaluate delinquency prevention—may reflect influences unconnected with those of organized programs and are difficult to define and measure.[8]

The point here is that in a carefully worked out plan based upon an empirically contructed theory it is difficult to determine what has been achieved. One can hazard the observation that if this is true with respect to delinquent behavior where mounting evidence has always supported the idea that its roots are deeply enmeshed in the network of social relationships, how much more difficult it will be in the field of psychiatry to make an assessment in preventive efforts when we are much more uncertain concerning the etiological foundations of those cases which appear in psychiatric offices, clinics, and hospitals.

The well-known Cambridge-Summerville Youth Study[9] provides the second example of a delinquency prevention program. While this study did not focus upon the community as such but rather on certain persons therein, it did proceed from a conception of a relationship between a person's needs and a treatment framework for administering to those needs. In this study an attempt was made to provide a warm, human, and continuing relationship between an assigned counsellor and a sample of delinquents and to withhold this relationship from another comparable matched sample. These relationships with most of the boys in the treatment group lasted for approximately eight years. At the conclusion of the experiment there was an attempt to assess the results. These were mainly negative. The number of boys in the treatment group appearing before the crime prevention bureau of the police department was slightly in excess of the number of boys making such appearances in the control group. The only positive note was that the boys in the control group were somewhat more active as recidivists than were the boys in the treatment group.

Although the results of this study were inconclusive and told us nothing particularly about the communities to which these boys were reacting, they did document the failure of one type of relationship therapy to reduce delinquency. While these results provide no final word they do point up the necessity for the various techniques in psychiatry to first acquire a far greater effectiveness than they now possess before starting to operate on a community level where there will be a great deal of fumbling in the dark before knowing exactly what to do.

It seems most appropriate in the light of the task envisioned for community psychiatry to call attention to the professional excitement that was engendered when the Commonwealth

Fund inaugurated a child-guidance program in 1922. The Child Guidance Clinic was hailed as a step that eventually should have far-reaching consequences. For who saw fit to deny at that time in the light of certain prevailing theories and the optimism provided by the cultural ethos of the United States that if emotional, mental, and behavioral disturbances were ever to be arrested and prevented at the adult level it would be necessary to arrest these tendencies at their incipient stage, namely, in childhood. This all appears most logical and reasonable. However, 40 years after the opening of the first child guidance clinic we have such clinics in almost every state and they are very much utilized as evidenced by the long waiting lists. Nevertheless, not only does juvenile delinquency remain a continuing community problem but also the adult incidence rates of at least the major psychoses appear to remain approximately constant during this period, especially if the study by Goldhamer and Marshall[10] is accepted as valid.

I cite these three different kinds of experience primarily for the purpose of emphasizing the necessity to review our past efforts in attacking certain behavioral problems at a community level and also to point to some of the difficulties that are inherent in any proposal that emphasizes the development of psychiatric treatment techniques for the "collective level."

The Widening Definition of Mental Illness

Efforts in the direction of carving out a subspecialty of psychiatry known as community psychiatry take place in a cultural atmosphere which has seen a definite attempt to widen the definition of what constitutes mental illness. This is shown by the tendency in our society to place any recognized behavior deviant into the sick role. By doing this we not only supposedly understand them, but also we can point to therapies which will be appropriate for their treatment. Thus, the past two decades have witnessed attempts to place in the sick role delinquents, sex offenders, alcoholics, drug addicts, beatniks, communists, the racially prejudiced, and, in fact, practically all persons who do not fit into the prevailing togetherness that we like to think characterizes middle-class American life. The danger here is that we only add to our state of confusion because the line between who is sick and who is well becomes increasingly a waving, uncertain one. Thus, we appear to be constantly moving the cutting point toward the end of the continuum that would include those persons who in some subcultural milieus are accepted as normal.

There is much current statistical evidence that supports this notion of a widening definition for mental illness. For example, if one examines the community epidemiological surveys of mental illness in the 1930's and compares them with the community epidemiological surveys in the 1950's one is struck with the fact that four to five times more cases are reported in the latter years.[11] In my own epidemiological study of schizophrenia, where I have examined many epidemiological studies from all over the world I have noted the great differences that are reported with respect to total mental disorders in the surveys, a marked decrease in the differences between the surveys when only psychoses are reported and a still further decrease in the rate variations when the reports are based upon only one mental disorder, namely, schizophrenia. In this latter case, the variations are slight and all of the rates are quite close together. One might point to the Midtown Manhattan Survey[12] where two psychiatrists reviewing symptom schedules on a sample population as collected by field workers found that approximately 80 percent of the sample were suffering from some type of psychiatric symptom. This extreme figure can be contrasted with the 20 percent reported as incapacitated. The providing of adequate psychiatric services for even the latter figure would place an impossible burden on any community.

Several factors help to explain this widening definition of mental illness which has been so apparent during the past two decades. One factor, of course, has been the adaptation of psychiatry to office practice following World War II.[13] Another factor is that the mounting frustration resulting from the failures to achieve therapeutic results with the bona fide psychotics has led to a widening of the psychiatric net in order to include those persons with minor emotional disturbances who are more responsive to existing treatment techniques. These people are suffering from what has been termed "problems of living," and they do not represent the bona fide mentally ill cases.[14] In this connection it is interesting to note that George W. Albee, at an American Medical Association meeting in Chicago, stated:

> What we clearly do not need more of in the mental health profession are people who go into private practice of psychotherapy with middle-aged neurotics in high income suburbs. While there are humanitarian and ethical reasons for offering all the help we possibly can to individuals afflicted with mental disorders, it seems unlikely that we will ever have the manpower to offer individual care on any kind of manageable ratio of therapists to sufferers.[15]

In the light of Albee's observation it is instructive to note Paul Hoch's evaluation[16] of the therapeutic accomplishments of mental health clinics in New York State. With respect to psychotherapeutic techniques he states:

> I do not mean to deny that psychotherapy brings relief to those suffering from emotional disorders or that it may not be the treatment of choice in certain cases. What I am questioning is the preoccupation with intensive psychotherapy in clinics which are part of the community health program. After more than fifty years of its utilization we still have no certain knowledge of its effectiveness, of its superiority over other forms of

treatment, or even that a long term is better than brief psychotherapy.[17]

He goes on to point out that while in the previous year 30,000 patients were released from the state hospital, nevertheless, only 8 percent of the cases that were terminated by psychiatric clinics came from inpatient facilities. He notes also that the volume of patients being treated in the state hospitals is greater than ever before, in spite of an almost unanimous need to develop alternatives to state hospital care. His evidence supports this contention of a widening definition of mental illness, implying that the outpatient clinics are not treating cases that are likely to need hospital care but are treating numerous cases that are experiencing emotional problems. These are, for the most part, tied up with the daily round of human existence and can never be completely eliminated except in a societal utopia. One conclusion appears inescapable—the more clinics, the more patients. In addition, this widening definition of mental illness has served as a type of fuel for the development of the idea of a community psychiatry.

Historical and Cultural Influences

There is the problem as every historian recognizes of how far back one should go in enumerating those events which helped to shape a present situation, because every historical event is both a consequence of some previous happening and a cause of something that is to take place in the future. However, I begin my history of the proposal for a community psychiatry with the accumulated psychiatric experience which came out of World War II. Psychiatric experience during the war showed that a large number of inductees were afflicted with various types of neuropsychiatric disorders. This finding was reported by Dr. William Meninger, head of psychiatric services of the United States Armed Forces, in a book dealing with his war experience and anticipating the uses to which psychiatry might be put in meeting the new problems and tensions that were arising in American society and in the societies throughout the world. In this volume Meninger[18] asks if psychiatry after the war is to continue its preoccupation with the end results of mental disease or is "to discover how it can contribute to the problems of the average man and to the larger social issues in which he is involved." Thus, Meninger anticipated that the new role for psychiatry would be expanded to deal with family problems, industrial conflict, community conflict, and in fact, any situation where conflict, difficulties, and tensions arise between people. Thus, the publication of this work seemed to play a role in turning psychiatry away from its traditional concerns and in directing its attention to problems of the community.

The work of Meninger, Thompson[19] and others tended to anticipate a more positive and frontal attack upon mental health problems in American society. The writings of these men set the stage for the passage of the National Mental Health Act in 1948 which has played a significant role in stimulating professional training, research, and treatment programs in psychiatry and its allied fields. After the passage of this act which raised mental health to the status of a public health problem numerous events followed swiftly. Certainly the new monies available through the Federal Government and foundations made it possible for scholars from all over the United States and Europe to meet more often to deal with specific problems in the mental health field. This exchange of scholars acquainted psychiatric workers in the United States with the various programs and plans that were being carried on in Europe for handling mental health problems, such as Querido's program for community psychiatry in Amsterdam, the development of the open door hospital in England, auxiliary psychiatric units such as night- and day-hospitals, rehabilitation houses, and various kinds of industrial units to train the mental convalescent for jobs. All of these developments proved most exciting and interesting, stimulated thinking, broke through conventional and traditional notions of the past, and paved the way for taking many new looks as to how we could more adequately treat the mentally ill in order to more quickly return them to their families and communities.

In fact, these developments began to undercut various conceptions of chronicity and we recognized that hospitalization for mental illness need not be a lifetime affair. We should call attention also to the research on the mental hospital conducted by social scientists that provided a rationale for the hospital as a therapeutic community, a development that Maxwell Jones[20] in his work in England has already anticipated. However, these studies that came during the 1950's in the work of Stanton and Schwartz,[21] Dunham and Weinberg,[22] Belknap,[23] John and Elaine Cumming,[24] and W. Caudill[25] increasingly began to pose the issue as to whether the therapeutic community could be considered as a real factor in the treatment process. These studies further called attention to the rigid traditional structure of the state hospital and how it actually contained within itself those cultural forms that tended to discourage patients towards moving to a level of acceptable behavior. Finally, there came the report of a Joint Commission on Mental Illness and Health[26] in 1961, along with the Surgeon General's recommendation in January, 1962 that the states explore a more complete utilization of all community resources dealing with the mentally ill towards achieving a maximum in the prevention and treatment of such illnesses. And as a final stimulus came the speech of the late President Kennedy[27] to Congress in October of 1963 in which he outlined a broad program with respect to community centered hospitals, research and training, covering both mental illness and mental retardation.

In the above account I have attempted a cursory examination of the central historical events that have led to the development of community psychiatry. However, in a broader perspective these events can be regarded as the consequences of the cultural forces embodied in certain beliefs and traditions that are deeply embedded in the texture of American society. In a sense the emergence of community psychiatry as a subspecialty of psychiatry is a reflection of the cherished American belief that all problems are capable of solution if we can just discover the key by means of the scientific methodology at our disposal. The ever-multiplying programs of health insurance during the past 20 years have also laid an economic foundation making it possible to bring mental patients out in the open instead of hiding them away as we have done in the past. Under these conditions the essential qualities of American culture, individualism, optimism, humanism, and equalitarianism have merely provided the additional push for the emergence of community psychiatry.

Some Hidden Aspects for the Future Role of Psychiatry

In this account I have pointed to the several conceptions that seem to be implied in the development of a community psychiatry. I have emphasized that the tying of community psychiatry with the several evolving plans throughout the country to reorganize the mental health facilities toward the end of maximizing treatment potential is a significant move. While there is the question as to whether community psychiatry extends beyond current psychiatric practices there may be a gain in identifying the psychiatrist more closely with the different community services and breaking down the isolation in which both the psychoanalytic practitioner and the hospital practicing psychiatrist have been enmeshed. This would move the psychiatrist not only closer to the patient but what is more important, closer to the entire network of interpersonal relationships of the family and the community in which the patient is involved.

However, it is in the other visions that have been held up for community psychiatry wherein I think, as I have indicated, great difficulties are in the offing. Here I am most skeptical concerning the adequacy of our knowledge to develop significant techniques for treating social collectivities or for developing techniques on the community level that will really result in a reduction of mental disturbances in the community. It seems that such expectations are likely to remove the psychiatrist still further from the more bona fide cases of mental illnesses that develop within the community context. Much of his effort will be spent on dealing with the noncritical cases. This trend has already been going on for some time as I have indicated in discussing the widening definition of mental illness. Until we have a more sound knowledge which will indicate that the minor emotional disturbances are likely to develop into the more serious types of mental disturbances we will be dissipating much of our collective psychiatric efforts.

Then, too, there is another hidden aspect of these projected conceptions of community psychiatry which deserves careful exploration. I refer to the implication that the psychiatrist will be able to move into the ongoing power structure of a community. The profession must confront the issue as to whether its effectiveness will be less or greater if some of its members should succeed in obtaining roles within the power structure of any community. Here, I would suggest that such a psychiatrist would find himself in a system where his professional effectiveness would be considerably reduced because he would be involved in a series of mutual obligations and expectations in relation to the other persons composing the power structure. He would thus lose the role that in general characterizes the professional in other areas, that of being an adviser and a consultant with respect to any psychiatric problems or issues that the groups, institutions, and associations of the community confront. What I am trying to indicate is that in becoming a part of the power structure he is likely to lose more than he gains. That is, his gains would be in respect to power, personal prestige, and recognition but his losses would be in the growing rustiness of his diagnostic and therapeutic skills with patients.

Another implication of these aspects of community psychiatry is the fact that psychiatrists are being pushed in a direction not entirely of their own making. The national efforts and monies that are being directed to the states and communities for the reorganization of the mental health facilities have engendered a high degree of excitement among professional social workers, mental health educators, psychiatric nurses, and numerous well-intentioned persons who see new professional opportunities for service and careers. Thus, the psychiatrist is led to think, because of these pressures, that he should prepare himself with new skills in order to provide the required leadership to these various professionals who are planning to work towards this new vision to maximize the treatment potential in the community for the mentally ill.

Finally, there is the implication that psychiatry is being utilized to move us closer in the direction of the welfare state. This may not be undesirable in itself but it seems most essential that psychiatrists should be aware of the role that they are asked to play. We can anticipate that while the doctor-patient relationship will still be paramount in most medical practice the psychiatrist is likely to move into roles unforeseen but which will be required by the new structural organization of psychiatric facilities with the proposal for a community psychiatry. In such new roles the psychiatrists may become agents for social control, thus sacrificing the main task for which their education has fitted them.

In this paper I have attempted to show the link between community psychiatry and the new evolving community mental health programs. While one can see in this linkage a most significant development I am somewhat skeptical toward those emphases in community psychiatry that aim at the development of treatment techniques on the community level. In discussing the widening definition of mental illness I have tried to show that this is one of the crucial factors that has accounted for this movement towards a new type of psychiatric specialty. I have seen, in this widening definition, an opportunity to overcome a frustration that engulfs psychiatrists with respect to their inability to make much therapeutic headway with the traditional mental cases. Finally, I have attempted to consider some of the hidden implications for psychiatry in the proposal for this new psychiatric specialty.*

* Thanks for critical comments on the manuscript are extended to the following colleagues at Lafayette Clinic; Jacques Gottlieb, MD, Director of Lafayette Clinic; Elliott Luby, MD, Assistant Director in Charge of Clinical Services; Paul Lowinger, MD, Chief, Adult Out-Patient Services; Garfield Tourney, MD, Assistant Director in Charge of Education.

Chapter 10

Psychosocial Forces and Public Health Problems

THOMAS F. A. PLAUT

THIS PAPER IS DIVIDED INTO FOUR MAJOR PARTS. THE FIRST presents findings on the relation of social and psychological forces to the aetiology and development of health problems. Second comes a discussion of certain determinants of persons' attitudes and behaviour in relation to their health. Next, two major types of public health activity—directed at bringing about individual and community action—are examined within a social science framework. Finally, I look at public health agencies operating in the community.

Role of Social and Psychological Factors in the Aetiology of Illness

Few illnesses are randomly distributed throughout the population. Plotting of cases on a map almost always shows clusters in certain areas. Such clusterings may be related to a variety of factors—the physical environment, genetic tendencies or characteristics of the "agent." Knowledge of the role of these factors has often led to programs of control and prevention. To deal with contemporary health problems—particularly chronic disease and the "behavioural disorders"—the impact of social and psychological forces on the development and course of these conditions must be understood.

I shall give several examples to show the extent of the relationship between social factors and illness. Infant mortality rates, as is well known, are highly correlated with social class. That is, deaths in early infancy occur at a higher rate among the poor than among the well-to-do. However, the effect of social factors is not restricted to conditions where personal health care is obviously a major factor. A recent (1949–51) analysis of mortality data in Houston, Texas, indicates that socioeconomic status is associated with mortality for the seven leading causes of death.[1] This applies to chronic conditions such as cancer and heart disease as well as to tuberculosis and pneumonia although the association with socioeconomic status is greater among the infectious diseases. Motor vehicle accidents—now a major cause of death among males in the age group 20 to 45—also occur at a higher rate among the poor than among any other income groups.[2]

It is not enough to demonstrate that there is an association between socioeconomic class and illness. What is it about poverty, for example, that leads to higher rates of most diseases? Many factors need to be considered. Among those suggested in the past are the following: nutrition, characteristics of the physical environment, working conditions, low intelligence, and genetic constitution. Recently, emphasis has been placed on "life style" or general behaviour patterns as crucial factors mediating between the socioeconomic conditions and the high rate of illness. Hours of sleep, level and nature of psychological tension may well be related to greater risk of certain conditions. Patterns of interpersonal relationships (psychological closeness or distance, mode of expressing hostility and responding to it, etc.) probably are closely linked to many elements of personal health. The nature of the "value" or "belief system" in any group often is highly correlated with many aspects of behaviour. It defines what is right and wrong, it sets expectations, and it assists individuals in making the myriad of decisions with which each of us is daily confronted.

The characteristics of life rather than the poverty itself may be the crucial factor. For example, in the early years of this century, infant mortality rates were far lower in Jewish groups than in other groups that had the same income levels, lived under equally crowded conditions and had comparable family size.[3] There was probably, then, something about the patterns of infant and maternal care that strikingly distinguished this cultural group from others.

There are marked differences in rates of various types of cancer among ethnic groups. For example, cancer of the lung occurs three times more often among Polish-born American males than among Italian-born ones.[4] On the other hand, cancer of the bladder and colon occurs more often in the Italian population. Again, while it is possible that ethnic constitutional factors may account for these differences, this does not seem likely. There are variations in customs—for example, in relation to diet, hygiene religion, family relationships—between ethnic groups. Such cultural practices may predispose the individual to or protect him from a given disease.

A factor not necessarily associated with social class is "stress." This term, as generally used, refers to unusual pressures on the individual or group. It has been found to be associated with both the appearance and the disappearance of certain conditions. A Dutch physician reported on the experiences of some of his Jewish patients during the days of the German occupation in World War II. These men, mainly wealthy merchants, had serious stomach ulcers before the war. During the early part of the occupation, they continued to live in the community. Their diets were very meagre—often they were on the verge of starvation. The physician maintained contact with many of these men and found no appreciable change in their ulcerative condition. Subsequently, most of the men were sent to concentration camps. While in these inhuman settings, the men totally lost all symptoms of the ulcer of their stomachs. When the war ended, they returned to more or less normal lives in their home communities and the ulcers returned![5] Several American missionaries who were working in Korea when captured by the Japanese stated that their severe headaches disappeared completely while they were in the prison camps. These headaches, which they had had for years prior to the war, returned once the men were released and again resumed their regular duties in the U.S.[6] An epidemiological study of the relation between stress and mental illness was undertaken in Stirling County of Nova Scotia. The major finding of this investigation was the existence of a substantial association between "social disintegration" and the prevalence of psychiatric disorders. The authors conclude that "disintegrated social systems produce disintegrated personalities."[7]

Role of Social and Psychological Factors in Persons' Health-Related Behaviour

There is much emphasis in public health on influencing individuals' behaviour regarding their own health. This is central to the work of public health nurses and of health educators. Before such efforts can be successful there must be an understanding of the meaning of health and illnesses to different groups of persons. A principal factor related to persons' views of themselves—including their reactions to symptoms in themselves and others—is social class.

While economic indices are often used to determine social class, the essential differences between class groups may relate not to material wealth, nor to education or employment, but to general styles of life, to values, to ways of viewing oneself and the world. To highlight the differences between some aspects of middle class and lower class culture, I shall summarize the observations of two social scientists[8] who contrast between the principal "focal concerns" of youth in these two cultural groups. In the middle class the emphasis is on: (1)

the deferment of immediate pleasure and gain for the attainment of future goals, (2) the accumulation of material goods and the maintenance of property, (3) achievement through directed work effort, (4) education and intellectual improvement, (5) ambition to "get ahead," and (6) heavy stress on child-rearing and the maintenance of the stable two-parent household. In the lower class, the "focal concerns" of youth are as follows: (1) "getting into" and "staying out of" trouble, (2) being tough, (3) being "smart" i.e., possessing the ability to dupe and outsmart others, (4) excitement—the search for thrill and stimulation, (5) fate—belief in luck, (6) autonomy —both the explicit assertion of a desire not to be "bossed" and the implicit wish to seek stable sources of dependency. Much of the behaviour of lower class individuals, adults as well as youngsters, can be understood in the context of this type of picture of the total cultural pattern. Lower class behaviour has long seemed quite unintelligible and "irrational" to professional workers who evaluate it in terms of the middle class norms most familiar to them.

Many different approaches have been used to describe dimensions along which class groups differ. For example, some have stressed differences in "time-orientation."[9] Most lower class persons are more oriented to the immediate present than is true for middle class individuals. Planning for the future, postponing present gains for the sake of future ones is a strongly middle class characteristic.

Certain of the characteristics of the lower class culture have great bearing on persons' responses to signs of ill-health and on their relationship with health workers and health services. Physical symptoms that would lead most middle class persons to define themselves as "sick" and immediately call a doctor are not so viewed by many lower class individuals.[10] In many instances the symptoms are noticed, but lower class persons find it far more difficult to assume the role of a patient. Often this may be because taking on the "sickrole" involves giving up a much needed self-image or because the reality situation is such that the person cannot drop his responsibility as a contributing member of his family. Further, if there has been little prior experience with the sick role and with obtaining medical help there is still greater likelihood that the definition of oneself as sick will be postponed as long as possible. Of course, if medical care is not available, for financial or other reasons, this only increases the difficulty in labelling oneself as ill.

The sick person, by virtue of his illness, is exempted in varying degrees and for varying periods of time, from his normal role and task obligations. He is not expected to be as autonomous or as contributory to family and community welfare as when he is well. Generally the sick person is not held "personally responsible" for his illness—he cannot be expected to overcome his incapacity on his own. We expect the sick individual to realize that it is inherently undesirable to be ill, that he has an obligation to get well and to cooperate with others in achieving this.[11]

The way in which a particular illness is viewed will have a considerable impact on the reactions of persons to having this illness. The ostracism and stigma attached to psychiatric disorders in our society make it more difficult for patients to accept the "sick-role" in relation to this illness and this often complicates the recovery of the patient. Among the Hutterites of Western Canada and U.S.[12] a type of serious emotional depression frequently found is labelled as "Anfechtung" (literally, "attack" or possession by the devil). Because all Hutterites view themselves as having to contend with bad impulses (the devil) within themselves there is great sympathy for the person going through this type of depression. Individuals recovering from the illness may have a higher status because of their having successfully coped with this challenge.

Persons in different cultural groups may respond quite differently to pain.[13] For example, the reactions to pain among Jews and Italians were compared. These two groups are generally described as being emotional in their responses. Physicians often say that both Jews and Italians have low pain thresholds or that they exaggerate their pain experiences. However, on closer examination some major differences emerge. For the Italian, it is the pain as such that bothers him. The Jewish patient, on the other hand, is concerned far more about the symptomatic meaning of the pain—to him it is an indicator that his health is threatened. This concerns him because of the possible impact on his own—and his family's—health and welfare. Medication will often completely relieve the Italian patient, but it does not reassure the Jew since he is still concerned about the possible longer-range consequences of his illness. In relation to something as specific as pain, it is relatively easy to be aware of cultural differences. In other areas of health, the impact of differences in values and norms may be less evident, but they nevertheless have their effect.

Socio-Psychological Factors and Public Health Programmes and Activities

Influencing Individual Action

Health education is often directed at getting persons to take action in relation to their own health. In recent years, social scientists have sought to determine why health education campaigns often are not successful. Hochbaum has studied reasons for participation and nonparticipation in chest X-ray programmes. He found that persons were most likely to have voluntary X-rays when the following three sets of beliefs were present: (1) that one could contract tuberculosis, (2) that one cannot rely on the absence of symptoms as an index of health and (3) that early detection will be helpful. The most crucial factor appeared to be the second one. An implication of this is that educational campaigns must stress that asymptomatic individuals may actually have tuberculosis. Hochbaum also sought to determine why some persons who accepted all three of the propositions nevertheless did not have the X-rays. He found that many of these individuals failed to take action because they did not relate the information to themselves. They felt that having tuberculosis would lead to serious consequences for their role as a husband, a father, a jobholder and as a person with social prestige and position in the community. Thus the possibility of discovering that they had the disease seemed so overwhelming, so catastrophic that they preferred to reject this possibility and, therefore, they were unwilling to undergo the diagnostic procedure.

The tasks that the health educator asks of his audience usually are much more complex—and sometimes they also are inconvenient, painful, time-consuming and difficult to perform.[14] Often in education approaches we have expected too much, that is, we have not realized that the mass media are only one of many influences that are acting upon the individual or group. Usually mass media will have an effect only if other circumstances are unusually favourable.

Perhaps we have placed too much reliance on education as a means of bringing about changes in the field of health. The behaviour of persons can often be radically influenced by the way in which certain institutions and structures are organized. For example, it was long felt that the type of alcoholics who appear in the emergency wards of general hospitals are simply "not sufficiently motivated" to utilize the services of outpatient alcoholism clinics. In one study[15] it was found that usually less than 5 percent of the patients initially seen in the emergency unit ever made their way to the alcoholism clinic and practically no patients ever returned to the alcoholism clinic for as many as five visits. When the reasons for this poor record were examined, it was discovered that alcoholics had to "get by" many different professional and clerical personnel in moving from the initial entrance into the emergency area to a treatment relationship in the alcoholism clinic. After personnel of the alcoholism clinic were assigned to the emergency ward so that they could see the alcoholics at the time of initial contact with the hospital, the proportion of patients who visited the clinic increased from 5 percent to 65 percent and the proportion who stayed for at least five visits increased from 1 percent to 42 percent. When patients do not respond the way we expect them to, or wish them to, it is very easy to place the blame on them, to define them as nonresponsive or "beyond reach." In at least some instances this is an abdication of responsibility, since the professional workers have not been sufficiently imaginative to experiment with other approaches.

While there has been increasing interest in applying public health concepts to the field of mental health, the possibilities of reducing rates of psychiatric disorders by "administrative actions" has not been sufficiently explored.[16] The purpose of such actions is to improve the psychological experiences of many persons in the population. It is hoped that this will have a positive impact on mental health functioning. For example, the British Ministry of Health decided that hospitals should greatly extend the visiting hours for patients in the pediatric wards. This was based on the belief that mother-child separation at the time of this crisis can be particularly damaging to the psychological well-being of the child. Since a sizeable proportion of all youngsters are hospitalized at some time in their youth, the potential long range impact of such a policy change might be quite great.

Another suggestion for health-related "administrative action" has been made in relation to public housing. Most public housing projects have strict eligibility requirements and families are required to move out when their income reaches a certain level. Since financial need often is associated with other social problems, one result of this policy is that families with the greatest problems are constantly moving into these projects and those who are just beginning to manage better are required to move out. Thus there is little opportunity for the development of a stable core group of reasonably well-functioning families in most projects. This may well be one reason that many public housing units present such problems for welfare, school, and police department. Perhaps consideration should be given to permitting a certain proportion of the families in each unit to remain in the project even when their income exceeds the allowable maximum. Such a policy could have a major impact on the total social and psychological climate within the housing project and thus contribute to the present and future mental health of its occupants.

Influencing Community Action

An important activity of many health workers is that of securing community actions on matters related to public health. This may consist of community organization efforts by health educators or activities by health officers to secure a coordinated attack on a major health problem or it may take the form of trying to obtain approval for the support of a new programme. Such activities require an understanding of basic social and psychological forces operating in communities.

Public health leaders often wish to develop citizens' organizations as part of educational campaigns to bring about the improvement of local conditions or to create public support for a health programme or activity. In some instances such efforts fail because the potential "recruits" to the association or group lack familiarity with the procedures and organizational structures involved. While health workers and other middle class persons are accustomed to activities such as attending meetings, discussing policy, electing officers, and formulating bylaws, these may seem very strange and irrelevant to individuals in other cultural and social groups. For example, an effort to set up a prepaid medical care cooperative in

Colorado failed, in part at least, because the Spanish-American population of that area was accustomed to different modes of solving community problems.[17] They were accustomed to authoritarian rather than democratic approaches to problems; they relied on traditional rather than elected leaders. Also important is the fact that the health association was based on the principle of prepayment and this required a "future-time" orientation, which was alien to the Spanish-Americans who were far more "present-time" oriented.[18]

In the U.S. and Canada the term "community power structure" has become part of the vocabulary of both professional workers and lay persons. Recently a San Francisco newspaper had a front-page story with a headline saying that the civil rights groups were demanding meetings with the city's power structure! While it is obviously true that "power" is not equally distributed among all persons in the community it is erroneous to believe that there is any individual or even any group of individuals who have unlimited power. Persons who can influence action in one area of community activity may be very different from those who have "power" in another. Action on specific issues is frequently accomplished by an amorphous fleeting coalition of certain individuals.

> It is necessary to distinguish between economic, political and social power and to decide which combination of these is most important for the promotion of the health sub-system in which one is interested. When the major concern is political, there is little point in enlisting the support of businessmen who may have no standing with those making political decisions; when the major concern is fund-raising, the help of political leaders—who may be prevented by law from using public funds for the cause—may be less important than one might at first imagine.[19]

What actually is meant by "leadership"? Are leaders those who participate in making decisions? Participants in a decision may not necessarily be those who most influenced the outcome.

It has also been suggested that persons with formal authority are the leaders. However, individuals outside such institutions often have a major impact on decision-making. One group of American sociologists[20] describes three basic types of community leaders: (1) The *institutional leaders*—these are the persons who are the heads of the largest business, industrial, governmental, political and other organizations. Usually these leaders are not active participants in community affairs. Often there is no evidence that they have had any direct impact on the decisions made. Perhaps their main function is to make it possible for their underlings to have access to the decision-making structure. (2) The *effectors*—these are the employees or subordinates of the institutional leaders just referred to. The effectors appear to be active workers in the actual process of community decision-making. While they sometimes are guided by the specific instructions of their employers often they seem to be pretty much on their own. (3) The *activists*—these persons, usually members of voluntary organizations, are frequently very involved in the making of decisions. They have neither the positional stature in organizations nor the power base of the effectors, but at the same time just by their sheer level of activity they do help to shape the decisions made by the community.

Studies of the decision-making process in Chicago[21] graphically demonstrates that no single person or even group of persons has the ability to force their decisions on others. The outcome of community controversy is often either no action on the proposed change or a compromise solution. Both of these outcomes suggest that many constraints operate in large communities to greatly reduce the freedom of any group or organization. Banfield stresses that the major "actors" in the community decision-making process are not individuals but large formal organizations—governmental as well as private. The leaders of each of these structures generally are more concerned about the position and the future viability of their organizations than about the issue at hand.

> Civic controversies in Chicago are not generated by the efforts of politicians to win votes, by differences of ideology or group interest, or by the behind-the-scenes efforts of a power elite. They arise, instead, out of the maintenance and enhancement needs of large formal organizations. The heads of an organization see some advantage to be gained by changing the situation. They propose changes. Other large organizations are threatened. They oppose, and a civic controversy takes place.[22]

While any given leader (political or otherwise) may have a great deal of influence or power he is not likely to exercise a substantial amount of it on any one occasion. Persons in such positions tend to marshal, to conserve their power. It is like capital that is better to "invest" than to "spend." If a leader uses his influence to obtain certain ends he will be making demands on other powerful individuals and as a result will be more beholden to them. For this reason, any leader, political or other, is likely to be very cautious about his exertion of power. What emerges then is a picture of power vested in the leaders of major organizations and institutions who place high priority on the maintenance and survival of these institutions. Certainly in larger communities it is a mistake to imagine that there is a single power elite that generally controls the decision-making process.

Often it is not realized that groups and communities have self-protective techniques which are roughly analogous to the personal defence mechanisms. An intensive mental health education campaign was conducted in a western Canadian community to convince people that there is a continuum from normal psychological functioning to severe psychiatric disorders and to make people aware of the fact that the nearby mental hospital badly needed improvement. Much to the surprise of the workers this campaign aroused great resentment in the community.[23] How can this reaction be understood? In this community, and probably in many others also, the people classed a broad range of behaviour as "normal"; that is, there was little tendency to label strange behaviour as deviant. However, when the behaviour became too bizarre, the individual was defined as "outside the fold." If this occurred a pattern of "denial and isolation" came into play which required the physical and psychological removal of the person from the community. "The community, in order to maintain the sanity and balance of its members, must dissociate itself from the now dangerous deviant."[24] The mental health workers' view that all psychological behaviour is on a continuum thus ran counter to the community's traditional way of handling this situation. Further, the suggestion that the mental hospital did not offer adequate care was very threatening to the townsfolk because it destroyed ". . . the device people used to assuage their guilt over having exiled their relatives."[25] Undoubtedly there are other situations in which health educational campaigns may be threatening the protective beliefs of a community.

Public Health as a Major Community System

A "community system" is a set of agencies and institutions that relate to a particular area, i.e., health, the economy, religion or education. Each such system can be described in terms of its structure (i.e., the organizations that make it up), its manifest and latent functions, its functionaries (i.e., the equipment and material resources) and its linkages with other systems in the community.[26] It may be useful for persons to analyze both their own agency and others in terms of such characteristics. For example, in the larger health system there are at least five separate (although often related) parts. There are: (1) the private office practice of professional health persons—particularly physicians, (2) group health care—medical and health services set up in factories, business or governmental agencies, schools, labour unions, etc., (3) hospitals, clinics and health agencies, (4) public health, and (5) pharmacists and others who sell materials and supplies to patients. There is not always agreement between these subsystems regarding the responsibilities of each. The physician and the medical society will usually see the doctor as the natural leader in the field of health. The health officer may feel that the health department should have this responsibility. And hospital leaders see their facility as the logical place for the coordination of all health services in the community.[27] Persons working in the field of public health need to understand the structures, functions, and linkages of each of these subsystems.

It is generally agreed that better coordination of health and medical services is urgently needed. Usually, however, such coordination is extremely difficult to achieve. Factors often listed as barriers include the following: lack of knowledge about the work and objectives of other agencies, personality conflicts, differences in professional philosophy, and "vested interests."[28] In the area of delinquency control and prevention, there has been a very cogent analysis of the impediments to interagency cooperation.[29] Courts, police, correctional institutions, social and psychiatric agencies find it difficult to work together on delinquency because of differences regarding: (1) the aetiology of crime (morality versus pathology and individual versus social locus); (2) methods of dealing with offenders (restriction versus rehabilitation); (3) priorities of approach (action versus research); (4) methods of organizing programmes of control (localization versus centralization), and (5) appropriate types of personnel (lay versus professional). Similar disagreements exist in other areas.

Contemporary health problems are deeply embedded in many aspects of community life. Often it is difficult if not impossible to disentangle a problem in physical health from one in mental health. Economic insecurity and poverty cannot be separated from health problems. As public welfare moves from a primary concern with financial maintenance to focus on remedial action and on the ultimate prevention of the conditions that produce indigency, the interdependence of public health and welfare activities becomes clearer. Many nongovernmental agencies are deeply involved in the field of health.[30] Public health workers in the future will need to work more with other types of community agencies and institutions than has been true in the past. This may well bring the differing ideologies and value systems into the open. For example, maximization of pleasure is often not consistent with the promotion of health. Persons or institutions principally concerned with the former may find themselves in conflict with health workers. Health as a goal may be in conflict with the goal of financial profit. This latter can perhaps already be observed in relation to alcohol, tobacco and motor vehicles. Choices among these goals cannot be made on a scientific basis—they represent disagreements about values, about what is right and wrong, about how man should live or about how society should be organized.

Alfred North Whitehead has said, "Knowledge unapplied is knowledge shorn of its meaning." In the fields of public health and medical care there is much scientific and technical knowledge. It is our skills in application of this knowledge that have lagged behind. Further understanding of social and psychological factors should speed up the closing of this gap.

Chapter 11

*Maintenance Drug Therapy: The Schizophrenic Patient in the Community**

DAVID M. ENGELHARDT AND NORBERT FREEDMAN

IN 1957 THE PSYCHOPHARMACOLOGY TREATMENT AND RE-search Unit of the Department of Psychiatry at the State University of New York Downstate Medical Center undertook a study of the feasibility of maintaining chronic schizophrenic patients in the community on a program of drug treatment and minimal supportive psychotherapy. Intimately related to this pilot clinical project was a broad-based research effort aimed at a systematic study of the changes under long-term treatment and of the factors influencing these changes. The clinical goal of this long-term maintenance program was three-fold: first, prevention of hospitalization; second, sustained and stable symptom modification; and third, reduction in social dysfunctioning. A body of literature reporting on the effects of ataractic therapy on inpatient schizophrenics suggested that the goals we set for outpatient schizophrenics were potentially realizable. Because the focus of our treatment program was on community

* The research reported in this paper was supported in part by a grant (MY-1983) from the National Institute of Mental Health, U.S. Public Health Service. The authors would like to express their appreciation to Dr. Reuben Margolis, Assistant Director of the Research Unit, and to Dr. David Mann, whose work has been basic to some of the findings reported here.

adaptation, we included in our levels of observation not only the patient's psychological status but also his performance at home and in the community.

At the time we admitted our first patient, there was mounting evidence that the use of tranquilizers such as chlorpromazine with hospitalized schizophrenic patients resulted in reduction in psychotic symptomatology and improved social behavior. The reports in the literature dealt almost exclusively with acute hospitalized patients and short-term clinical effects. In time, interest in the tranquilizers spread to their effect on hospitalized chronic schizophrenic patients. More recently, the increasing number of patients discharged from state hospitals "on drugs" led to inquiries into the effects of drug treatment on the post-hospitalized schizophrenic patient. The number and quality of studies reporting on the effect of drugs on hospitalized and post-hospitalized schizophrenic patients have grown steadily. However, despite the ever-widening use of psychopharmacological agents at the outpatient level, there have been few attempts to validate this treatment procedure, especially in its long-term application.

This chapter is a report on our observations and findings over the past seven years on the long-term maintenance drug treatment of schizophrenic outpatients. Involved are 500 patients admitted to the research clinic between 1957 and 1963. We are concerned not only with identifying the effect of drugs on the schizophrenic patient in terms of the clinical areas already outlined, but also to trace these effects over a significant period of time. Observations on the patient's psychopathology and his community adjustment have been made over periods in excess of three years.

It is our ultimate hope that we will be able to describe a significant sample of the life spans of particular schizophrenic patients in the community as they may be affected or modified by drug treatment. Some of our more recent findings have suggested the presence of a variety of specific adaptive mechanisms among schizophrenic outpatients. These will be sketched briefly toward the end of the discussion.

To place our observations in their proper perspective, it is necessary to indicate our particular philosophy of maintenance treatment. The organization of our treatment program reflects not only our particular research interests in long-term effects, but also specific theoretical and clinical biases relative to the response potential and treatment needs of the schizophrenic patient in the community. We consider the chronic schizophrenic patient as in need of *continuous treatment* in a *stable treatment setting*. Emphasis is placed on the supportive role of the doctor-patient relationship and on the clinic milieu. (The psychiatrist's role here is perhaps more that of the family physician than that of the psychodynamically oriented psychotherapist.) The treatment objective sought is the attainment of "maximum clinic benefit" with emphasis thereafter on maintenance of the improvement attained. Maintenance treatment thus aims at both maintenance of community status and maintenance of an improved clinical condition. Drug treatment is perceived as functioning in a dual role. In addition to the chemotherapeutic effect, the administration of a "pill" has a symbolic effect which reinforces the doctor-patient relationship and defines the supporting role of the doctor. In this respect, the administration by the doctor of a "placebo" in a double-blind design, as if it were active medication, within the context of a supportive clinical program, cannot be designated as "no treatment."

The majority of our patients were drawn from the intake of the Mental Health Clinic of the Kings County Hospital Center in Brooklyn, New York. The population includes both males and females, whites and Negroes, between the ages of 18 and 44. All patients had to have a primary diagnosis of schizophrenia and there had to be evidence that the patient had been ill for at least one year. The patients were chronically ill with more than half having been ill 10 years or more. While our population was clearly schizophrenic and clearly chronic, they varied considerably in the amount of previous treatment received. Ten percent of the patients had never received any psychiatric treatment prior to admission to the clinic, 8½ percent had received only outpatient treatment; 31 percent had been in the hospital only briefly for observation purposes and their aggregate hospitalization prior to admission to the clinic did not exceed three months. Thus, one half of our patients had essentially maintained an ambulatory mode of adjustment throughout their life. Only one quarter of our patients had an aggregate history of hospitalization exceeding one year. The basic diagnostic categories represented were Chronic Undifferentiated Schizophrenia and Paranoid Type of Schizophrenia, with the ratio being four to one in favor of the Chronic Undifferentiated patients. The mean age of our population was 30. More than half had never completed high school and the vast majority fell into Hollinghead's Social Classes 4 and 5, that is, they tended to represent the lower socioeconomic groups.

On admission to the research clinic, patients were randomly assigned to chlorpromazine, promazine, or placebo treatment, administered under double-blind conditions. Medication was in the form of pink #2 capsules available in 50 mg. and 100 mg. strengths and dosage schedules were flexible. The mean dosage for drugs was approximately 200 mg. daily, and for placebo the mean dosage was consistently higher, being the equivalent of 350 mg. a day. Chlorpromazine, promazine, and placebo were chosen because clinically they represented an ordinal scale of drug effectiveness. Promazine did, in fact, maintain an "intermediate" position on a large variety of outcome measures. The intensity of the clinical effect of promazine, however, was highly variable, at times resembling that of placebo, at times approaching that of chlorpromazine.*

* The inclusion of promazine in the treatment design proved fortuitous in a number of ways. The consistent ordinal scale of drug responses served as an independent validation of the fact that our patients were, indeed, taking their prescribed medication, an important consideration in outpatient chemotherapy. In addition, the variable clinical effect of promazine, alluded to

Once the patient enters treatment he remains on the same drug for the duration of his clinic attendance; thus treatment continues indefinitely. Patients are retained in the clinic regardless of degree of improvement attained so that at present some patients have been in treatment in excess of five years. However, when patients drop out of treatment spontaneously, no pressure is exerted to have them return to the clinic.

The treatment program was organized to maximize the doctor-patient relationship through regularly scheduled monthly visits. Thus, the patients were seen once a week for the first four weeks, biweekly for the next two months, and once a month thereafter. Visits usually lasted no more than 20 minutes except for the initial and quarterly major evaluations. No attempt was made to offer the patient or family any other support such as might be rendered by a social worker working with the family of the patient.* Contacts with a key family member were maintained on a monthly basis but only for the purpose of assessing change in the patient's behavior in the community. (A condition for acceptance in the clinic was the availability of a cooperative relative willing to participate in the project.)

Between 1957 and 1963 over 750 patients were admitted to the clinic. The sample of 750 patients was divided into two parts for research purposes. The first 500 patients admitted represent the basic treatment and research population. The remaining 250 patients, who were admitted under identical intake criteria and exposed to identical treatment conditions, serve as a population on whom findings obtained on the first 500 patients will be replicated.

Because the patients were free to leave the clinic program at

---

previously, tended to confuse our doctors as to which drug the patient was receiving. Thus the inclusion of promazine as a third and "intermediate" agent had the additional merit of protecting the double-blind nature of the research design.

* From a public health point of view we were interested in ascertaining whether a treatment program such as ours, with its economy in dollars and professional manpower, could effectively serve the needs of the larger number of schizophrenic patients in the community.

will, we were in a position to obtain information on dropouts from treatment. In our group of schizophrenic outpatients the dropout rates from treatment proved to be high. (To be considered as having entered the project, the patient was required to have had at least two weeks of drug treatment prior to dropout.) By the end of three months, 77 percent of the patients were still in treatment. At six months, the percentage remaining was 60 percent; at nine months the percentage remaining had dropped to 46 percent; and by the end of one year, only 39 percent of the original cohort were still in treatment. In considering these attrition rates, it should be recognized that they stem from three sources: the first is "spontaneous dropouts," that is, the patient's failure to return to treatment; the second refers to "protocol dropouts," that is, the patient is dropped from the project for failure to abide by the requirements of the research protocol; the third refers to "hospitalization." These sources of dropout are not just research artifacts. They represent important types of treatment effects, each deserving separate study. Only the third type of dropout, that due to hospitalization, is described in this chapter in detail.

From the description given of our population, treatment regimen, and research design, it is now possible to present our long-term outpatient studies in the proper perspective, especially in relation to a number of other systematic investigations into the effects of pharmacologic therapy on schizophrenic outpatients. Another group of investigations has focused on the treatment of the post-hospitalized patient. In addition to the differences in setting, treatment program, and research design, the investigations into the effect of drugs in the after-care population differ from ours in one radical respect. Our patients are characterized by a basically ambulatory mode of adjustment to their illness while the after-care populations are generally characterized by frequent and often prolonged hospitalizations. While our patients seek treatment voluntarily and are free to leave at will, the after-care patients' attendance is compulsory and failure to attend may result in rehospitalization. Since hospitalization often reflects a decision on the part of the patient's family, it is likely that the home environment as well of our patients is different from that of the after-care patient. Our findings on outpatient maintenance therapy, therefore, cannot be readily equated with the findings reported by such investigators as Gross, Kris, Pasamanick, and Tuteur.

A variant of the after-care investigation is represented by the study of Wold. More appropriately it may be termed a "crisis avoidance" regimen. The patient is seen over sustained periods of time with active drug given and withdrawn. Active drug is reinstituted at the point of crisis. This type of investigation has the specific advantage of showing the efficacy of drug in a crisis situation, but if the interest is the observation of drugs on continuance maintenance therapy, this research design would not be appropriate. A third type of outpatient investigation is represented by the V.A. Cooperative Outpatient Study. This investigation was carried on in V.A. mental hygiene clinics all over the country and usually included patients also in psychotherapy. The population differed from the after-care population in that the patients exhibited a more ambulatory mode of adjustment. The V.A. study represents another variant of outpatient treatment investigation.

We believe that the observations we are about to report reflect more closely the responses to long-term drug treatment of a cross-section of schizophrenic patients present in the community. By working in a free community clinic, and with large numbers of patients, it was possible to collect observations on schizophrenic patients representing varying modes of adjustment: patients whose typical adjustment has been hospitalization and patients for whom the decision of hospitalization was never a critical one. Using such a community panel, it is now possible to subdivide one's observations into various relevant criterion groups.

Despite these apparent differences in population, it is important to note that there is a considerable body of agreement between our findings and the findings of other investigators, particularly with reference to early treatment effects. As regards the short-term treatment effects (within three months or less) there is a consensus of findings both as to quality and intensity of response to psychotropic agents in schizophrenic patients. The issues of treatment regimen and type of population become important only when one starts examining individual aspects of treatment outcome and in particular the effects of treatment over prolonged periods of time.

Prevention of Hospitalization

In May 1960 we published our first findings on the role of phenothiazines in the prevention of hospitalization among schizophrenic outpatients. These findings applied to the first 18 months of operation of the special clinic, during which time 173 patients had been treated and studied for variable periods of time ranging from 2 weeks to 18 months. The findings of the report were striking. Of the 56 patients treated with placebo, 28.6 percent had been hospitalized, while only 4.8 percent of the 62 patients treated with chlorpromazine had been hospitalized. The effectiveness of chlorpromazine in preventing hospitalization among outpatient schizophrenics was impressive.

When we reexamined the data in 1963 on a larger sample of 445 consecutive admissions, important qualifications appeared to be necessary. The prevalence of hospitalization for the placebo group was 29.6 percent and 19.0 percent for patients on chlorpromazine. While the difference between the two extremes (chlorpromazine and placebo) still attained statistical significance ($P < .05$), this finding is in marked contrast to the difference obtained in the earlier sample ($P < .001$). While placebo hospitalization rates remained relatively constant, the rate of hospitalization on chlorpromazine had increased considerably. As we looked at these data, it became evident that an important parameter had been introduced. Not only were we studying a larger sample, but the patients studied had had a greater opportunity to become hospitalized. While the patients in the 1960 sample had a maximum of 18 months and a minimum of 2 weeks of possible treatment exposure, the patients in the 1963 sample had a maximum of 61 months and a minimum of 15 months of possible treatment exposure. Length of treatment was clearly a significant parameter affecting outcome.

To test the time factor more directly, we examined our data with the time dimension clearly controlled. (We were now in a position to observe a substantial panel of patients under continuous treatment for 12 months and beyond.) When patients with treatment exposure of 6 months or less were studied the differential rates for chlorpromazine and placebo were again demonstrated. Hospitalization rates were 21.1 percent for placebo-treated patients and 8.5 percent for chlorpromazine treated patients ($P < .01$). When we studied the hospitalization rate of patients exposed to 6 to 12 months of treatment, a drug-placebo differential was no longer evident. Thus, our findings indicated that chlorpromazine treatment was effective in reducing the incidence of hospitalization during the first six months only. Thereafter, it was no more effective than placebo. The questions raised by these findings were critical to our interest in long-term outpatient maintenance therapy. Was the effect of chlorpromazine one of preventing hospitalization, or was its effect merely one of delaying hospitalization?

We next sought to trace the differential rates of hospitalization for drug and placebo treatments as a function of duration of treatment. A separate analysis of the cumulative hospitalization rates of the three drug groups for successive periods of treatment was made. Figure 1 shows the prevalence of hospitalization at successive three-month periods of treatment exposure up to 15 months and the rate after 15 months. As

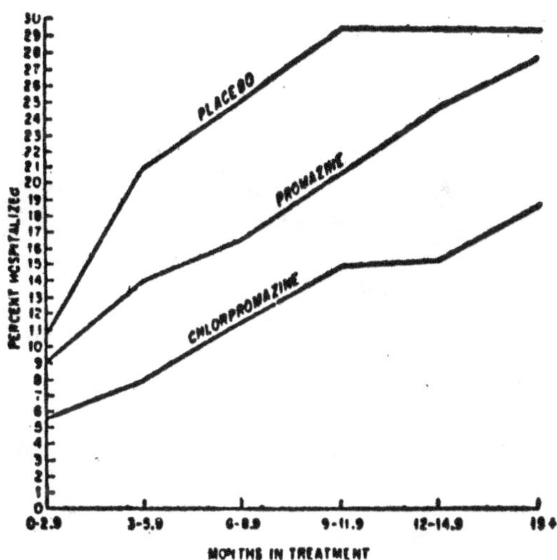

FIGURE 1. Cumulative hospitalization rates by drug treatment.

can be seen, the placebo rate increases faster than that of the other two groups during the first six months of treatment. After the first six months, however, the rate of increase of the placebo curve declines and becomes comparable to the rate of increase of the other two curves. At one year the placebo curve reached a plateau; that is, there is no further hospitalization on placebo. The phenothiazine treated groups show a steady cumulative increase beyond one year and hence the distance between the phenothiazine curves and the placebo curve decreases. The rates of increase for the two phenothiazine-treated groups are fairly consistent throughout.

A statistical comparison of the cumulative hospitalization

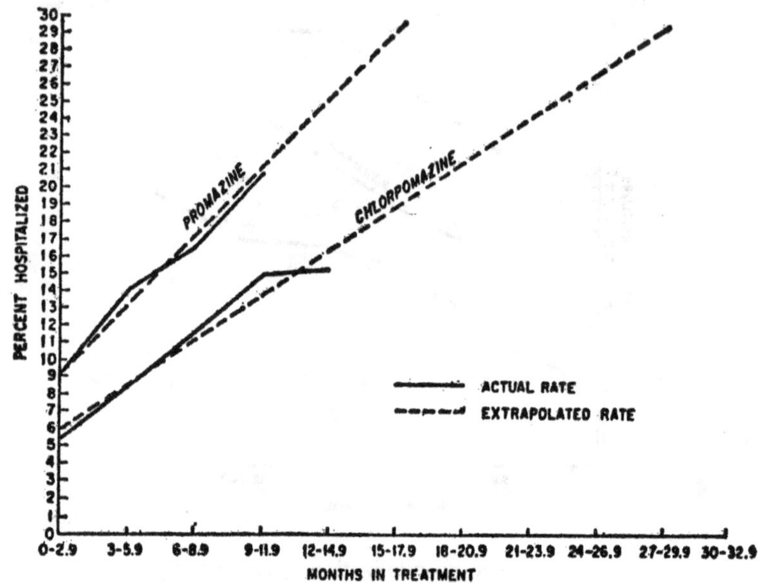

FIGURE 2. Extrapolated cumulative hospitalization rates by drug treatment.

rates for successive periods of treatment exposure, as reflected in Figure 1, revealed that from 3 months and up to 15 months of treatment, the cumulative hospitalization rate for chlorpromazine treatment was significantly lower than that occurring in the placebo treated group ($P < .01$). Even after 15 months of treatment, the difference between placebo and chlorpromazine remained significant (29.6 percent vs. 19.0 percent, $P < .05$). In no instance could the hospitalization rate for the promazine-treated group be differentiated statistically from that of the other two treatment conditions.

The convergence of the chlorpromazine and placebo curves led us to extrapolate the incidence of hospitalization beyond 15 months for active drug (see Figure 2). These extrapolation curves suggest that for promazine the cumulative hospitalization rate was equivalent to that of placebo at 17 months, while for chlorpromazine the rate was equivalent to that of placebo at 30 months.* While the data in Figure 2 indicate an end-point at which the hospitalization prevention effect of chlorpromazine ceases, this period of delay is appreciable and clearly represents a major clinical achievement attributable to drug.

In evaluating the significance of this finding, it should be borne in mind that our population of schizophrenic patients represented a cross-section drawn from the community at large and contained within it patients with differing histories of hospitalization. The nature of the placebo curve with a 30 percent hospitalization rate within 12 months and no hospitalizations thereafter suggests that we were studying a group with mixed hospitalization potential. As will be seen later when the patients are subdivided on the basis of potential for hospitalization, the hospitalization rate under placebo is found to be considerably higher and the action of drug in preventing hospitalization emerges with greater clarity.

From a research point of view, the most startling information in Figure 1 is the nature of the placebo curve. After 12 months, no patient continuing on placebo treatment becomes hospitalized. The placebo curve suggests the possibility that within our placebo group there is a subgroup of patients highly vulnerable to hospitalization, a group we might designate as "hospitalization prone," and a group with relatively little tendency to hospitalization who may be designated as "nonhospitalization prone." The identification of subgroups of schizophrenic outpatients in terms of their hospitalization proneness is, of

* Subsequent to the derivation of these extrapolated curves, two additional patients on chlorpromazine (treated beyond 15 months) were hospitalized. These additional hospitalized cases confirmed the trends indicated by extrapolation.

course, only possible when there is available for analysis a random community sample of patients treated on placebo over sustained periods of time. In view of the difficulty of obtaining "drug-free" schizophrenic patients for study, we consider ourselves most fortunate in having a large sample of such patients available for investigation.

We consider our findings on the pattern of hospitalization under "no drug" treatment an important one. We will return to the problem of prevention of hospitalization under phenothiazine treatment later. For the present, we would simply indicate that prevention of hospitalization under drug treatment cannot be studied without reference to the problem of length of treatment or without reference to the particular characteristics of the schizophrenic patients receiving treatment. These two considerations have clear practical implications and must be considered in any evaluation of a maintenance treatment program.

Control of Psychotic Symptomatology

Maintenance therapy as it applies to the control of psychotic symptomatology must take into consideration the speed with which symptom alteration takes place, whether this alteration is sustained over time, the stability of the symptom modification (visit to visit), and whether further improvement takes place after initial improvement. One of our early findings in the area of psychopharmacological treatment of chronic schizophrenic outpatients was that phenothiazine treatment was effective in the control of psychotic symptomatology. A variety of psychopathological features appeared to be responsive to treatment including formal aspects of schizophrenic thinking, hallucinations and delusions, paranoid thinking, obsessive compulsive features, incoherent and blocked speech, all derived from a psychiatric rating scale and combined into an overall morbidity index. The data thus closely parallel the observations of other investigations, particularly those of the Cooperative V.A. Inpatient Study. More recently, we have been able to confirm this observation on a much larger sample, comprising 360 patients exposed to three months of treatment and 270 patients exposed to six months of treatment. What emerged, however, was that the overall morbidity index was much less discriminating but we were able to narrow down the specific treatment effect to a single symptom area, namely, paranoid thought. This effect of drug treatment on paranoid symptomatology, which will be discussed later, may have important implications for the patient's functioning in the community and the maintenance of his outpatient status.

The more interesting aspects of the issue of controlling psychotic symptomatology, however, concern the dimension of time. Our first long-term observation of phenothiazine action on outpatients was reported in 1962. In this study we departed from the usual "prepast" evaluation and attempted to compare the clinical course of each of 12 matched pairs of patients over periods of time ranging from 12 to 51 months.*

As expected, within three months the chlorpromazine-treated patients showed significantly greater reduction in psychotic symptomatology in comparison with placebo-treated patients, and this superiority could be observed up to 24 months of therapy.

Qualitatively, the chlorpromazine-treated member of each pair showed greater stability of clinical improvement from

* Twelve patients on chlorpromazine and placebo were selected and matched on sex and severity of psychotic symptomatology at intake. The criteria for selection of the 24 patients were presence of severe psychotic symptomatology at intake and continued treatment in the clinic for at least 12 months. (The range of clinic attendance was from 12 to 51 months with an average of 27 months.) Patients were rated and compared not only on the usual prepast status but more specifically on their pattern of clinical course. Clinical course was charted graphically for each matched pair, plotting the severity score at intake and at three-month intervals thereafter. Symptom modification was defined as a minimum four-point drop in the severity score relative to intake. The median severity score of the clinic sample as a whole was 10 and this score was used as the minimum for inclusion of a patient in the sample.

visit to visit and a pattern of clinical course in which relapse was minimal. For example, while in eight of the chlorpromazine-treated patients the severity score remained consistently at least four points below the intake score, this was true only of two placebo-treated patients. Another important aspect of the long-term treatment effect was reflected in the increment of improvement beyond the initial three-month treatment effect. It was observed that chlorpromazine-treated patients showed a further improvement between three months and one year, an effect not observed with placebo treatment. The findings of this study lend support to the effectiveness of chlorpromazine maintenance therapy.

Changes in Social Behavior

Improvement in social behavior among hospitalized schizophrenic patients was one of the earliest observed and reported effects of phenothiazine treatment. The early enthusiastic response to the introduction of these drugs into psychiatric treatment was to a great extent related to the observation that drugs altered the behavior of psychiatric patients, making them more "manageable" on the ward and more "accessible to treatment."

In evaluating the effect of phenothiazines on the social behavior of schizophrenic outpatients, a number of questions present themselves: Is the quality of change in social behavior in outpatients treated with phenothiazines comparable to that observed among inpatients? Can improvement in social behavior be discerned or gauged reliably by a relative? Are changes in social behavior as observed by the relative related to changes in psychopathology as observed by the psychiatrist?

Our first attempt was to evaluate changes in social behavior in a global way, using a checklist of 15 items describing clearly dysfunctional social behavior. This checklist was imbedded in an intensive, open-ended social behavior interview. Information was obtained on a regular once-a-month basis from a relative having close personal contact with the patient.

We found that patients treated with chlorpromazine, promazine, and placebo, respectively, showed very different rates of improved social functioning over six months of outpatient treatment. The incidence of improvement at six months as perceived by the family is significantly greater for patients on phenothiazines than on placebo: 46 percent of the patients on chlorpromazine and 33 percent of the patients on promazine were improved, as opposed to 8 percent on placebo. Observations on the incidence of worsening of the patient's condition reinforce these findings. At six months the proportion of patients rated as "worse" was 54 percent for placebo, 30 percent for promazine, and 14 percent for chlorpromazine.

As in the psychiatric evaluation where an overall morbidity index discriminated between drug and placebo, an overall social pathology checklist demonstrated drug-associated changes. While the relative's ability to discriminate changes in the patient's deviant behavior at home was demonstrated, it was found that the changes observed were generally unrelated to changes in psychopathology observed by the psychiatrist. Thus, it would appear that both the psychiatrist and the patient's relative are important observers who, independent of each other, are able to discern drug-associated changes in the patient's condition. Each apparently picks up different aspects of the patient's behavior.

As part of our analysis of social behavior, we attempted to obtain additional qualitative descriptions of the patient's transactions with a significant relative. At specified time points over the course of treatment, we obtained behavior descriptions of the patient's typical daily activity with his relative (housekeeping habits, eating habits, leisure and work habits). From these descriptions, certain scalable social traits could be derived. Of the various social traits, the most consistent and specific findings obtained were in the area of social isolation and in the area of social aggression, particularly the type of social aggression which the relative experienced as directly oppositional to his wishes.*

Examination of changes in social traits reveals a significant reduction in social aggressiveness or belligerence as reported by the relative in patients receiving phenothiazine treatment. There is also a trend for certain patients to become more withdrawn and more solitary in their social behavior. Finally, the relatives also report changes in the patient's work adjustment. Work adjustment changes were studied only for males and involved rating the patient's work record on such items as number of jobs held, amount of time worked, days missed, etc., during a given time period. Essentially we obtained an index of the stability of the work record. The impact of drugs on "productive" social behavior is a complex one. There appears to be a trend under phenothiazine treatment for patients having a typically low work adjustment history and having certain psychological attributes to show an increase in productivity. Conversely, there is evidence that patients whose typical work adjustment has been "high" suffer a reduction in productivity when treated with chlorpromazine.

The improvement in social behavior observed over the first six months of treatment parallels closely those observed for psychotic symptomatology and for incidence of hospitalization. In this "relatively" early phase of treatment, social behavior is altered in a meaningful way by the intervention of phenothiazines. When treatment effects on social behavior were

* In defining these social traits initially, we were cautious to assign meaning to them. Thus, it had been our feeling that these traits may be descriptive of the particular relationship that exists between the patient and his respondent. More recently, as a result of further data analysis, we have come to the conclusion that these traits, which certainly are derived from the interaction of two participants, do in fact represent to some extent qualities which are specifically attributable to the patient's behavior. This type of inference makes it much more possible to speak of an alteration within the patient as well as an alteration in a relationship.

observed for a period exceeding six months—for example, 9 and 12 months—the discrimination between drug and placebo was no longer evident. The failure to observe a significant difference between drug and placebo at 12 months does not represent a deterioration in the drug-treated patients. The initial gains in social behavior under phenothiazine treatment are maintained. Rather, we tend to note a cumulative effect of placebo treatment which narrows the differential between the two treatments leading to nonsignificant differences.

The Patient as a Variable in Treatment Outcome

It is difficult to say to what extent one may generalize from the findings just presented. Our data apply to a special population of chronic schizophrenic outpatients who have maintained essentially an ambulatory type of community adjustment and who therefore differ from the inpatient and after-care populations described in the literature. Furthermore, our findings apply to a specific treatment program in which drug treatment is imbedded in a matrix of supportive therapy and is continued indefinitely regardless of the patient's changing condition. Finally, the different effects of treatment that we have just outlined, even though they all occur in schizophrenic outpatients, do not all occur in the same patient. The patients showing reduced psychoticism or whose hospitalization has been prevented, or those who show changes in social behavior and work adjustment are often different individuals. In a sense, this is our most important finding: the effects observed under phenothiazine treatment do not apply equally to all patients and that the patient in treatment is himself a critical variable in outcome.

The material to be presented now is tentative compared to the findings that we have reported so far. What follows is a first report of our attempts to identify specific patient attributes or characteristics which can be meaningfully related to the outcome measures that we have studied. Our present effort is concerned with identification of discrete panels of patients who are likely to be hospitalized, show change in psychopathology, or show changes in social behavior and work productivity.

Identifying responders and nonresponders to drug treatment is guided by the "placebo model." A specific outcome variable, such as hospitalization, is selected for study and the response of all placebo-treated patients is used as a criterion to separate responders from nonresponders. Responders and nonresponders are next identified in terms of a number of descriptive attributes and the predictive profiles on placebo are cross-validated. Next, the fate of the drug-treated patients having the profile attributes of responders and nonresponders is traced.

We are currently attempting to identify the characteristics of patients who are likely to be hospitalized and the characteristics of patients who are likely to show an alteration in their psychotic state. The data of the long-term treatment effects by relevant patient panels have only barely begun and we can only sketch these effects in rough outline. The issues of time and of specificity of treatment effect will occupy our interest increasingly over the coming years, since we consider these factors critical to the understanding of long-term drug maintenance therapy.

The Characteristics of the Hospitalization-Prone Patient

From our data on the cumulative incidence of hospitalization with placebo treatment, we were led to the supposition that in any given population of outpatient schizophrenics drawn from the community at large, there is a relatively finite group that is likely to be hospitalized. As indicated, we conceptualize this group of outpatient schizophrenics as being "hospitalization-prone." The placebo-treated patient in our clinic who does not get hospitalized, we consider to be "nonhospitalization-prone." We observed large numbers of schizophrenic patients in a drug-free state over relatively sustained periods of time and found that under these conditions all patients likely to become hospitalized were hospitalized within the first 12 months of treatment. We used the panels of hospitalized and nonhospitalized placebo patients as a basis for building up a profile of the hospitalization-prone patient as described previously. "Hospitalization-prone" is defined here as the patient who, in fact, becomes hospitalized on placebo within 12 months of intake.

Hospitalized and nonhospitalized patients were compared on some 80 different attributes. Of the 80 items, 13 clearly differentiated the two groups. Together the items appeared to form a rational or clinically meaningful pattern. A number of statistical criteria led us to reduce the 13 items to an 8-item "proneness" scale. The clinical meaning of this score could be defined by its correlation with "factor" scores descriptive of our population. There were three essential types of relationships: the first deals with the patient's social interaction patterns (a "prone" patient tended to be socially isolated and nonbelligerent); the second deals with the organization of psychological functions (a "prone" patient tended to show undifferentiated cognitive functioning and inefficiency in problem-solving tasks, such as the Porteus Maze Test); the third deals with socioeconomic factors (the "prone" patient tended to be lower in his educational and occupational status). It is noteworthy that nosological groups or symptomatology as evaluated by the psychiatrist failed to correlate with the scale. On the other hand, modes of psychological organization and social interaction appear to be a critical differentiating characteristic between prone and nonprone patients.

Using the hospitalization proneness scale, we stratified our drug-treated patients in terms of "proneness" to determine their incidence of hospitalization in long-term maintenance therapy. We were particularly interested in the issue of whether maintenance drug therapy would show a decreased differentiation between drug and placebo over time as had been observed previously. When we studied only the prone patients under the three drug conditions (placebo, promazine, and chlorpromazine), a clear drug effect was noted up to three years of continued therapy. As was to be expected, the differential between the three treatment conditions was greatest during the first 12 months of treatment (attributable to the high hospitalization rate on placebo); yet differences between both chlorpromazine and placebo, and promazine and placebo could be observed up to three years of treatment exposure. This finding would argue that up to at least 36 months of drug maintenance therapy *do have* a "prevention of hospitalization" effect for the "prone" patient.

Analysis of hospitalization rates for the "nonprone" patient presented a different picture. As expected, the overall hospitalization rates were significantly lower for the "nonprone" patients. At no point in treatment was it possible to observe a superiority of drug over placebo in the incidence of hospitalization. In fact, the hospitalization rates for the combined promazine- and chlorpromazine-treated patients were significantly higher than those for placebo. The possibility that maintenance phenothiazine therapy has an adverse effect on the ability of the "nonprone" patient to maintain outpatient status has to be kept in mind.

We have reason to believe that the characteristic of "proneness" may affect the clinical course of the schizophrenic outpatient in ways other than hospitalization. While 50 percent of the placebo-treated "prone" patients become hospitalized, there still remain 50 percent who are not hospitalized. What is the fate of the prone patient who succeeds in avoiding hospitalization? Our impression so far is that the prone patient who is not hospitalized especially under active drug treatment "fits" himself into treatment. After an initial positive treatment response within the first two or three sessions, he tends to show minimal symptomatic changes thereafter, although he tends to remain in treatment for substantial periods of time. It would thus appear that for the "prone" patient the predominant effect of phenothiazines is not symptom modification but facilitation or stabilization of his ambulatory status. For the "prone" patient the doctor-patient relationship appears to be critical.

Characteristics of the Patient with a Propensity for Symptom Modification

Following a procedure similar to that described for the identification of hospitalization proneness, we selected a panel of patients whose main characteristic was paranoid thought. The choice was guided by the observation mentioned earlier that in our population this symptom appeared to be most responsive to drug intervention. Starting again with a "placebo model," it was observed that on placebo, within three months, some patients showed a significant alteration in their paranoid symptomatology; others did not.

The characteristics of the patients with a propensity to respond (or not to respond) with modification in paranoid thought under placebo treatment were then identified. Again variables dealing with the patient's mode of social interaction and differentiation of cognitive functioning discriminated most sensitively. The placebo responder was characterized as socially isolated, nonaggressive, psychologically undifferentiated, and inefficient in problem-solving behavior. While the attributes are not identical, one gains a picture which is similar to the hospitalization-prone patient. In terms of type or prevalence of psychotic symptoms, responders and nonresponders could not be differentiated.

A propensity measure (combining the discriminating variables) was developed next. Higher propensity patients showed, of course, a significantly higher improvement rate within three months for placebo-treatment in contrast to low propensity patients. The reversal of improvement rates for high and low propensity patients upon introduction of drugs is of particular interest. For the patient with a propensity to respond to placebo, the effect produced by the addition of phenothiazines is minimal. The rate of improvement in paranoid thinking for all three treatment conditions is equivalent. These patients, like the hospitalization prone patients, once they remain in treatment tend to adapt easily to continued treatment. The addition of drug contributes little. An opposite picture is presented by the patient who does not show the propensity to respond to placebo treatment. With the introduction particularly of chlorpromazine, a dramatic difference in response is observed. As opposed to the placebo-treated patient, there is a significant alteration and reduction in paranoid symptomatology.

Other panels being investigated have to do with propensity to change in social isolation, in social aggressiveness, in anxiety, and in productivity. However, these findings are so preliminary that they do not warrant presentation. There appears to be a common theme running across the data: nosology and symptomatology are poor predictors while certain psychological and social indices appear to be meaningful predictors of change. We are not asserting that the "response" groups are equivalent in psychopathology. One would have to assume that "isolated" and "nonisolated" paranoid patients represent very different pathological pictures. However, they could not be discriminated on the usual items descriptive of psychopathology. In fact, one of the goals which we expect to pursue intensively is to discover differences between "isolated" and "nonisolated," "differentiated" and "nondifferentiated" paranoid patients.

What appears to emerge from our recent studies are patient-response potentials describable along cognitive and social dimensions. Although our cognitive and social interaction variables are not correlated with each other, they appear to effect treatment outcome in a functionally equivalent manner. The hypothesis suggests itself that they may represent aspects of a common process. At one end of the continuum is the patient characterized by social isolation, absence of belligerence, and low cognitive differentiation; at the other end is the patient characterized by relatively higher social participation, overt belligerence, and higher cognitive differentiation. In view of the critical position of the social participation variable, we tend to think that the dimension reflects differences in the degree to which the patient's activities are committed to his environmental "space" in the sense of "retrenchment" from or "expansion" into the social environment.

The patient's position on the cognitive or social dimensions may then determine a number of significant events in the course of treatment including the patient's response to drug or placebo. Most generally, the undifferentiated and socially retrenched patient is prone to hospitalization, but under drug his hospitalization is prevented and he exhibits a facility to fit into treatment and to remain in treatment for prolonged periods of time. For the differentiated, expanded patient, there is a lesser likelihood of hospitalization and evidence of a negative symptomatic response to placebo. With drug treatment, however, there is a marked reduction of paranoid thought and belligerence. It is, of course, inviting to speculate on the underlying adaptive mechanisms and processes in the genesis of the illness that may be implicated by these response patterns. Such speculation must await more intensive study of the patient panels.

Summary and Critique

We may best summarize our findings on long-term maintenance drug therapy around the concept of community adaptation and stabilization. Our experience over the past years leads us to believe that drugs such as chlorpromazine can contribute in a meaningful way not only toward keeping the chronic schizophrenic patient out of the hospital but also toward improving his adjustment in the community. There seems to be a drug effect (not easily identifiable by rating scales), which facilitates the patient's ability to "fit into" both the treatment and home situation. While we do not as yet understand the nature of this effect, we consider the stabilizing effect achieved by drug a new and important finding.

Earlier in this chapter we stressed the importance of the doctor-patient relationship in long-term psychopharmacological treatment of chronic schizophrenic outpatients. Implicit in this statement is the view that with our present drugs and crude methods of identifying patients, "drugs" alone do not suffice to maintain the patient in the community. There is some suggestion in our more recent work that with more refined methods of classification, schizophrenic patients may be identified for whom this may no longer be true.

In the dosages given, both chlorpromazine and promazine are well tolerated by our patients over prolonged periods of time and are free of serious toxicity. While our dosages may be viewed as low by some clinicians, we have no reason to believe that they were inadequate. The possibility exists, nonetheless, that under a higher (or lower!) dosage schedule our patients may have fared better. The same would apply to the possible effect of more intensive psychotherapy or more frequent visits.

Our positive impressions of the effectiveness of maintenance drug therapy in schizophrenic outpatients should not hide from the reader the limitations of this form of treatment evidenced in our findings. At this time, our conclusions are based essentially on the action of two drugs, chlorpromazine and promazine, and on periods of observation of one to three years. We can say nothing definite about treatment periods in excess of those given. In their excellent review of long-term effects of psychotropic drugs, Gittelman et al. call attention to Staudt and Zubin's review of the long-term effects of "nondrug" somatic treatments (ECT, insulin, psychosurgery). These authors found that while at two years a treatment differential could be observed between treated and untreated patients, the difference between the two patient groups was no longer visible at three years. It may very well be that many of our patients are "coasting" on the initial treatment impact and that with additional time the drug effect will cease to be visible.

Equally important is the limited effect of drug on the more formal aspects of psychopathology and the more subtle aspects of social participation. While there is some evidence of increased productivity in some patients under drug, the overall effectiveness of the patient and his usefulness to the community fall far short of the desired goal and call for novel forms of intervention.

Throughout our research we have been acutely aware of the difficulties involved in pursuing a long-term controlled outpatient study. The most serious problem we have encountered is that of population attrition. We have tried to compensate for this somewhat by collecting a fairly large study sample and a second sample for replication of findings. (Planned for the future is a "field trial" in our community clinic of the more clinically significant replicated findings.) However, the progressive shrinkage of our study sample limits the generalization we are able to make.

Nonetheless, we feel encouraged by our experiences so far. We are fairly confident that the research protocol, as far as drug intake and double-blind design are concerned, has been maintained. Our instruments have been adequate to describe qualitative aspects of the treatment effect and to permit both the doctor and the patient's relative to distinguish between drug and placebo. Finally, we have had encouraging results in our attempts to attain greater specificity in identifying "sub-groups" of schizophrenic patients in terms of their selective response to phenothiazines. In the case of certain treatment targets (prevention of hospitalization and work adjustment) this has resulted in identifying the potential hazard of phenothiazine treatment in certain schizophrenic patients.

The spectrum of drug effects observed under phenothiazine treatment is a kaleidoscope, true for the group but not for the individual. In the absence of greater knowledge about schizophrenia and with the presently available drugs, we feel that the identification of drug-patient interaction panels for specific treatment targets is the most useful clinical and research approach open to us. However, to assess properly the value of the new psychopharmacological agents in outpatient maintenance therapy will require the development of new methods of classification of patients permitting greater specificity in prediction of outcome with drug treatment. Identification of the schizophrenic patient will have to concern itself not only with nosology, symptomatology, age, sex, race, and education, but more directly with his characteristic modes of adjustment to his psychosis, his patterns of social interaction, and his cognitive organization.

Chapter 12

*British Experience in Community Care**

KATHLEEN JONES

When the history of the world mental health movement comes to be written—and there is a task here worthy of a new Arnold Toynbee or a future Max Weber—one of the fundamental themes must be the development of the concept of community care. By a long process of evolution and a few imaginative leaps in the dark, we have progressed from a belief in a limited and somewhat monolithic mental hospital service to a vision of a flexible and diversified service which will represent society's changing response to the changing needs of psychiatric patients. Stereotyped habits of thought have been replaced by fresh, empirical thinking about clinical care, about administrative methods, and about the basic philosophy which underlies both.

In this field, the Dutch are the acknowledged pioneers, and it is particularly fitting that we should be discussing this subject in Amsterdam, where Prof. Arie Querido's work and that of his colleagues has been an inspiration to psychiatrists and administrators from so many countries. Perhaps the most impressive characteristic of this work has been the humility of approach: the insistence on starting from an actual situation and investigating it in depth by means of a variety of research techniques.

* Presented at the Sixteenth Annual Meeting, World Federation for Mental Health, Amsterdam, the Netherlands, August, 1963.

Professor Querido's recent book *The Efficiency of Medical Care*[1] illustrates this view by its careful and scholarly refusal to theorize about the situation until detailed investigations have shown its nature and characteristics. I should like to proceed with similar caution, by first outlining the present situation in Britain and then discussing some of its problems and potentialities. Some of our problems will be relevant to those of other countries, and some may be international problems in the true sense, that is, problems common to all countries; but in the present state of our knowledge it would probably be unwise to try to distinguish these in any detail.

In Britain, the view that the institution was the right place for the mentally disordered, both for their own protection and for that of society, was dominant right through the nineteenth century. Mental hospitals were constructed in three great waves of building development, following the County Asylums Act of 1808, the Lunatics Act of 1845, and the Lunacy Act of 1890. They were usually sited several miles distant from the town that formed their main catchment area, partly because rural land was cheaper than town land and partly because there was a rejection mechanism at work, the patients being literally as well as metaphorically rejected by the society from which they came.

Until 1913, the law made no clear distinction between the mentally ill and the subnormal; but when a separate service was instituted for subnormal patients, a new principle emerged. Hospitals, or "colonies," as they were then called, were to care for the low-grade patients and for those whose home background had been found unsuitable; but there were provisions for the care and supervision of patients who remained in their own homes. The care of the mentally ill and that of the subnormal were administratively separated, and there was nothing equivalent to the new system for the mentally ill.

In the 1920s, however, outpatient clinics began to develop. This was a major breakthrough: the first means of treating patients without committing them to the mental hospital under certification. In 1930, mental hospitals were empowered to take voluntary patients. The huge chronic populations remained, but a new category of short-stay patients appeared and the question of aftercare became an urgent one. Hospitals began to appoint social workers, and the nucleus of a hospital-based psychiatric service developed.

After World War II, the institution of the "welfare state" brought radical changes. A variety of locally based services for the care of underprivileged or handicapped groups in the community developed. Mental health departments were organized as subsections of local public health departments.

The development of these new services was inevitably uneven. Some local authorities were quick to grasp the implications of their new position and began to experiment with community services. Others did very little apart from their statutory duties: the supervision of subnormals in the community and the conveyance of the mentally ill to the mental hospital. In a few cases (Worthing is probably the best known) the hospital took the initiative in providing a community service; but the relation between the role of the local authority and that of the hospital was obscure, and quite often the work went by default, neither body taking the initiative.

The Mental Health Act of 1959 changed the situation decisively. This act was the result of a royal commission that saw a great and expanding future for community care and a dwindling role for the hospital. Even while its discussions were taking place, there were new developments: the day hospital movement began to spread; mental hospitals, realizing the dangers of "institutional neurosis" so ably described by Dr. W. Russell Barton,[2] began to experiment with the idea of the "therapeutic community" and to open their doors; and local authorities began to test the potentialities of hostels for those who had no settled homes and sheltered workshops for those who could not be fully absorbed into industry.

By 1959, the idea of a diversified system of care was widely accepted, though the place of the inpatient hospital was (and still is) the subject of much debate. The official policy of the Ministry of Health[3] since 1961 has been based on a statistical projection from trends in the years from 1954 to 1959 which suggested a possible reduction in inpatient beds from 3.3 to 1.8 per 1,000 population within fifteen years. This policy has been criticized on the following grounds:

1. A long-term projection cannot be adequately based on a short-term trend.

2. The decline in mental hospital populations between 1954 and 1959 was marginal and is unlikely to continue indefinitely of its own momentum.

3. This decline resulted from a change in administrative policy rather than from a clinical advance.

4. There is a need for local variation in provision according to local need.

5. Any decision about the future of the mental hospital population is premature until the potentialities and limitations of community care have been more thoroughly explored.[4]

In recent months, the argument concerning institutional or community care has widened to include other forms of provision—homes for old people and epileptic colonies, for instance—and two main points of view have emerged. One is that the institution is a relic of custodialism, necessary enough when other services were not available but now outmoded. The second view is that although the institution is now only one among a number of means of social care, it still possesses a useful function for people whose disabilities are so great that they need a sheltered environment.

The argument is very largely one of degree, for very few people are prepared to push either view to its logical extremes by contending that all institutions should be abolished or that all patients now in institutions should stay there. The question is how many can be rehabilitated by modern methods of care and under what circumstances. A preliminary and necessary step is to ascertain what kinds of patients are at present in the institutions under review and to assess how far they would be capable of rehabilitation under existing conditions of community care. As Professor Querido has shown, such arguments need to be tied to what is possible and practicable now if they are to retain any contact with reality.

With these considerations in mind, a patient census of 10,000 psychiatric beds in the Leeds region has been mounted as a result of cooperation between the regional hospital board and the University of Manchester. We hope that the first results of our analysis will be available in the near future.

This controversy concerning institutional or community care may be a peculiarly British one, but the basic question underlying it is one of *balance* between the different parts of a diversified service. It seems likely that other countries will have encountered this question, though possibly framed in different terms, according to local tradition and needs. It is allied to two other questions, those of dimension and finance.

The problem of *dimension* arises from the fact that psychiatric need is difficult to estimate or delimit. Epidemiologic work is an urgent necessity; but while there is little argument about the extent of the field in other areas of epidemiology (we can establish clearly who suffers from typhus or smallpox), the need for psychiatric care must always be based on a multiple assessment. It is a matter not simply of disease or handicap but of disease or handicap plus social factors: no home, a poor home background, relatives who cannot cope with the patient, inability to hold down a job, and so on.

Mental disorder is still to some extent a submerged problem. We can measure the number of patients who come forward for treatment and construct incidence rates and prevalence rates, but we have no way of knowing how many more would come forward if the conditions of treatment were more acceptable.

British experience is that increased provision has always resulted in increased demand. In the early days of outpatient clinics, it was thought that they would reduce the need for inpatient beds, but in fact they provided a supplementary service rather than an alternative one. Day hospitals have similarly tended to draw greater numbers of people into the orbit of the mental health services rather than providing a new means of catering for those already under care. The size of the problem is conditioned by the services we are prepared to offer. Presumably there is a limit to this process somewhere, but it is doubtful whether any country has yet made sufficient psychiatric provision to reach it. As Prof. P. Sivadon said recently, where mental health is concerned, all countries are "developing" countries.[5]

There is thus no clear answer to the problems of dimension. If one asks "How good a mental health service must we provide?" the answer must be "the best one we can afford."

The question of *finance* is basically one of allocating scarce resources among apparently bottomless needs. It seems to be a fundamental law of any society that this allocation will favor those who serve society best. Thus primitive societies have been known to abandon the old or expose the sick in time of famine or attack, concentrating food supplies on the working and fighting population (who guarantee the present survival of the group) and the children (who guarantee its future survival). It seems likely that this law holds good in more complex societies also. It is much easier to get money and equipment for a social service which will restore workers to productive employment or benefit children than to obtain these things for the mentally ill, the subnormal, or the old.

It seems likely that those who administer the mental health services will always have difficulty in securing the share of the national resources which social justice demands. The proper care of psychiatric patients costs a good deal of money, and it is difficult to demonstrate an adequate return on investments. A proportion of mental health work is, and perhaps always must be, economically unproductive.

Much of the opposition to adequate financing is not rationally expressed. If it were, it would be easier to combat, but it takes the form of agreeing that provision is necessary sometime and then putting it off indefinitely; or claiming that it will be sufficient to enlarge an existing building, when the real need is for another building elsewhere; or expecting one psychiatrist "temporarily" to do the work of two, or one nurse or social worker to do the work of four; or arguing that it is "good for the patient" to receive only minimal care, when the real benefit is to the taxpayer's pocket.

There are, of course, times when financial saving and therapeutic advantage do genuinely go hand in hand—when an authority can save money and at the same time produce a better service; but the occasions when this is possible are probably rarer than we care to think. An expensive service is no guarantee of quality, because the money can be spent unwisely, but a cheap service is rarely anything but an indication of inferior standards.

It is often claimed that day hospitals and other community care agencies can provide a cheaper service than that of the mental hospital. This may be so, but there is an urgent need for a full-scale costing study to prove it. The claims which are made for day hospitals sometimes ignore four important points:

1. The difference between capital and maintenance cost. A day hospital is cheaper to build but might be more expensive to maintain if it required a higher staff ratio.

2. The difference between marginal cost and average cost. Calculations are sometimes based on the additional cost of the day unit to the cost of a parent inpatient unit. This is marginal

costing. To give a reasonable figure, the cost of facilities used jointly by the day hospital and the inpatient hospital should be split between them.

3. Transferred cost. Day hospitals may be dependent on services paid for by some other authority—e.g., in England, ambulance and social work services, which are paid for by local authorities. These costs should be included.

4. Submerged cost. Day hospital care might result in a longer average stay than inpatient care or in a higher relapse rate.

Psychiatrists sometimes feel impatient at the mention of cost and financing, arguing that cost does not matter as long as the patient gets the best possible service. I think this is unrealistic. Just because it is difficult to get a fair share of the community's resources for psychiatric patients, it is important that psychiatrists should give consideration to these issues and put their claims in terms which politicians and government servants can understand. For instance, a study of mental hospital costs in the north of England[6] showed that, of three hospitals studied, the one with the highest weekly cost and the most intensive medical care actually had the lowest cost per case, because patients were discharged more quickly and did not relapse more often. Good care may be cheaper than minimal care in the long run. I think facts of this kind are worth demonstrating. Certainly studies in efficiency, whether linked to cost or organized on some other basis, may be crucial to development.

A further problem raised by the advent of community care is that of *selection of service.* When the traditional mental hospital was the only means of treatment, the question was simply whether the patient should enter the hospital or stay at home. When there is a diversified service, a day hospital, an outpatient clinic, a halfway house, and an inpatient ward all offer different types of care at different levels of intensity, appropriate for different needs. Each has a distinct function, and they are not necessarily interchangeable. From a whole range of services, the doctor must choose the one appropriate to his patient's needs. This involves a skilled assessment, based on two kinds of knowledge: (1) knowledge of the patient's condition and his environment; and (2) knowledge of the varied resources of the community, so that needs and resources can be matched. The kind of administrative knowledge necessary for an assessment of resources has rarely been included in medical curricula, but several British universities are now including some teaching (whether described as "social administration" or "social psychiatry") for medical students or postgraduate students in psychiatry.

Where some of the newer agencies for community care are concerned, the question of *function* is still being debated. Five years ago, we were arguing about the function of the day hospital. Did it provide the first stage in aftercare for those who had had inpatient treatment? Did it provide alternative care—a means of reducing the inpatient population? Did it provide supplmentary care, drawing on a new and hitherto untreated population? The answer seems to lie somewhere among the three views, but there are still many local differences. We may use the same term "day hospital" for agencies serving different and even mutually exclusive purposes.

Since the Mental Health Act envisaged the development of hostel facilities, there has been a corresponding debate on the function of the hostel. Should it be of the halfway house type for patients in the process of rehabilitation? Should it provide a home for the chronic patient with no family who no longer needs the full resources of the mental hospital? Should it provide for patients who can go out to work on a full-time basis or those who cannot work at all? Should it mix patients with different needs and, if so, in what proportions? Doubtless some large authorities will be able to provide specialized hostels for different types of patients, but for the smaller towns and the rural areas the solution is not so easy. Some local authorities appear to be constructing hostels because this is official policy, with no clear idea of what patients they would like to take but with a strong suspicion that, whatever their preferences, they will eventually have to deal with unemployable, elderly, and chronic patients.

This would be very undesirable. Hostel accommodation for patients who stay only a few weeks or who are out all day may be quite satisfactory; but we have as yet few trained hostel staff, and hostels cannot provide all the facilities for socialization which a mental hospital has: the workshops, the sports fields, the cinema shows and entertainments, the libraries, the education classes. Such facilities could not be provided economically for ten or twenty patients. It is not community care to take an elderly and chronic patient away from the active social life of the hospital he knows and to place him in strange surroundings (however modern and near the shops) where he has nothing to do all day.

Perhaps we should think seriously about defining "community care," because it is evident that the phrase is being used in many different ways. In fact, it is seldom defined at all; it is usually denoted: "Community care means day hospitals, night hospitals, outpatient clinics, day hospitals, and so on." It is much more difficult to describe its attributes.

It is, of course, possible to define community care negatively, by saying that it means any kind of care apart from that provided by the institution, the mental hospital; but this may be a false dichotomy. A good mental hospital is part of the community, anxious to keep its patients in touch with community life and to be "a flowing stream rather than a stagnant lake." It is not longer in most cases what it was in the nineteenth century: an isolated, forbidding institution for society's rejects.

I suggest the following attributes as being essential to a reasonable standard of community care:

1. *Diversity*—there must be several different types of care.
2. *Flexibility*—the system must fit the patients, and not

vice versa. Transfer from one type of agency to another should be as easy as possible.

3. *Adequacy*—the care offered must be at least as adequate as that offered by the traditional type of psychiatric hospital service. It is not community care to send an old man out of the hospital to live alone or in unfriendly lodgings, with only an occasional visit from a harassed general practitioner or a social worker. It is not community care to send a severely subnormal girl back to a family which neither understands nor wants her unless someone has the time to foster supportive family attitudes.

4. *Ability to facilitate social relationships*—the patient should have at least as active a social life as in the psychiatric hospital.

It is on factors such as these, rather than on the size of the unit or its siting, that community care depends.

Good community care is expensive. It is probably more expensive in running costs (though not in capital outlay) than good hospital care, because the services which the hospital would concentrate have to be diffused over an area. Even in England, where roads are reasonably good and the distances involved in traveling to outpatient clinics or domiciliary visits in the catchment area are rarely more than twenty or thirty miles, traveling time and mileage costs may be considerable.

In other spheres, we take it for granted that concentration is more efficient than dispersal. We do not expect the general practitioner to visit all his patients in their own homes, because it is more economical in time and effort for the patients to come to the doctor. We concentrate children in schools, students in laboratories and lecture rooms, and workers in factories for the same reason. If we disperse our resources for the treatment of mental disorder—and this is what community care means—we need more money, more workers, and more equipment than would be necessary for a centralized service. Community care may be better for many patients, but it is not a cheap alternative. The capital costs are lower than those of building new modern mental hospitals; the maintenance costs will almost inevitably be higher unless there is a drop in standards.

If I lay stress on the importance of maintaining standards, it is because they are very easily lowered, with often the best of intentions and the finest of descriptive phrases. Reform in the British mental health services has a curious cyclical movement: progress never follows a straight line, and the downward trend often seems to start from the moment of greatest success. There was a great step forward at the beginning of the nineteenth century, when the system of "moral management" used at the York Retreat by the Tuke family became well known.[7] The new county asylums provided a fresh start in care and treatment, and it was common practice for their staff to be sent to study the new methods at the retreat before taking up their appointments; yet the county asylums settled into an institutional mold, and the system of moral management was never widely applied.

In 1845, a burst of optimism followed the passing of Lord Shaftesbury's Lunatics Act and the introduction of the "non-restraint system" by John Conolly and Gardiner Hill. Conolly realized that the abolition of restraint was not enough in itself and that the corollaries of this reform were the improvement of standards among nurses and new forms of activity for patients; yet his plans for a nurses' training school and a school for patients were frustrated by a parsimonious committee. Half a century of neglect and indifference followed.

Such examples could be multiplied to show that the bright promise of one decade may be the lost cause of the next. It seems likely that this is not a specifically British phenomenon, for the American report *Action for Mental Health*[8] comments on a similar pattern in the United States. The report speaks of reform as coming in waves and adds that each wave is "quickly followed by apathy, loss of momentum and professional backsliding." It would be interesting to know if historians in other countries had found a similar movement, because this may be a pattern conditioned by the community's attitude to mental health problems.

Here is one explanation: the community at large is highly ambivalent to mental disorder. The general public will readily assent to the proposition that the mental health services should be improved or that psychiatric patients should be treated with kindness, but lip service does not lead to action. Intellect pulls one way; emotion, the other. This is where the stigma of mental disorder begins. Fear of becoming abnormal, of losing the power of responsible action and rational judgment, supersedes rational assent. Fear may be projected in the form of aggression against those who provoke it: the patient, the therapist, the institution. Sometimes laughter and ridicule take the place of open aggression. Thus, in the eighteenth century, young dandies in London paid twopence to see the lunatics in Bedlam; today, when we are too polite to laugh at the patients, there are plenty of jokes about psychiatrists and mental hospitals. Sometimes the reaction is a mental block: the whole problem is pushed out of the conscious mind as if it did not exist; hence the "conspiracy of silence."

May I suggest one more escape route? It is also possible to deal with this fear by becoming overarticulate about the problem. Catch phrases—"community care," "supportive therapy," "public tolerance," and the rest—can become almost a defense against the reality if used often enough, a kind of incantation. We define the problems of the day hospital when we ought to be building one or urging other people to build one. The case conference, instead of being a spur to action, becomes an excuse for a little dilettante speculation. Perhaps those of us who work in universities are particularly prone to taking refuge in verbalization, to thinking that we have dealt with a problem when we have merely described or defined it.

To sum up, I have tried to indicate some of the main problem areas in the community care field in the light of British experience: the questions of balance, dimension, finance and efficiency, selection, and function. I have suggested a definition of community care based on four attributes: diversity, flexibility, adequacy, and ability to facilitate social relationships; and I have offered a few comments on the cyclical nature of mental health reform as observed in England and the United States, with the sobering thought that the downward trend could happen again.

Perhaps I ought to end by saying, like Thomas Carlyle, "Brothers, I am sorry, but I have got no Morrison's Pill for curing the maladies of society." I suppose Morrison's Pill was some nineteenth-century panacea, some cure-all that failed to fulfill all the claims made for it. It is up to us to see that community care does not suffer the same fate.

PART IV

Social Problems

Introduction

PSYCHIATRY IS BECOMING INCREASINGLY INVOLVED IN BROAD social issues. The psychiatrist is being consulted for his knowledge of techniques for tackling and preventing social problems. The articles in this section, which are but a small portion of the literature of social problems, deal with advancing technology and the changing home; both of these topics have broad implications for the mental health of people in all parts of the world.

Michael's article deals with the social impact of technology and social engineering, two fields which have the greatest implications for the nature of society in the next two decades. We face moral, ethnical, psychological as well as political issues in the engineering of man's biological self. Developments in the areas of biological and chemical warfare, psychopharmacology, birth control, and transplants present very real problems for society. How does society decide who has access to the new information? Then too, who actually decides priorities?

Michael next turns his attention to the effect of technology on the social psychology of the individual. Automation threatens the status and security of an individual and affects the sense of self, thus causing varied responses such as selective involvement, withdrawal, or protest. The implications of technology for society are far-reaching in terms of the various role changes that will undoubtedly occur due to new types of employment, such as men's involving themselves in service-oriented jobs traditionally considered to be for women.

Social engineering, designed to guide, stimulate, motivate, and manipulate society raises numerous ethical problems. Imagine, for example the potential invasion of privacy that could occur with the increased collection and storage of masses of data. Michael contends that unless we can effectively minimize these dangers we will never enjoy the advantages derived from technological growth. The tasks to be faced themselves need the advantage of these new techniques. Programs must be planned, institutions must change at ever-increasing rates, and people must be able to shift perspective at a rate commensurate with technological change. The role of the psychiatrist will be increasingly important, for technological growth affects not only the very essence of our social foundation, but specific individuals as well.

The 1965 CIBA Foundation Symposium on transcultural psychiatry considered the prevalence and manifestation of psychiatric disorders, cross-cultural differences, varying treatment approaches, and the effects of social and cultural change on the vulnerabilities of specific population subgroups. Hes's article taken from the proceeding is a critical review of the literature on housing and mental health. Some studies have noted that change of living quarters is associated with an increased incidence of psychiatric disturbance, while others have reported a decreased incidence. A number of illustrative cases report the psychodynamic significance of home upon the formation of interpersonal relationships, the prevention of undesirable marriages, the cohesion of primary families and the resolution of major family problems.

The symposium discussion of Hes's paper offered a forum for the exchange of a wide range of information pertaining to cross-cultural differences in attitudes and customs influencing types of homes. The discussion concerned comparisons of cultures and pointed to the importance of early attitudes towards the home, for such attitudes have a direct relationship to mental health. Various conflicts in family relationships are acted out in this "container" or house that has different meanings depending on the culture under consideration. Caudill, for example examined and discussed the nature of the various sleeping arrangements and differences in maternal care that exist in Japan compared with those in the United States. He related this to different infant responses and also to different attitudes towards the home in both groups.

Fried's article calls attention to the far-reaching social and psychological problems pursuant to urban renewal and dislocation of the home. In his article, he likens the intense reaction of displaced people to that of a "grief response" as if they were mourning the loss of a loved one. He emphasizes the often ignored fact that individuals may feel at home in their slum communities, and that to change from the familiar to what is thought more desirable by urban planners may be indeed folly from a human viewpoint. Thus, the author feels that the degree to which one has deep commitments to an area in the form of good feelings about the physical aspects as well as familiarity with the area, numerous social ties, friends, relatives, etc., is reflected in the intensity of grief felt by the loss of a home through relocation. Actually either this "spatial identity" or "group identity," an aspect of feeling part of the group, having shared interests, similarity in life style, philosophy, etc., can be the cause for loss of continuity and can therefore lead to grief. A combination of these conditions only seems to intensify the grief response.

Of interest is Fried's proposal to examine slum areas more carefully before changing them and to analyze the physical and spatial arrangements that the dwellers of this community already consider gratifying and conducive to good community relations. "The problem is large," states the author. One has only to look at the data on urban growth and the need for slum renovation to begin to contemplate the magnitude of this problem for all urban areas in the years to come.

Chapter 13

Some Speculations on the Social Impact of Technology

DONALD N. MICHAEL

I WANT TO DRAW YOUR ATTENTION TO WHAT I THINK ARE THE important aspects of the social impact of technology that we have so far ignored or attended to only in passing. I do not intend to convince anyone of anything: I am not sure what the questions are in this area—much less what the answers might be. Rather, I want to sketch a variety of perspectives and circumstances that I think merit attention, so that you may determine whether or not these are significant issues for scholars and actionists concerned with the impact of technology on society on more than an occasional basis. These are issues that we ought to be concerned with at least as much as we have been with productivity, investment policies, employment, and so on.

Let me begin by making it clear that I am not asserting that technology is a villain, or that technology is a saviour. The problem is not that simple. The positive and negative interplay between technology and social processes is much too complicated to comprehend if only one aspect, technology, rather than technology in the context of society as a whole is dealt with. In no sense am I insensitive to or unappreciative of the great opportunities implicit in technology, particularly in the new technologies. Nor may the odds on adverse consequences from these technologies be any higher than on favorable ones.

But I believe that the consequences themselves, favorable or unfavorable, are of such magnitude that if they are negative, they will bring upon us much more serious trouble than we would have had in the past, in simpler days, when technologies had fewer derivative implications, and affected fewer people in a smaller area over a longer period of time.

Let me also make clear that I do not believe that the solutions to the problems we will discuss are to be found, by and large, in a moratorium on technological development. Such is the social environment technology has already produced that, unless we are to change our value system and way of life totally, we must use more technology to make an adequate environment out of the circumstances technology has already brought about. I fully expect the technologies to help deal with the problems the technologies produce. I also fully expect that unless we take a larger and deeper view of the social implications of technology than we have so far, we will not use our technologies or other resources sufficiently to protect us from the enormous potential for social disruption and disaster implicit in these technologies. Hence, I am going to emphasize aspects of the social impact of technology that I believe present problems which must be solved if we are to enjoy the advantages the technologies can provide. I think we can expect in our type of society, and in a society as rich as ours, that the opportunities will take care of themselves. Put another way, the opportunities do not need to be optimized, but the dangers, I think, must not be minimized.

Sketchy and impressionistic as these observations will be, I have tried to organize them into three general categories. First, I shall make some observations on the general considerations that should be applied to any estimate of the present and contemplated social impact of technology. Then, I want to mention three technologies that I expect will have a wide social impact in the next two decades or so, and which by their characteristics imply a far broader range of social impact than we have felt so far, certainly than we have studied so far. And finally, I will set out some examples of aspects of social impact that should be studied intensively now, if we are to be prepared to use the results of such studies for guiding the felicitous integration of technology and society in the years ahead.

Let me say something else by way of introduction. In many ways I will be implying that the methods and knowledge of our various disciplines are inadequate or nonexistent and, therefore, cannot help us understand what is happening to society vis-à-vis technology. I hope I shall be able to imply convincingly that many, probably most, of what may be the significant issues are *not* being explored effectively and on a scale and with the attention they deserve. If I "get to you" I will thereby, inevitably, threaten our various senses of self and status and purpose; I will question who we are, what we do, why we are what we are, and how important we are to ourselves and to others.

There are typical ways to defend oneself against such threats: by "not hearing" or misunderstanding the speaker's choice of points of emphasis and context of qualifying remarks; by translating and transforming what he emphasizes into a problem or a syntax with which the auditor is comfortable and familiar, thereby shifting the plane of discourse; by attending to the speaker's mood rather than to what he says, and so on. Inevitably, these defenses will operate here just as they do throughout the community of persons and institutions whose favored perspectives, and, thereby, senses of self, are challenged by the interplay of technology and society that makes obsolete or inadequate the conventional techniques for perceiving the society and dealing with it. Indeed, this type of threat to self and these responses to it, produced by a changed and changing world, conveyed from one person to another through the different perspectives of those involved, are in themselves important social impacts of technology about which we know too little, and which we need to understand much better.

With this forewarning, let me now turn to some general considerations on understanding the relationship between technology and society, which I think are too seldom appreciated or made central to the context when specific issues are explored.

1. It is important to remember that some of the significant impacts of technology derive from the accumulated effects of technological changes that have been under way for some time. Let me remind you of three examples: the population explosion, a direct product of medical technology initiated some years ago; the urban chaos that has been fundamentally exacerbated by transportation technology in the form of the private car; and the distortion and disruption of ecology in local areas and, probably, in much larger areas by the wholesale application of pesticides and fungicides, to say nothing of the continental pollution of the ecology by the waste products of many technologies. In the future some of these accumulated consequences will become more emphatic and complex, when the new technologies contribute their consequences too. The technologies we have to be concerned with thus include some older ones as well as the new ones. This is important: we do not have to wait for the new technologies to improve our concepts and methods for understanding their impact. All we have to do is recognize our ignorance and indifference regarding the present social impact—and do something about it.

2. A major purpose of our preoccupation with technology and social change is to prepare for the future. But doing so is going to to be very difficult. There are some social consequences of technology for which we should have begun to prepare yesterday. For example, the type of education appropriate for a rapidly changing work force and for substantial increases in leisure probably requires fundamentally different attitudes and approaches by the teachers in primary and secondary

schools than the present ones. But recruiting the teachers and teaching the teachers requires changes at least in the schools of education and in teachers colleges, and all such sequential changes take time to introduce. The upshot is that most of those teaching today's youngsters and imbuing them with the values and attitudes they will carry into their lives tomorrow are probably conveying the wrong things, because the teachers were wrongly trained and perhaps, in part, wrongly selected. Similarly, problem-solving investigations in the area of urban affairs must be undertaken long in advance of the actual reconstruction and reorganization of our cities. The riots in Los Angeles and the water shortage in New York may be mild precursors of the potential disasters that may otherwise overtake us.

In general, we do not understand and appreciate, and thereby tend to overlook, the nature of the time lag between recognition of a problem and the development of techniques for dealing with it.

We do not allow for—often we do not know how to allow for—the needed intervening period to accumulate knowledge and understanding. I suspect that over the next couple of decades or so, this gap between problem recognition and the development of solutions, or approximate solutions, is going to become increasingly serious: problems will confront us before we are able to deal with them knowledgeably. The integration of technology with other social processes and the felicitous sequencing of contingent social actions to accomplish the integration is going to be much more difficult than it has been in the past.

3. Value conflicts and tensions between generations will very likely increase, especially between the new generation that is moving into political and professional power and is using new types of operational and substantive expertise, and the older generations already occupying the field. These conflicts and their various expressions in differing values and op-

erating techniques will mean that both the pressures and the inhibitions to make the kind of social and technological changes that we are going to need are certain to be very great. As the distinguished public servant, systems theorist, and student of decision processes, Sir Geoffrey Vickers, puts it:

> In the transitional period from the conditions of free fall to those of regulation (at whatever level), political and social life is bound, I think, to become much more collectivist or much more anarchic or—almost certainly—both. Communities national, subnational and even supranational will become more closely knit in so far as they can handle the political, social and psychological problems involved and more violent in their mutual rejections in so far as they cannot. The loyalties we accept will impose wider obligations and more comprehensive acceptance. The loyalties we reject will separate us by wider gulfs from those who accept them and will involve us in fiercer and more unqualified struggles.[1]

What the resolution or stalemate will be between the old and new approaches to the uses of knowledge and power via technology remains to be seen, but an understanding of this conflict in approaches will be prerequisite to an understanding of the social impact of technology.

4. Under what circumstances does an issue become significant or critical? What determines when small percents, such as the unemployment rate, become sufficiently large in absolute numbers to become a major issue? When does indifference become transformed into action, as for example, in the poverty program? When does the ability to extrapolate trends begin to carry real significance in terms of program implementation, as, for example, in the moon program, where the ability to use computer technology to predict whether we could succeed was an important factor in the decision to go ahead.

Understanding the general principles of when, or how, or

why issues become important and become recognized as issues, would be essential for estimating the seriousness of or coping with, among other things, the gap between posing a problem about and finding a solution to an impact of technology on society.

5. Often interpretations of the past are called upon to help interpret the present and to suggest solutions to expected problems in the future. By and large I think these interpretations have been inadequate. First of all, there is often only a surface similarity: the presumed analogy is based on a partial or on a misunderstood picture of the past. A prime example of this is the frequent submission of the Periclean age of Greece as evidence of what our future leisure patterns should or could be. That the "leisured" society of Greece numbered only in the tens of thousands, that it spent much of its time warring or doing those political tasks we have professionalized, that no women were involved, that the system lasted only a couple of generations and then decayed, all such considerations are left out of the supposed apt and happy analogy.

Or consider the argument that since we mastered the first Industrial Revolution, we will not have any enduring trouble with the second industrial revolution that the new technologies represent. But we have not mastered the first Industrial Revolution. Let me mention three social consequences of the first Industrial Revolution that are increasingly acute. While other factors have contributed to them and while in some form or another they may have existed previous to the first Industrial Revolution, undoubtedly our inability to deal with the consequences of that revolution have enormously exacerbated these conditions. The first is the increasing gap between the developed nations and the have-not nations that was widened by the technological prowess of the developed nations, and by their inability to share their technology with the underdeveloped nations. The second example is the persistence—the growth, in some cases—of slums and poverty. This peculiar type of degrading, enclaved existence was the direct result of the first Industrial Revolution's concentration of factory technology, and the resulting transfer of manpower from the farms to the factories. The third example is the alienation from and breakdown of earlier, more stable, systems of value and faith. There are very few students of this problem who feel that the Industrial Revolution has not contributed enormously to the complexity and persistence of the problem.

Another inadequacy in appealing to the past is that even if there is more than a surface similarity in the particular social processes involved, there usually are differences in the surrounding social or physical circumstances, which imply very different consequences than those occurring in the past. Two very important examples of such differences are worth mentioning.

First, never before in history has any nation had such a complex technology combined with a population as large as that of the U.S., now and as it will be—230 million around 1975, 250 million around 1980. Those who assert that because thus and such a technological consequence was coped with in the past, or that a specific social consequence is not new and neither, by implication, are its future consequences, have to consider whether the multiple social and physical consequences of a population of such huge size carry significantly different implications for the future.

The second difference, which we tend to overlook, is that today there very probably are different expectations than there were in the past of what the implications of technology on society will be. Because people are different today, they expect different things to happen to them as a result of technology than people did in the past. It does not help to say, "Their beliefs do not really jibe with the facts." (Especially since we probably do not know the facts.) If they think, for example, that technological change is galloping along at a rate never before equalled, then this results in various reactions by business executives, scientists, pundits, and government officials—to say nothing of the man in the street. These reactions, very likely, are significantly different from those in the past, when this kind of issue did not cross most people's minds. For example, I strongly suspect (but we have not bothered to find out) that a recent major social consequence of the interaction of several technologies is that more types of people are concerned about the future social impact of technology, and more different viewpoints have arisen regarding it, and that these in turn are initiating other social consequences.

Let me now turn to three technologies, biological technology, cybernation, and social engineering. I expect these will, over the next two decades, have very great implications for the nature of society and for the place of the individual in it. I want to emphasize those implications that go beyond those we have tended to preoccupy ourselves with, not because I think they have been unimportant, but because I believe the ones I want to mention are equally important, perhaps more so. Let me again make clear that I recognize that many of the impacts will not be new in kind. However, I do believe that it is likely that the scale and scope, the potency, of their impact, as they interact with an already huge and enormously complex society, will be of an unprecedented order of magnitude. In that potency of impact lie many exciting opportunities, and some very profound problems having to do with the place the individual has in a democractic society, and the way we conduct our lives. Again, I will emphasize problems not because I am certain that they will outrun the opportunities, but rather because I feel that if the problems are not dealt with effectively, the consequences may be so disastrous that we shall never enjoy the opportunities—at least not within the format of presently preferred values. (Of course, a different set of values may be all right or even better than the present ones. But what I want to emphasize is the kind of confrontations these technologies are to our present values, if only to indicate the necessity for understanding the social impact of technology better, so that we may invent or respond to a more appropriate set of values.)

Perhaps the fundamental question that the potency of these technologies raises is how do we deliberately decide how we are going to balance the social costs and social benefits; obviously I mean infinitely more here than the dollar costs and benefits. I think we must do much more than hope for the best or retreat behind some inhuman "averaging out" philosophy. But what do we do if, as I believe they will, the consequences of these technologies will be upon us before we accumulate the understanding needed to establish such a balance—if we ever can accumulate such understanding?

In the application of biological technology—the engineering of man's biological self and his biological enviroment—we will face moral, ethical, psychological, and political issues, which will make those faced by the atomic scientists look like child's play. Biological and chemical warfare will very likely be used much more in local wars, even perhaps in the pacification activities of international police forces. But whether it is used to kill, hurt, nauseate, paralyze, cause hallucination, or to terrify military personel and civilians, the systematic use of biological and chemical warfare will require the resolution of major moral and ethical problems—especially since the most likely victims will be nonwhites in Asia and Africa.

Psychopharmacology is another aspect of biological technology already beginning to confront us with interesting issues. What is to be the role of hallucinogenic chemicals in society? There are two schools of thought on this—even the theologians seem to have taken sides. One is that these chemicals represent sin and corruption; the other, that they are exciting means for enlarging emotional or aesthetic or religious experience. Moreover, new drugs will permit many people, who otherwise would be in mental institutions, to walk the streets and to engage in regular social activities. Questions arise about the "nature" of the individual. How do we judge the extent to which a person is "responsible" for himself in such circumstances? For, while the chemical affects the individual, the person is significant to himself and to society in his *social* context—at work, at home, at play. The consequences are social consequences. In deciding how to deal with such alterers of the ego and of experience (and consequently alterers of the personality after the experience), and in deciding how to deal with the "changed" human beings, we will have to face new questions such as, "Who am I?" "When am I who?" "Who are *they* in relation to me?"

As far as the hallucinogenic agents are concerned, how will we judge whether people, just because they want it, are entitled to a risky if richer emotional experience than that provided by their everyday life? Are these decisions to be left to the individual, like skiing or surfboarding, or will they need legal restrictions like homosexual liaisons or the present use of nonhabitforming marijuana? In general, will "multiple" personalities and increasing amounts of idosyncratic behavior simply be absorbed into the already proliferating scale of novelties, sensations, and leisure-time pursuits, or will they have to be controlled to facilitate the functioning of a stable society? Whatever way is chosen, what are the ethical, legal, political, and psychological considerations needed to help us understand the implications of such altered egos and their control?

A related aspect of biological technology merits mention here: with the increasing dissemination of birth control information and technology, we can expect the pressures on the poor to limit family size to become greater. Though such pressure already exists, in the form of inadequate housing for large, poor families, the pressure may well become more explicit as the "excuses" for having large families inadvertently are eliminated by the pervasive availability of birth control methods. If our laws and ways of operating come to condone this invasion of the right of couples to choose the number of children they want, then a new ethical issue will arise and it will reverberate into other areas of private affairs, conduct, and choice.

A third area in biological technology has to do with organ transplants. Some top research people in this area are convinced that in a few years techniques will have improved substantially. The problem then arises, Who is entitled to what transplant under what criteria of priority? We will have to do better than "women and children first." This situation already exists on a tiny scale with regard to the use of scarce kidney-substitute machines. Difficult as the decisions are now, they will become more difficult and more socially consequential when more people compete for more organs.

Though it is unlikely that organ transplantation will be available to such an extent as to increase substantially the number of people who will live longer, it is likely that developments in the technology of preventing and treating malignant diseases, will mean that there will be still more older people in this society, which has not yet learned to deal humanely with the older population it now has. Thus, developments in biological technology, combined with those from cybernation, in particular, will add to the numbers and to the social problems of older people. The accumulated social impact on our political system, and thereby on our social priorities, will undoubtedly be substantial as the old become a larger proportion of the voting public. Here, too, our understanding of the situation is much too slight at present to give us the knowledge we need to plan effectively for this growing population.

Finally, there is the question of genetic engineering: the deliberate controlled alteration of human inheritance. Late in the next couple of decades, either the capability to do so will exist or almost certainly it will become clear that soon thereafter the capability will exist. Indeed, there are already expressions of exuberant optimism, as well as sober concern, about the possibilities this presents. The optimists, typically, are concerned with technological manipulation, pointing out that maybe we could give everybody an IQ of 140 and eliminate all inherited human "inadequacies." The concerned, typically, look at the looming social and ethical issues that arise from such actions. For example, what are the psychological and, therefore, social consequences of producing a generation of adults who, as youngsters, shared little with their parents because their IQs were so much higher? And who is to decide when an inherited "inadequacy" is one that should be eliminated by genetic engineering? Who will decide where the line is to be drawn on the definition of "inadequacy"? Fundamentally, who will make what decisions about which human beings are to be changed before they are born, and in what way? Or, for that matter, who will determine that we will not use the technology with its implicit potentialities for improving the race?

Cybernation—the application of automation to material processes and the application of computers to symbols—is the second technology I want to mention. I shall not dwell on the usual questions about cybernation's impact on employment: they have been discussed amply enough to demonstrate our awareness of the matter as a social impact—even if we are unclear on what the impact is, much less what it will be. (Indeed, I suspect we put so much of our emphasis on the employment effects of cybernation simply because, having some figures and concepts available, it is psychologically more comfortable to emphasize this narrow aspect of the issue than to struggle with the clear evidence of our wider ignorance.) However, two aspects of cybernation's effects on employment should be mentioned here to broaden the picture.

Substantial numbers of the relatively skilled, including the middle-level manager and the middle-level engineer, are going to be displaced; *Business Week, Newsweek,* and *Time*—a little late—acknowledge this.[2] The competences that have made these people economically valuable in the past will increasingly be made obsolete, either because cybernation, particularly computers, can do the job better, or because the process of rationalizing the overall activity in which they were involved will eliminate, or substantially reduce, the need for humans to do the tasks. Here we have members of a career-oriented, affluent segment of society, who were brought up to believe they possessed all the credentials for a lifetime of advancement, now forced to find another job, or to go back to school and learn something new. They are now perpetually under the threat of being displaced by younger men and by more sophisticated machines. Many of these people are already anxious and insecure personalities—as well as substantially in debt. It is likely, then, that they and their families will suffer considerable disruption as they revise their images of themselves; who they are, what they might become, and how others see them. What will happen to these ex-cynosures, to their aspirations, and to their way of living? And what political action will they take in response to the threats to their status and security?

There is another economic and emotional problem that cybernation's impact on employment level and employment changes will pose: What is to be the future of unskilled women in the work force? In the work force, of which one third are women, about 80 percent are no more than semiskilled; many of them do the clerical and routine service jobs, which cybernation will replace as its application is accelerated by the increasing size of organizations responding to the increasing population. Now, about 60 percent of the $9,000 to $15,000 a year incomes in this country are those of families in which both spouses work. If the unskilled women lose their jobs, there will be less family income, less consumption. And there is also the question of psychic income; many women work for other reasons than to earn money. What will provide this psychic income?

Doubtless, many jobs could be invented, particularly in the human services area, which trained women could fill and which, because of the interpersonal nature of the task, no machine could do. As it now stands, however, and the poverty program demonstrates this, we are neither seriously inventing these jobs nor making the elaborate affort needed to motivate young women so that we can retrain them, and older women, for such jobs. It is likely that this problem will be upon us before techniques for job-producing, motivating, recruiting, and training are sufficiently developed, in which case there will be serious social consequences. But if we do develop such techniques, society will become significantly different from today's, because the roles of so many women will be so different from what they traditionally have been.

This leads me to the third technology: social engineering. I yield to no one in my reservations about the ability of the behavioral sciences to deal with complex issues at the present time, but the evidence to date indicates that this situation will very likely change dramatically in the next two decades. The combination of large research funds and the computer provides the social scientist with both the incentive and the technique to do two things he has always needed to do and never been able to do in order to develop a deep understanding of and technology for the manipulation of social processes.

On the one hand, the computer provides the means for combining in complex models as many variables as the social scientist wants in order to simulate the behavior of men and institutions. In the past, the behavioral scientist simply could not deal with all the many important variables that would help him understand and predict human behavior. Now he can. (This is not to say that everything that is important about the human condition can be so formulated, but much that is important can be put in these terms; almost certainly enough to bring about substantial improvements in our ability to understand and predict behavior.) And then the social scientist can test these models against conditions representing "real life." For, on the other hand, the computer has a unique capacity for collecting and processing enormous amounts of data about the state of individuals and of society today—not that of ten years ago. Thus, the behavioral scientist not only can know the state of society *now,* as represented by these data, but he can use them to test and refine his theoretical models. The convergence of government programs and the computer is of critical importance; it will result in an efflorescence of longitudinal studies of individual and institutional change as functions of the changes in the social and physical environment. Such knowledge, now essentially nonexistent, will inevitably increase our ability to effect social change. And given the convergence of the powerful technologies and our already enormously complex and huge society, it would seem that social manipulation will be necessary if we are to introduce appropriate changes in society at the appropriate times. The problem, of course, is: Who is to make the decision who is to be manipulated and for what ends?

Let me now turn to some general questions regarding the social impact of technology—questions that to some extent refer to circumstances already with us, and which seem to me to be greatly in need of serious and extensive study. Let me hasten to add that I am certain that in many cases we do not at present know how to study these problems, but if we do not start now to try to invent means for doing so, we shall be in a far worse position when the time comes for us to understand these issues better. Again, the time lag problem bedevils us.

What happens to the sense of self in a world of giant and pervasive man-made events, especially when, at the same time, we insist on emphasizing the autonomy of the individual? We talk about the importance of the individual and of the wealth of options this world offers him. Yet, we have surrounded him with pollution, radiation, megalopolis, etc., which, though man-made, may appear to many people to be of such power and scale as to dominate them like "acts of God." How does a man see himself in relation to his espoused ideal of individual autonomy when he also sees other *men* and man-made circumstances, as awesome and implacable and often as impersonal as "acts of God," framing his destiny?

What kind of personalities live most fully in the midst of

multiple and simultaneous change? Daniel Bell has pointed out that we are experiencing the end of the rational vision, that events today (and more so tomorrow) do not have simple cause and effect sequences, that, instead, events all happen at once and in circular and probabilistic ways.[3] What kind of person can live meaningfully in that type of world, and can keep in touch with it?

I suspect three kinds of responses will have increasing social implications as technology alters the scale of events that define the individual to himself—and thereby the ways in which he responds to the world.

One response is that of "selective involvement." People pick the issues and things they are going to respond to and be responsible about, and ignore the rest. We know people do this now, deliberately or, more often, unconsciously: there are limits to the amount of information humans can process in a given amount of time.

Therefore, it behooves us to examine carefully the degree of validity, as measured by actual behavior, of the statement that a benefit of technology will be to increase the number of options and alternatives the individual can choose from. In principle, it could; in fact, the individual may use any number of psychological devices to avoid the discomfort of information overload, and thereby keep the range of alternatives to which he responds much narrower than that which technology in principle makes available to him.

Another type of response, now evident among returned Peace Corps volunteers, college students, and some executives, is withdrawal—pulling out of the big system, looking for environments in which one can have face-to-face relationships in a simple, less technologized, more direct world.

A third response, protest, is exemplified by such things as the urban race riots and the Berkeley demonstrations. Here, the individual responds to overwhelming complexity by sidestepping the legal or ethical constraints that sustain or are at least associated with the complexity. (It is worth noting that a battle cry in the Berkeley protests was "Put your body where your punch card is!" It was one of the chief reasons for the sit-in in Spraoul Hall.) I suspect that these attempts, these experiments, to simplify an increasingly complex world will have very important social consequences, produced, in part, by a proliferating technology. If these responses are important in the future, we need to know much more about them, at least as responses to technology, than we do now.

Another way to look at the implications of technology for the individual is to consider the roles he plays. Two examples typify the unanswered and, for the most part, unstudied, questions in this area. The psychatrist Robert Rieff has suggested that to the extent that tomorrow's society is service-oriented (material productivity becoming increasingly cybernated), many men will play roles that traditionally, in our society, have been women's roles, i.e., person-to-person helping roles. What, then, happens to the image and conduct of men? What happens to the relation between the sexes, as the hard won pattern of women competing with men for "male" jobs is reversed, and men begin to compete with women for "female" jobs?

A second role implication: as society puts more and more emphasis on rationalization, logic, science, and technology, and as our educational system reflects this emphasis from the lower grades on, what will be the role of the mother—the female—in preserving the ineffable, the intuitive, and the aesthetic in the basic learning experiences of the young? This, traditionally, has been what we expect of women, but traditionally we have deprecated those contributions, at least out of one side of our mouth. Will we come to appreciate this contribution more? Will we insist that women fulfill this role more effectively, or will we further deprecate its utility in a society oriented toward technology? And what effect will our choice have on our way of life and on societal goals?

The opportunities and problems that increased leisure—resulting from the increased productivity of the new technologies—provides, to help individuals find themselves or to extend the means by which they lose themselves, have been commented on extensively and, to my mind, unimaginatively and unperceptively. I will not explore the issue here. A couple of observations, however, are in order.

An increasing number of theologians and religious denominations are becoming concerned with this problem. Their theologies assert that it is through work that man gains his salvation and fulfills himself. If work is to be a much less significant part of life for more people, what are the revisions in theology and the revisions in religious bureaucracies required to cope with this? On the other hand, the Protestant ethic, in its original form, may not be so pervasive as we have surmised, or at least its modes of implementation may be changing. Instead of leisure being a reward for hard work, we "travel first and pay later"—which may mean, of course, that work is now a "punishment" for taking the leisure first. Or, of course, it may mean that many people no longer need the justification of work to comfortably enjoy a vacation.

We can assume that leisure should have meaning in addition to that associated with recreation and hobbies, as is now taught. But it is hard to see how the state of mind required for this is to be conveyed to young people in an educational system stressing efficiency, and by adults who themselves are products of the Protestant ethic. Tranquility, contemplation, loafing, the cultivation of self, require a different school and different teachers. Just how real or serious would be the variety of social consequences implicit in these observations remains to be seen. Again we have not studied and again we have not tried to lay out the implications in a sufficiently elaborate social and technological context.

What *is* to be the relationship between the churches and an increasingly rationalized and technologized society? In a society preoccupied with dealing with the average, with the mass of the population, with grandiose schemes for remaking man and his environment (often accompanied by an arrogance indistinguishable from *hubris*), will it be the role of the churches to insist on another set of values for judging the direction and purpose of man, to protect the ideal of the individual and the validity of extralogical and transcendent motives and experiences? Here, indeed, a profound confrontation between two cultures *may* occur or, perhaps, one may absorb the other. Whatever the case may be, the consequences of the new technologies for the churches are bound to be great.

Consider the changing role of the scientist and the scientist-engineer. The symbiosis between science and technology has, as we all know, evolved into big science and big technology, and these two, in turn, are dependent on big money, which inevitably means big politics. The result, as a Report of the Committee on Science in the Promotion of Human Welfare of the American Association for the Advancement of Science argues, is that the integrity of science has been eroded and that in the absence of procedures (which have not been invented, much less implemented) the erosion of the integrity of science will very likely increase in the future.[4] In part, this is because in the future still bigger technological investments in science and engineering will be needed. Hence, still more funds will have to be raised, and political methods will have to be used still more often to mediate between the needs of technology, the other needs of society, and the needs of competing groups within the science and engineering communities. Inevitably, there will be persistent, very likely increasing, confusion between the political and rhetorical validity and utility of scientific knowledge and its inherent scientific validity and utility. For not only will scientists and engineers turn to politics to get the technology they want in the first place, but they will use politics to praise, apologize for, or criticize the social consequences of that technology when they happen.

> [The] combination of esoteric knowledge and political power alters the function and character of the scientific elites. They no longer merely advise on the basis of expert knowledge, but they are also the champions of policies promoted with unrivaled authority and frequently determined by virtue of it. In the eyes both of the political authorities and the public at large, the scientific elites appear as the guardians of the *arcana imperii,* the secret remedies for public ills.
>
> As the nature and importance of scientific knowledge transform the nature and functions of the scientific elites, the availability of democratic control becomes extinguished. Scientific knowledge is by its very nature esoteric knowledge; since it is inaccessible to the public at large, it is bound to be secret. The public finds itself in the same position vis-à-vis scientific advice as do the political authorities: unable to retrace the arguments underlying the scientific advice, it must take that advice on faith.[5]

The growing potency of social engineering will become a crucial ethical issue for the behavioral scientist. Whether he is working for the government, for business, for Madison Avenue, for the CIA, for the Poverty Program, or is doing basic research, the results of his work are going to be used to "guide," "stimulate," "motivate," and "manipulate" society. Again, it is the potency of the technology, its capacity to do wonderful good or monstrous evil, that will make the situation in the future different from the past.

This ethical problem: whether to assist in the growth of social engineering, is going to become ever more serious as the potency of social engineering increases. And right now we have no ethical or scientific models for dealing with this problem. One example of this dilemma: The Job Corps trainees will have very elaborate computerized reports prepared about them, to cover their whole social and psychological background, their experience in the Job Corps, and what happens to them for several years after they have left the Job Corps. The reason for these records is a very good one—they will improve the selection and training techniques. However, such a record also means that the Job Corps trainee will no longer have a private life: once recorded, his life history will always be available in this form. The dilemma that faces the social scientist is that on the one hand he needs this kind of information to improve the Job Corps, and that, on the other hand, so much personal information made available to as yet unspecified people, may completely undermine the conventional privilege and social advantages of privacy.

Underlying these issues is the profoundly important one: what are the implications, for the form and conduct of democratic political processes, of the complex social issues that technology generates and of the esoteric methods technology provides, for dealing with these complex issues? The increasing complexity of social problems and of the techniques for dealing with them will mean that the average well-educated person—to say nothing of the man in the street—will no longer be able to understand what the issues and the alternatives are.

This will be partly a matter of the complexity of the issues and of the technologies for defining, interpreting, planning for, and then dealing with, them. It will be partly a matter of the partial availability of knowledge. Often the issues will be politically sensitive and, as now, the interested parties will release only what they wish to release. Moreover, laymen able to use the knowledge, if they did have it, would need reasoning abilities which most people now lack. They would have to understand that the world picture is in most critical cases a statistical one, not black or white. These laymen would have to be comfortable dealing with multivariable problems operating in multiple feedback processes, where cause and effect are inextricably intermixed, and where it is often meaningless to try to differentiate one from the other. And they would have to be comfortable with making judgment based on a much longer time perspective than most people are used to now. They would have to be able to think ahead ten and twenty years, and make their judgments accordingly. These are not characteristics we are going to find in large numbers in our population: our educational system simply does not mass-produce such people—and evidently will not do so for some years to come. But if we are to operate a democracy, the need for such reasoning abilities will be upon us sooner than that. Indeed, it is already upon us. The political scientist and pundit, Joseph Kraft, recently observed:

> To apply common sense to what is visible on the surface is to be almost always wrong; it produces about as good an idea of how the world goes round as that afforded by the Ptolemaic system. A true grasp of even the slightest transaction requires special knowledge and the ability to use abstractions which, like the Copernican system, are at odds with common-sense impressions. Without this kind of knowledge, it is difficult to know what to think about even such prominent matters as the United Nations financing problem, or the bombing of North Vietnam, or the farm program, or the federal budget—which is one reason that most people don't know what they think about these questions. The simple fact is that the stuff of public life eludes the grasp of the ordinary man. Events have become professionalized.[6]

Moreover, the problems, whether they be urban renewal, air pollution, education for the new age, Medicare, international development programs, the exploitation of the oceans, assigning technology development priorities, etc., will be too complicated to be dealt with effectively by the techniques that have characterized our society to date. And the issues will be too critical, the potentials for and scale of disaster too great to stake our social survival upon conventional approaches—even when they are undertaken (as they rarely are) with the best of disinterested goodwill. All we have to do is to look at the looming disaster our cities represent, to recognize that we are going to have to do much better.

The tasks we face, then, will require the full use of whatever rationalized techniques we have, and these techniques will proliferate in the years ahead with advances in the social sciences, with increasing use of computers, data banks, simulation, system analyses, operations research, and so on.

In consequence, planners and decision makers will be confronted with a set of circumstances that will also suggest important changes in the democratic process. The competing demands for human and physical resources, necessarily expended over long periods of time, will require the development of ways to assign priorities and to revise costly efforts, even if it is politically uncomfortable and institutionally disruptive. At present we have neither the priority scheme nor the means for efficiently and reliably transcending conventional and institutional restraints. Yet, obviously, we will have to be able to choose between major technological and social developments, and we will have to be able to maintain or alter these decisions more in the light of their real accomplishments, rather than in the light of political commitments. Furthermore, because of the massive needs of the society, there will be a tendency to respond to average human and social requirements, rather than to the needs of the individual qua individual. This tendency will be exacerbated by the inherent characteristics of technologies, of systems analysis, and of operations research and computer simulation. The pressures to value those things most about the society that can be described and dealt with in terms of the techniques available, and the pressures to deal with the massive needs of the society will make it especially difficult for the policy maker and decision maker to preserve a sensitivity for and responsibility toward the idea of the idiosyncratic and extrarational needs of the individual.

If, then, we are to preserve the ideal of the cherished individual we will need wise men more than we will need technically skilled men, though obviously we will need the technically skilled men too. As it is, we do not know how to produce wise men, and we do not know how to provide them with an environment that will encourage their wisdom to blossom and act. Yet without wise men, the chances are that the democratic concept and the Judeo-Christian tradition built around the obligations and rights of the individual will be lost under the crush of the vast needs of the society and the enormous potency of the technologies put into operation in a massive society to meet those needs. How shall we prepare for and invent the new forms of democracy and the new roles to be played by citizen and leader in such a system?

Above, I implied the need for the ability to change institutions rapidly. This, too, is a consequence of the impact of technologies on society, for through their effects technologies make the mandates of institutions, and the validity of the operating styles within the mandates, obsolete. Yet institutions persist and change only slowly and usually reluctantly—barring some kind of disaster. Some observers have pointed out the potentialities for society if we apply our technologies. They then bemoan the apathy of the public and the ineffectualness of institutions because they do not take advantage of the technologies. The usual interpretation of this state of affairs is that we lack "leadership." But this is a naïve solution and a premature definition of the problem. The question really is how to change institutions so that leadership arises in a given situation and then acts. Here our formal knowledge, limited as it is, makes it clear that this is an extremely difficult condition to deal with expeditiously.

As institutions produce and use the new technologies, they inevitably will have to change at a rate concomitant with the changes produced in the society by the very technologies they have encouraged and applied. But getting institutions or, rather, the people in them, to shift their perspectives radically as technology radically alters reality; getting the members of institutions to risk statuses, self-images, empires, in order to prepare for future needs, is an enormously difficult task, usually only successfully accomplished after a major institutional disaster has occurred. Over the years we can expect that the social sciences will provide us with more knowledge about how to make these changes quickly (or perhaps provide us with an understanding of why, if we want to preserve a humanitarian set of values, institutions cannot be changed quickly). But even if we assume the former, there are still many years ahead in which institutions will lag behind in their ability to respond to the real environment as it is altered by technologies, and this lag will become increasingly dangerous. What we do now and in the long run about this impact of technology is a matter that I believe deserves intensive attention.

Perhaps we might do well to spend some significant portion of our professional time stockpiling solutions to social problems, which we cannot hope to get into our social system now, but which we can reasonably expect to apply if some of these problems back up on us to the point where we cannot cope with them within the present social format. It is after disasters that institutions can most easily be changed.

Let me close with some comments on the special social impact on scholars or action-oriented professionals of the very *question* of the social impact of technology. One direct effect of the new technologies is to challenge deeply the adequacy of our academic disciplines for dealing with the kind of world they are producing. We sit here and talk learnedly about economic and social processes—rates of change, institutional process, etc.—but my impression is that few of our disciplines or techniques are now really adequate. Even in the well-studied area of productivity and technological change we cannot be sanguine about our methods. As Solomon Fabricant recently said, "The problem of measurement has not yet been solved. . . . There are competing and widely differing measurements of technological change. . . . I'm afraid that people talk about both the past and the future . . . with more confidence than is warranted by the available knowledge about technological change."[7] In the few cases where our techniques are adequate, they are not being used broadly or intensively enough to deal with the multiple issues that must be understood if we are going to secure the advantages these new technologies possess.

If my impression is accurate, we face some very uncomfortable questions, which, as scholars and professionals, we are morally bound to wrestle with far more than we have until now. What about our research techniques? What must we do—and what must we abandon of what we now take status and comfort in—to get methods that adequately tackle the issues? We must find out what we should really be studying, even if it means breaking down cherished disciplinary barriers and repudiating the importance of the issues we have studied up to now? Over the next few decades many of our techniques are likely to become much more adequate, but what is our role until then? It seems to me that we belong to one of the institutions of society whose members and operating styles need to be shaken up quickly—we need to have our awarenesses of reality enlarged and refined and revised if we are to make our contribution in good conscience and with significant effect.

One might decide, of course, that even with all these conflicts and changes and even without the participation of the scholars, some kind of accommodation will be worked out. Probably so, but there is the possibility that the accommodation will be one we will not like. And there is also the possibility that there will be no accommodation. Certainly ours would not be the first society that disappeared because it could not find a way to accommodate in time to changes generated within it by its own momentum and style.

Chapter 14

Housing and Mental Health in Developing Countries

JOSEF PH. HES

A PRACTICAL PROBLEM THAT AROUSED OUR INTEREST IN THIS subject. Many of the hypochondriacal patients under treatment in our clinic apply to us for recommendations that will enable them to acquire new flats. These patients complain that their mental condition is influenced by their poor housing and they are convinced that their health will improve with a change of abode.

We decided to investigate this problem from three angles:

(1) The literature on the influence of change of abode on mental condition.
(2) Man's attitude to his home.
(3) Study of our own cases.

Study of the Literature

Grootenboer[1] demonstrated a connexion between housing conditions and behavioural disturbances. Before the second world war young couples started their conjugal life in a separate flat away from their parents. Due to a shortage in the post-war period young couples had to live with their parents. In several cases the removal of the young couple to a separate new apartment relieved tensions between grandparents and parents. On the other hand it was frequently found that the first child born to a couple during their stay with the parents served as a kind of reminder of this unhappy time. This child would find difficulties in adapting itself to the new home and would yearn for the coddling and attention provided by the grandparents. As a result of the parents' rejection of the child in whom they saw a remnant of their past sufferings, and because of the inaccessibility of the grandparents' love, behavioural disturbances developed in the children observed in this research that found their expression in the home and at school. In such cases a change of abode reduced parental tensions, but created mental problems in certain of the children.

Martin, Brotherson and Chave[2] found a negative relationship between housing conditions and mental pathology in a study from England. It was found that the number of psychiatric hospitalizations in a new housing estate was from 23 percent to 74 percent higher than the expected number when compared to the average number of hospitalizations in England and Wales. The greatest abnormality was shown by the fifty-five and over age group. Women of forty-five years and over, who made up only 13 percent of the population of a development town, formed 55 percent of the admissions of the psychiatric hospital. Martin concluded that change of abode had constituted a serious psychological stress and caused mental breakdown particularly in the case of aging women.

An additional finding in this study was that the rates for neurosis and ill-defined nervous conditions from records of general practitioners greatly exceeded the rates found by Logan.[3]

Mention should be made here of the work done by Tyhurst[4] that stresses the appearance of depressive-paranoid patterns after a change of abode and after a change in social strata.

A most impressive piece of research by Wilner and co-workers[5] investigated a thousand families (four hundred experimental families and six hundred control families) and examined the influence of change of abode upon the general and mental health of the subjects. The investigators interviewed the families eleven times over a period of three years, and one of the interviews took place before the move. One of the most outstanding findings of this work is the discovery of a rise in morbidity in the under-twenty age-group during the first five months after the move. A further finding was the even higher morbidity in the thirty-five to thirty-nine age-group, which was, however, found to be due to a small group of subjects who had suffered from chronic diseases before the move. This work teaches us not to draw hasty conclusions from the effects of moving. General and mental health is liable to change after the move has taken place. The authors close their work with the statement that no drastic changes take place from a statistical point of view, on moving house, but that there is a tendency to improvement in general and mental health after a period of one year.

This is not a comprehensive review, but is intended to emphasize various aspects of the problem of the connexion between change of abode and mental health.

Man's Attitude to His Home

What do we know of man's attitude to his home? The information at our disposal is drawn from various sources including psycho-analytical research,[6] projective tests,[7] and phenomenological studies.[8]

Man's first home is his mother's womb. From the day of his birth to the day when he enters his own dwelling as a grown man, there unfolds a long series of developments. On the one hand the child is bound to, and dependent upon his mother, while on the other hand he feels the urge to break away from her, and to experience his own individuality. This development covers the differentiation of the self from the object world and reaches its peak in the successful solution of the Oedipus situation, when the male child finds himself capable of discarding the mother as a sexual object.

Langeveld, who describes this development from the phenomenological aspect, draws our attention to the child's need for a hiding place. Children love to hide in cupboards, and there is no doubt that this lure of the cupboard represents a regression to the mother's body, and the need for privacy, at one and the same time. Importance is also attributed to the lookout, which allows the child to participate in activities and occasions from which his age should preclude him. The author stresses the stages of development in this need of a hiding place in the life of the child. The tiny child is satisfied with his place behind the furniture or the curtain where he can be alone yet close to the rest of the family. The school child isolates himself further afield and creates a place for himself in the garden, in the woods, and elsewhere. In adolescence, boys and girls find such hiding places unsatisfying and desire a private room of their own. The adult lives in his own house and does not relate to it purely as a place of abode, for this place is also significant as a status symbol.

This development applies to children of Western cultures, which stress the importance of the child's independence. We have insufficient knowledge of the function of the home in the development of the nonwestern child who has been reared in a large extended family where no importance is given to independence and individuality.

The projective tests which were brought into daily psychological use by Buck[9] emphasize the fact that man expresses himself in the drawing of a picture of a house. In the house-tree-person test, the house represents femininity and the tree masculinity. Tree and house also represent father and mother or the masculine and feminine aspects of man himself.

Illustrative Case Reports

I will now describe some cases from our clinic which illustrate certain aspects of the problem of housing and mental health.

(A) Simcha, A., female, aged 40 years, born in Morocco, referred to our clinic for mental tension, social withdrawal, and hypochondriacal complaints. The patient is dissatisfied with her present home. During the intake process it emerged that she had moved to this apartment at her own volition, to avoid contact between her daughter and a neighbour of the previous home. When, however, her daughter persisted in this relationship with the man of her choice and indeed became his wife, our patient grew exceedingly dissatisfied with her new home. This had disappointed her as she had expected it to prevent her daughter's undesirable marriage. It had also separated her from her relatives who lived close to her former home.

(B) Sason, E., male, aged 40 years, born in Iraq. The patient is of medium intelligence with antisocial behaviour, referred to our clinic for depression. Preliminary talks revealed that the patient's family, consisting of himself, his wife and six children, existed in wretched living conditions. The wife endured great hardship, as all six of her children had had rheumatic fever and her husband was frequently unemployed. As a result of intervention by the Anti-Rheumatic Fever League, this family was allotted an apartment in a residential area on the easiest terms. The patient's wife, the pillar of the family, had been able to bear the burden of her children's sickness and her husband's unemployment because of the proximity and support of her relations; she was broken since moving away from them. The father of the family, a passive and weak personality, was sent to the clinic for treatment after the collapse of the wife who had been his support until the change of abode.

This case stresses the importance of the extended family

unit in the maintenance of balance between the roles of husband and wife in Oriental communities.

(C) Nissim, M., male, aged 32 years, born in Morocco. This head of the family was referred to our clinic for stomach pains, nervousness and excessive smoking. The patient is fourth in a family of ten children, very dependent upon his parents, and incapable of expressing anger—"Eats himself up inside." There is no verbal communication between husband and wife. In the event of family conflicts the husband flees to his parents who reside in the south of the country and the wife turns to the social service bureau to complain about her husband. The wife is the youngest of seven children, and her mother died when she was six months old. The wife has a domineering and demanding personality while the husband is of a passive and dependent nature. When both husband and wife are invited to the clinic the husband sits on one bench in the waiting room while his wife sits on another as far away from him as possible. When they come for a joint discussion the husband is mute and the wife does the talking. The wife makes many demands including different work for her husband, financial support from the social services, an apartment closer to her husband's place of work, and transfer of the family to where her parents-in-law reside. The wife has great expectations of this move, since her father moved from Rabat to Casablanca at a time of great financial hardship and thus improved his family's condition: "change of place, change of luck."

Particularly in patients from nonwestern communities who have married by family decree and not by mutual choice, we find a tendency to seek family support when friction arises between man and wife. In this present case, the family quarrel was caused by the conflicting personalities of husband and wife. She saw the solution of their strife in the experience of her childhood when a change of abode had brought a change for the better.

Discussion

When we examined the case records of patients who turned to our clinic for help in their housing situation, we were impressed with the fact that not a single family returned to the clinic to report the favourable results of the move. If we wish to learn which factors are operating in cases of improvement in the general and mental health condition after moving to a different apartment and/or a different residential area, we will have to invite these patients for a follow-up study. It is clear from our material, and from Wilner's study,[10] that an evaluation of the effects of housing on mental functioning is a costly and time-consuming enterprise with many pitfalls.

The preponderance in our material of non-Western patients, that is, those from Mediterranean countries such as North Africa, Iraq, and Turkey, was the second phenomenon to draw our attention. We suggest as a speculative explanation of this phenomenon that families of European background know ways and means for improving their housing situation.

In the value system of western immigrants the house occupies a different position from that of their nonwestern neighbours. In the western family, the home is a place for the nuclear family exclusively and stands also as a status symbol. Emphasis on hospitality and food are predominant in nonwestern families and housing itself seems to fulfil a secondary need. Of course these categorical statements do not hold in our present society influx, in which many nonwestern families pattern their lives according to European standards.

In this paper I have not paid attention to the importance of the neighbourhood, to moving within the neighbourhood and moving to a different residential area. There are many studies on the influence of slums and crowding on mental health, criminal behaviour, and the like, but these are mainly of a sociological nature and would not add much to the solution of our problem of the vicissitudes of housing and mental health.

Study of our cases showed us that the unrealistic expectations characterized the problem of Mrs. Simcha. She did not suffer from crowding or a bad neighbourhood, but regarded the move as a last resource to solve the problem of the undesirable relationship of her daughter and a neighbour. After the move proved unsuccessful the patient became very dissatisfied with her new apartment that was far removed from her close relatives.

We learned from Mr. Sason's case that in recommending rehousing it is not just one factor such as the children's health that should be taken into account. A thorough study should be made of the family situation as a whole including the relationship of the head of the houshold and his wife and their specific needs, such as closeness to parents and relatives, proximity to the husband's job, and school for the children.

The last case, Mr. Nissim, emphasized the importance of the extended family but also underlined the role of childhood experiences, which determined the expectations about moving. When things went badly, the wife recalled a similar situation in her childhood, when her father had decided to move to a different city and conditions had improved.

In reviewing our cases we find that we do not know which factors in the move to a new apartment favour improvement in the mental state.

Particular aspects of this problem which seem to be of some importance and which might usefully be assessed in future studies are:

(A) The motives which lead a patient to apply for a recommendation for relocation.

(B) The patient's attitude towards his present living conditions: advantages, disadvantages, and unrealistic attitudes.

(C) The expectations he has about the new apartment.
(D) The dynamic structure and the social and ethnic affiliation of the family of the applicant and the differential needs of the various family members.
(E) Living conditions in childhood and the significance of previous moves.
(F) Attitudes towards parental figures of the applicant (especially mother).
(G) The place of the house in the value system of non-western patients.

Chapter 15

Grieving for a Lost Home

MARC FRIED

FOR SOME TIME WE HAVE KNOWN THAT THE FORCED DISlocation from an urban slum is a highly disruptive and disturbing experience. This is implicit in the strong, positive attachments to the former slum residential area—in the case of this study the West End of Boston—and in the continued attachment to the area among those who left before any imminent danger of eviction. Since we were observing people in the midst of a crisis, we were all too ready to modify our impressions and to conclude that these were likely to be transitory reactions. But the postrelocation experiences of a great many people have borne out their most pessimistic prerelocation expectations. There are wide variations in the success of postrelocation adjustment and considerable variability in the depth and quality of the loss experience. But for the majority it seems quite precise to speak of their reactions as expressions of *grief*. These are manifest in the feelings of painful loss, the continued longing, the general depressive tone, frequent symptoms of psychological or social or somatic distress, the active work required in adapting to the altered situation, the sense of helplessness, the occasional expressions of both direct and displaced anger, and tendencies to idealize the lost place.[1]

At their most extreme, these reactions of grief are intense, deeply felt, and, at times, overwhelming. In response to a series of questions concerning the feelings of sadness and depression which people experienced *after* moving, many replies were unambiguous: "I felt as though I had lost everything," "I felt like my heart was taken out of me," "I felt like taking the gaspipe," "I lost all the friends I knew," "I always felt I had to go home to the West End and even now I feel like crying when I pass by," "Something of me went with the West End," "I felt cheated," "What's the use of thinking about it," "I threw up a lot," "I had a nervous breakdown." Certainly, some people were overjoyed with the change and many felt no sense of loss. Among 250 women, however, 26 percent report that they still feel sad or depressed two years later, and another 20 percent report a long period (six months to two years) of sadness or depression. Altogether, therefore, at least 46 percent give evidence of a fairly severe grief reaction or worse. And among 316 men, the data show only a slightly smaller percentage (38 percent) with long-term grief reactions. The true proportion of depressive reactions is undoubtedly higher since many women and men who report no feelings of sadness or depression indicate clearly depressive responses to other questions.

In answer to another question, "How did you feel when you saw or heard that the building you had lived in was torn down?" a similar finding emerges. As in the previous instance, the responses are often quite extreme and most frequently quite pathetic. They range from those who replied: "I was glad because the building had rats," to moderate responses such as "the building was bad but I felt sorry," and "I didn't want to see it go," to the most frequent group comprising such reactions as "it was like a piece being taken from me," "I felt terrible," "I used to stare at the spot where the building stood," "I was sick to my stomach." This question in particular, by its evocative quality, seemed to stir up sad memories even among many persons who denied any feeling of sadness or depression. The difference from the previous result is indicated by the fact that 54 percent of the women and 46 percent of the men report severely depressed or disturbed reactions; 19 percent of the women and about 31 percent of the men report satisfaction or indifference; and 27 percent of the women and 23 percent of the men report moderately depressed or ambivalent feelings. Thus it is clear that, for the majority of those who were displaced from the West End, leaving their residential area involved a moderate or extreme sense of loss and an accompanying affective reaction of grief.

While these figures go beyond any expectation which we had or which is clearly implied in other studies, the realization that relocation was a crisis with potential danger to mental health for many people was one of the motivating factors for this investigation.* In studying the impact of relocation on the lives of a working-class population through a comparison of prerelocation and postrelocation interview data, a number of issues arise concerning the psychology of urban living which have received little systematic attention. Yet, if we are to understand the effects of relocation and the significance of the loss of a residential environment, it is essential that we have a deeper appreciation of the psychological implications of both physical and social aspects of residential experience. Thus we are led to formulations which deal with the functions and meanings of the residential area in the lives of working-class people.

The Nature of the Loss in Relocation: The Spatial Factor

Any severe loss may represent a disruption in one's relationship to the past, to the present, and to the future. Losses generally bring about fragmentation of routines, of relationships, and of expectations, and frequently imply an alteration in the world of physically available objects and spatially oriented action. It is a disruption in that sense of continuity which is ordinarily a taken-for-granted framework for functioning in a universe which has temporal, social, and spatial

* This is implicit in the prior work on "crisis" and situational predicaments by Dr. Erich Lindemann under whose initiative the current work was undertaken and carried out.

dimensions. From this point of view, the loss of an important place represents a change in a potentially significant component of the experience of continuity.

But why should the loss of a place, even a very important place, be so critical for the individual's sense of continuity; and why should grief at such loss be so widespread a phenomenon? To clarify this, it is necessary to consider the meaning which this area, the West End of Boston, had for the lives of its inhabitants. In an earlier paper we tried to assess this, and came to conclusions that corroborate, although they go further, the results from the few related studies.

> In studying the reasons for satisfaction that the majority of slum residents experience, two major components have emerged. On the one hand, the residential area is the region in which a vast and interlocking set of social networks is localized. And, on the other, the physical area has considerable meaning as an extension of home, in which various parts are delineated and structured on the basis of a sense of belonging. These two components provide the context in which the residential area may so easily be invested with considerable, multiple-determined meaning. . . . the greatest proportion of this working-class group . . . shows a fairly common experience and usage of the residential area . . . dominated by a conception of the local area beyond the dwelling unit as an integral part of home. This view of an area as home and the significance of local people and local places are so profoundly at variance with typical middle-class orientations that it is difficult to appreciate the intensity of meaning, the basic sense of identity involved in living in the particular area.[2]

Nor is the intense investment of a residential area, both as an important physical space and as the locus for meaningful interpersonal ties, limited to the West End.[3] What is common to a host of studies is the evidence for the integrity of the urban, working-class, slum community as a social and spatial unit. It is the sense of belonging someplace, in a particular place which is quite familiar and easily delineated, in a wide area in which one feels "at home." This is the core of meaning of the local area. And this applies for many people who have few close relationships within the area. Even familiar and expectable streets and houses, faces at the window, and people walking by, personal greetings and impersonal sounds may serve to designate the concrete foci of a sense of belonging somewhere and may provide special kinds of interpersonal and social meaning to a region one defines as "home."

It would be impossible to understand the reactions both to dislocation and to relocation and, particularly, the depth and frequency of grief responses without taking account of working-class orientations to residential areas. One of our primary theses is that the strength of the grief reaction to the loss of the West End is largely a function of prior orientations to the area. Thus, we certainly expect to find that the greater a person's prerelocation commitment to the area, the more likely he is to react with marked grief. This prediction is confirmed again and again by the data.* † For the women, among those

* The analysis involves a comparison of information from interviews administered *before* relocation with a depth of grief index derived from follow-up interviews approximately two years *after* relocation. The prerelocation interviews were administered to a randomly selected sample of 473 women from households in this area at the time the land was taken by the city. The postrelocation interviews were completed with 92 percent of the women who had given prerelocation interviews and with 87 percent of the men from those households in which there was a husband in the household. Primary emphasis will be given to the results with the women since we do not have as full a range of prerelocation information for the men. However, since a split schedule was used for the postrelocation interviews, the depth of grief index is available for only 259 women.

† Dr. Jason Aronson was largely responsible for developing the series of questions on grief. The opening question of the series was: Many people have told us that just after they moved they felt sad or depressed. Did you feel this way? This was followed by the three specific questions on which the index was based: (1) Would you describe how you felt? (2) How long did these feelings last? (3) How did you feel when you saw or heard that the building you had lived in was torn down? Each person was given a score

who had said they liked living in the West End *very much* during the prerelocation interviews, 73 percent evidence a severe postrelocation grief reaction; among those who had less extreme but positive feelings about living in the West End, 53 percent show a similar order of grief; and among those who were ambivalent or negative about the West End, only 34 percent show a severe grief reaction. Or, considering a more specific feature of our formulation, the prerelocation view of the West End as "home" shows an even stronger relationship to the depth of postrelocation grief. Among those women who said they had no real home, only 20 percent give evidence of severe grief; among those who claimed some other area as their real home, 34 percent fall into the severe grief category; but among the women for whom the *West End* was the real home, 68 percent report severe grief reactions. Although the data for the men are less complete, the results are substantially similar. It is also quite understandable that the length of West End residence should bear a strong relationship to the loss reaction, although it is less powerful than some of the other findings and almost certainly it is not the critical component.

More directly relevant to our emphasis on the importance of places, it is quite striking that the greater the area of the West End that was known, the more likely there is to be a severe grief response. Among the women who said they knew only their own block during the prerelocation interview, only 13

---

from 1 to 4 on the basis of the coded responses to these questions and the scores were summated. For purposes of analysis, we divided the final scores into three groups: minimal grief, moderate grief, and severe or marked grief. The phrasing of these questions appears to dispose the respondent to give a "grief" response. In fact, however, there is a tendency to reject the idea of "sadness" among many people who show other evidence of a grief response. In cross-tabulating the "grief" scores with a series of questions in which there is no suggestion of sadness, unhappiness, or dissatisfaction, it is clear that the grief index is the more severe criterion. Those who are classified in the severe grief category almost invariably show severe grief reactions by any of the other criteria; but many who are categorized as "minimal grief" on the index fall into the extremes of unhappiness or dissatisfaction on the other items.

percent report marked grief; at the other extreme, among those who knew most of the West End, 64 percent have a marked grief reaction. This relationship is maintained when a wide range of interrelated variables is held constant. Only in one instance, when there is a generally negative orientation to the West End, does more extensive knowledge of the area lead to a somewhat smaller proportion of severe grief responses. Thus, the wider an individual's familiarity with the local area, the greater his commitment to the locality. This wider familiarity evidently signifies a greater sense of the wholeness and integrity of the entire West End and, we would suggest, a more expanded sense of being "at home" throughout the entire local region. It is striking, too, that while familiarity with, use of, and comfort in the spatial regions of the residential area are closely related to extensiveness of personal contact, the spatial patterns have independent significance and represent an additional basis for a feeling of commitment to that larger, local region which is "home."

The Sense of Spatial Identity

In stressing the importance of places and access to local facilities, we wish only to redress the almost total neglect of spatial dimensions in dealing with human behavior. We certainly do not mean thereby to give too little emphasis to the fundamental importance of interpersonal relationships and social organization in defining the meaning of the area. Nor do we wish to underestimate the significance of cultural orientations and social organization in defining the character and importance of spatial dimensions. However, the crisis of loss of a residential area brings to the fore the importance of the local spatial region and alerts us to the greater generality of spatial conceptions as determinants of behavior. In fact, we might say that a *sense of spatial identity* is fundamental to human functioning. It represents a phenomenal or ideational integration of important experiences concerning environmental arrangements and contacts in relation to the individual's conception of his own body in space.* It is based on spatial memories, spatial imagery, the spatial framework of current activity, and the implicit spatial components of ideals and aspirations.

It appears to us also that these feelings of being at home and of belonging are, in the working class, integrally tied to a *specific* place. We would not expect similar effects or, at least, effects of similar proportion in a middle-class area. Generally speaking, an integrated sense of spatial identity in the middle class is not so contingent on the external stability of place or so dependent on the localization of social patterns, interpersonal relationships, and daily routines. In these data, in fact, there is a marked relationship between class status and depth of grief; the higher the status, by any of several indices, the smaller the proportions of severe grief. It is primarily in the working class, and largely because of the importance of external stability, that dislocation from a familiar residential area has so great an effect on fragmenting the sense of spatial identity.

External stability is also extremely important in interpersonal patterns within the working class. And dislocation and relocation involve a fragmentation of the external bases for interpersonal relationships and group networks. Thus, relocation undermines the established interpersonal relationships and group ties of the people involved and, in effect, destroys the sense of group identity of a great many individuals. "Group identity," a concept originally formulated by Erik Erikson,

* Erik Erikson[4] includes spatial components in discussing the sense of ego identity and his work has influenced the discussion of spatial variables. In distinguishing the sense of spatial identity from the sense of ego identity, I am suggesting that variations in spatial identity do not correspond exactly to variations in ego identity. By separating these concepts, it becomes possible to study their interrelationships empirically.

refers to the individual's sense of belonging, of being a part of larger human and social entities. It may include belonging to organizations or interpersonal networks with which a person is directly involved; and it may refer to "membership" in social groups with whom an individual has little overt contact, whether it be a family, a social class, an ethnic collectivity, a profession, or a group of people sharing a common ideology. What is common to these various patterns of group identity is that they represent an integrated sense of shared human qualities, of some sense of communality with other people which is essential for meaningful social functioning. Since, most notably in the working class, effective relationships with others are dependent upon a continuing sense of common group identity, the experience of loss and disruption of these affiliations is intense and frequently irrevocable. On the grounds, therefore, of both spatial and interpersonal orientations and commitments, dislocation from the residential area represents a particularly marked disruption in the sense of continuity for the majority of this group.

The Nature of the Loss in Relocation: Social and Personal Factors

Previously we said that by emphasizing the spatial dimension of the orientation to the West End, we did not mean to diminish the importance of social patterns in the experience of the local area and their effects on postrelocation loss reactions. Nor do we wish to neglect personality factors involved in the widespread grief reactions. It is quite clear that prerelocation social relationships and intrapsychic dispositions *do* affect the depth of grief in response to leaving the West End. The strongest of these patterns is based on the association between depth of grief and prerelocation feelings about neighbors. Among those women who had very positive feelings about their neighbors, 76 percent show severe grief reactions; among those who were positive but less extreme, 56 percent show severe grief; and among those who were relatively negative, 38 percent have marked grief responses. Similarly, among the women whose five closest friends lived in the West End, 67 percent show marked grief; among those whose friends were mostly in the West End or equally distributed inside and outside the area, 55 percent have severe grief reactions; and among those whose friends were mostly or all outside, 44 percent show severe grief.

The fact that these differences, although great, are not so consistently powerful as the differences relating to spatial use patterns does not necessarily imply the *greater* importance of spatial factors. If we hold the effect of spatial variables constant and examine the relationship between depth of grief and the interpersonal variables, it becomes apparent that the effect of interpersonal contacts on depth of grief is consistent regardless of differences in spatial orientation; and, likewise, the effect of spatial orientations on depth of grief is consistent regardless of differences in interpersonal relationships. Thus, each set of factors contributes independently to the depth of grief in spite of some degree of internal relationship. In short, we suggest that *either* spatial identity or group identity may be a critical focus of loss of continuity and thereby lead to severe grief; but if *both* bases for the sense of continuity are localized *within the residential area* the disruption of continuity is greater, and the proportions of marked grief correspondingly higher.

It is noteworthy that, apart from local interpersonal and social relationships and local spatial orientations and use (and variables that are closely related to these), there are few other social or personal factors in the prerelocation situation which are related to depth of grief. These negative findings are of particular importance in emphasizing that not all the variables which influence the grief reaction to dislocation are of equal importance. It should be added that a predisposition to depression markedly accentuates the depth of grief in response to the loss of one's residential area. But it is also clear that prior depressive orientations do not account for the entire relationship. The effects of the general depressive orientation and of the social, interpersonal, and spatial relationships within the West End are essentially additive; both sets of factors contribute markedly to the final result. Thus, among the women with a severe depressive orientation, an extremely large proportion (81 percent) of those who regarded the West End as their real home show marked grief. But among the women without a depressive orientation, only a moderate proportion (58 percent) of those who similarly viewed the West End as home show severe grief. On the other hand, when the West End is not seen as the person's real home, an increasing severity of general depressive orientation does *not* lead to an increased proportion of severe grief reactions.

The Nature of the Loss in Relocation: Case Analyses

The dependence of the sense of continuity on external resources in the working class, particularly on the availability and local presence of familiar places which have the character of "home," and of familiar people whose patterns of behavior and response are relatively predictable, does not account for all the reaction of grief to dislocation. In addition to these factors, which may be accentuated by depressive predispositions, it is quite evident that the realities of postrelocation experience are bound to affect the perpetuation, quality, and depth of grief. And, in fact, our data show that there is a strong association between positive or negative experiences in the postrelocation situation and the proportions who show severe grief. But this issue is complicated by two factors: (1) the extent to which potentially meaningful postrelocation circumstances can be a satisfying experience is *affected* by the degree and tenaciousness of previous commitments to the West End, and (2) the postrelocation "reality" is, in part, *selected* by the people who move and thus is a function of many personality factors, including the ability to anticipate needs, demands, and environmental opportunities.

In trying to understand the effects of prerelocation orientations and postrelocation experiences of grief, we must bear in mind that the grief reactions we have described and analyzed are based on responses given approximately two years after relocation. Most persons manage to achieve some adaptation to their experiences of loss and grief, and learn to deal with new situations and new experiences on their own terms. A wide variety of adaptive methods can be employed to salvage fragments of the sense of continuity, or to try to reestablish it on new grounds. Nonetheless, it is the tenaciousness of the imagery and affect of grief, despite these efforts at dealing with the altered reality, which is so strikingly similar to mourning for a lost person.

In coping with the sense of loss, some families tried to remain physically close to the area they knew, even though most of their close interpersonal relationships remain disrupted; and by this method, they appear often to have modified their feelings of grief. Other families try to move among relatives and maintain a sense of continuity through some degree of constancy in the external bases for their group identity. Yet others respond to the loss of place and people by accentuating the importance of those role relationships that remain. Thus, a number of women report increased closeness to their husbands, which they often explicitly relate to the decrease in the availability of other social relationships for both partners and that, in turn, modifies the severity of grief. To clarify some of the complexities of prerelocation orientations and of postrelocation adjustments most concretely, a review of several cases may prove to be instructive.

It is evident that a very strong positive prerelocation orientation to the West End is relatively infrequently associated with a complete absence of grief; and that, likewise, a negative prerelocation orientation to the area is infrequently associated with a strong grief response. The two types which are numerically dominant are, in terms of rational expectations, consistent: those with strong positive feelings about the West End and severe grief; and those with negative feelings about the West End and minimal or moderate grief. The two "deviant" types, by the same token, are both numerically smaller and inconsistent: those with strong positive prerelocation orientations and little grief; and those with negative prerelocation orientations and severe grief. A closer examination of those "deviant" cases with strong prerelocation commitment to the West End and minimal postrelocation grief often reveals either important reservations in their prior involvement with the West End or, more frequently, the denial or rejection of feelings of grief rather than their total absence. And the association of minimal prerelocation commitment to the West End with a severe grief response often proves on closer examination to be a function of a deep involvement in the West End which is modified by markedly ambivalent statements; or, more generally, the grief reaction itself is quite modest and tenuous or is even a pseudogrief that masks the primacy of dissatisfaction with the current area.

Grief Patterns: Case Examples

In turning to case analysis, we shall concentrate on the specific factors that operate in families of all four types, those representing the two dominant and those representing the two deviant patterns.

1. The Figella family exemplifies the association of strong positive prerelocation attachments to the West End and a severe grief reaction. This is the most frequent of all the pat-

terns and, although the Figella family is only one "type" among those who show this pattern, they are prototypical of a familiar West End constellation.

Both Mr. and Mrs. Figella are second-generation Americans who were born and brought up in the West End. In her pre-relocation interview, Mrs. Figella described her feelings about living in the West End unambiguously: "It's a wonderful place, the people are friendly." She "loves everything about it" and anticipates missing her relatives above all. She is satisfied with her dwelling: "It's comfortable, clean and warm." And the marriage appears to be deeply satisfying for both husband and wife. They share many household activities and have a warm family life with their three children.

Both Mr. and Mrs. Figella feel that their lives have changed a great deal since relocation. They are clearly referring, however, to the pattern and conditions of their relationships with other people. Their home life has changed little except that Mr. Figella is home more. He continues to work at the same job as a manual laborer with a modest but sufficient income. While they have many economic insecurities, the relocation has not produced any serious financial difficulty for them.

In relocating, the Figella family bought a house. Both husband and wife are quite satisfied with the physical arrangements but, all in all, they are dissatisfied with the move. When asked what she dislikes about her present dwelling, Mrs. Figella replied simply and pathetically: "It's in Arlington and I want to be in the West End." Both Mr. and Mrs. Figella are outgoing, friendly people with a very wide circle of social contacts. Although they still see their relatives often, they both feel isolated from them and they regret the loss of their friends. As Mr. Figella puts it: "I come home from work and that's it. I just plant myself in the house."

The Figella family is, in many respects, typical of a well-adjusted working-class family. They have relatively few ambitions for themselves or for their children. They continue in close contact with many people; but they no longer have the same extensiveness of mutual cooperation in household activities, they cannot "drop in" as casually as before, they do not have the sense of being surrounded by a familiar area and familiar people. Thus, while their objective situation is not dramatically altered, the changes do involve important elements of stability and continuity in their lives. They manifest the importance of externally available resources for an integral sense of spatial and group identity. However, they have always maintained a very close marital relationship, and their family provides a substantial basis for a sense of continuity. They can evidently cope with difficulties on the strength of their many internal and external resources. Nonetheless, they have suffered from the move, and find it extremely difficult to reorganize their lives completely in adapting to a new geographical situation and new patterns of social affiliation. Their grief for a lost home seems to be one form of maintaining continuity on the basis of memories. While it prevents a more wholehearted adjustment to their altered lives, such adjustments would imply forsaking the remaining fragments of a continuity which was central to their conceptions of themselves and of the world.

2. There are many similarities between the Figella family and the Giuliano family. But Mrs. Giuliano shows relatively little prerelocation commitment to the West End and little postrelocation grief. Mr. Giuliano was somewhat more deeply involved in the West End and, although satisfied with the change, feels that relocation was "like having the rug pulled out from under you." Mr. and Mrs. Giuliano are also second-generation Americans, of background similar to the Figellas'. But Mrs. Giuliano only moved to the West End at her marriage. Mrs. Giuliano had many objections to the area: "For me it is too congested. I never did care for it . . . too many barrooms, on every corner, too many families in one building. . . . The sidewalks are too narrow and the kids can't play outside." But she

does expect to miss the stores and many favorite places. Her housing ambitions go beyond West End standards and she wants more space inside and outside. She had no blood relatives in the West End but was close to her husband's family and had friends nearby.

Mr. Giuliano was born in the West End and he had many relatives in the area. He has a relatively high status manual job but only a modest income. His wife does not complain about this although she is only moderately satisfied with the marriage. In part she objected to the fact that they went out so little and that he spent too much time on the corner with his friends. His social networks in the West End were more extensive and involved than were Mrs. Giuliano's. And he missed the West End more than she did after the relocation. But even Mr. Giuliano says that, all in all, he is satisfied with the change.

Mrs. Giuliano feels the change is "wonderful." She missed her friends but got over it. And a few of Mr. Giuliano's hanging group live close by so they can continue to hang together. Both are satisfied with the house they bought although Mrs. Giuliano's ambitions have now gone beyond this. The post-relocation situation has led to an improved marital relationship: Mr. Giuliano is home more and they go out more together.

Mr. and Mrs. Giuliano exemplify a pattern that seems most likely to be associated with a beneficial experience from relocation. Unlike Mr. and Mrs. Figella, who completely accept their working-class status and are embedded in the social and cultural patterns of the working class, Mr. and Mrs. Giuliano show many evidences of social mobility. Mr. Giuliano's present job is, properly speaking, outside the working-class category because of its relatively high status and he himself does not "work with his hands." And Mrs. Giuliano's housing ambitions, preferences in social relationships, orientation to the class structure, and attitudes toward a variety of matters from shopping to child rearing are indications of a readiness to achieve middle-class status. Mr. Giuliano is prepared for and Mrs. Giuliano clearly desires "discontinuity" with some of the central bases for their former identity. Their present situation is, in fact, a transitional one that allows them to reintegrate their lives at a new and higher status level without too precipitate a change. And their marital relationship seems sufficiently meaningful to provide a significant core of continuity in the process of change in their patterns of social and cultural experience. The lack of grief in this case is quite understandable and appropriate to their patterns of social orientation and expectation.

3. Yet another pattern is introduced by the Borowski family, who had an intense prerelocation commitment to the West End and relatively little postrelocation grief. The Borowski's are both second-generation and have four children.

Mrs. Borowski was brought up in the West End but her husband has lived there only since the marriage (fifteen years before). Her feelings about living in the West End were clear: "I love it—it's the only home I've even known." She had reservations about the dirt in the area but loved the people, the places, and the convenience and maintained an extremely wide circle of friends. They had some relatives nearby but were primarily oriented towards friends, both within and outside the West End. Mr. Borowski, a highly skilled manual worker with a moderately high income, was as deeply attached to the West End as his wife.

Mr. Borowski missed the West End very much but was quite satisfied with their new situation and could anticipate feeling thoroughly at home in the new neighborhood. Mrs. Borowski proclaims that "home is where you hang your hat; it's up to you to make the adjustments." But she also says, "If I knew the people were coming back to the West End, I would pick up this little house and put it back on my corner." She claims she was not sad after relocation but, when asked how she felt when the building she lived in was torn down, a strangely morbid association is aroused: "It's just like a plant . . . when you tear up its roots, it dies! I didn't die but I felt kind of bad. It was home. . . . Don't look back, try to go ahead."

Despite evidences of underlying grief, both Mr. and Mrs. Borowski have already adjusted to the change with remarkable alacrity. They bought a one-family house and have many friends in the new area. They do not feel as close to their new neighbors as they did to their West End friends, and they still maintain extensive contact with the latter. They are comfortable and happy in their new surroundings and maintain the close, warm, and mutually appreciative marital relationship they formerly had.

Mr. and Mrs. Borowski, and particularly Mrs. Borowski, reveal a sense of loss which is largely submerged beneath active efforts to deal with the present. It was possible for them to do this both because of personality factors (that is, the ability to deny the intense affective meaning of the change and to detach themselves from highly "cathected" objects with relative ease) and because of prior social patterns and orientations. Not only is Mr. Borowski, by occupation, among the highest group of working-class status, but this family has been "transitional" for some time. Remaining in the West End was clearly a matter of preference for them. They could have moved out quite easily on the basis of income; and many of their friends were scattered throughout metropolitan Boston. But while they are less self-consciously mobile than the Giuliano's, they had already shifted to many patterns more typical of the middle class before leaving the West End. These ranged from their joint weekly shopping expeditions to their recreational patterns, which included such sports as boating and such regular plans as yearly vacations. They experienced a disruption in continuity by virtue of their former spatial and group identity. But the bases for maintaining this identity had undergone many changes over the years; and they had already established a feeling for places and people, for a potential redefinition of "home" that was less contingent on the immediate and local availability of familiar spaces and familiar friends. Despite their preparedness for the move by virtue of cultural orientation, social experience, and personal disposition, the change was a considerable wrench for them. But, to the extent that they can be categorized as "over-adjusters," the residue of their lives in the West End is primarily a matter of painful memories which are only occasionally reawakened.

4. The alternate deviant pattern, minimal prerelocation commitment associated with severe postrelocation grief, is manifested by Mr. and Mrs. Pagliuca. As in the previous case, this classification applies more fully to Mrs. Pagliuca, since Mr. Pagliuca appears to have had stronger ties to the West End. Mr. Pagliuca is a second-generation American but Mr. Pagliuca is first-generation from an urban European background. For both of them, however, there is some evidence that the sadness and regret about the loss of the West End should perhaps be designated as pseudogrief.

Mrs. Pagliuca had a difficult time in the West End. But she also had a difficult time before that. She moved into the West End when she got married. And she complains bitterly about her marriage, her husband's relatives, West Enders in general. She says of the West End: "I don't like it. The people . . . the buildings are full of rats. There are no places to play for the children." She liked the apartment but complained about the lady downstairs, the dirt, the repairs required, and the coldness during the winter. She also complains a great deal about lack of money. Her husband's wages are not too low but he seems to have periods of unemployment and often drinks his money away.

Mr. Pagliuca was attached to some of his friends and the bars in the West End. But he didn't like his housing situation there. And his reaction tends to be one of bitterness ("a rotten deal") rather than of sadness. Both Mr. and Mrs. Pagliuca are quite satisfied with their postrelocation apartment but are thoroughly dissatisfied with the area. They have had considerable difficulty with neighbors: ". . . I don't like this; people are mean here; my children get blamed for anything and everything; and there's no transportation near here." She now idealizes the West End and claims that she misses everything about it.

Mr. Pagliuca is an unskilled manual laborer. Financial problems create a constant focus for difficulty and arguments. But both Mr. and Mrs. Pagliuca appear more satisfied with one another than before relocation. They have four children, some of whom are in legal difficulty. There is also some evidence of past cruelty toward the children, at least on Mrs. Pagliuca's part.

It is evident from this summary that the Pagliuca family is deviant in a social as well as in a statistical sense. They show few signs of adjusting to the move or, for that matter, of any basic potential for successful adjustment to further moves (which they are now planning). It may be that families with such initial difficulties, with such a tenuous basis for maintaining a sense of continuity under any circumstances, suffer most acutely from disruption of these minimal ties. The Pagliuca family has few inner resources and, having lost the minimal external resources signified by a gross sense of belonging, of being tolerated if not accepted, they appear to be hopelessly at sea. Although we refer to their grief as "pseudogrief" on the basis of the shift from prerelocation to postrelocation statements, there is a sense in which it is quite real. Within the postrelocation interviews their responses are quite consistent; and a review of all the data suggests that, although their ties were quite modest, their current difficulties have revealed the importance of these meager involvements and the problems of reestablishing anew an equivalent basis for indentity formation. Thus, even for Mr. and Mrs. Pagliuca, we can speak of the disruption in the sense of continuity, although this continuity was based on a very fragile experience of minimal comfort, with familiar places and relatively tolerant people. Their grief reaction, pseudo or real, may further influence (and be influenced by) dissatisfactions with any new residential situation. The fact that it is based on an idealized past accentuates rather than minimizes its effect on current expectations and behavior.

Conclusions

Grieving for a lost home is evidently a widespread and serious social phenomenon following in the wake of urban dislocation. It is likely to increase social and psychological "pathology" in a limited number of instances; and it is also likely to create new opportunities for some, and to increase the rate of social mobility for others. For the greatest number, dislocation is unlikely to have either effect but does lead to intense personal suffering despite moderately successful adaptation to the total situation of relocation. Under these circumstances, it becomes most critical that we face the realities of the effects of relocation on working-class residents of slums and, on the basis of knowledge and understanding, that we learn to deal more effectively with the problems engendered.

In evaluating these data on the effect of prerelocation experiences on postrelocation reactions of grief, we have arrived at a number of conclusions:

1. The affective reaction to the loss of the West End can be quite precisely described as a grief response showing most of the characteristics of grief and mourning for a lost person.

2. One of the important components of the grief reaction is the fragmentation of the sense of spatial identity. This is manifest, not only in the prerelocation experience of the spatial area as an expanded "home," but in the varying degrees of grief following relocation, arising from variations in the prerelocation orientation to and use of local spatial regions.

3. Another component, of equal importance, is the dependence of the sense of group identity on stable, social networks. Dislocation necessarily led to the fragmentation of this group

identity which was based, to such a large extent, on the external availability and overt contact with familiar groups of people.

4. Associated with these "cognitive" components, described as the sense of spatial identity and the sense of group identity, are strong affective qualities. We have not tried to delineate them but they appear to fall into the realm of a feeling of security in and commitment to the external spatial and group patterns which are the tangible, visible aspects of these identity components. However, a predisposition to depressive reactions also markedly affects the depth of grief reaction.

5. Theoretically, we can speak of spatial and group identity as critical foci of the sense of continuity. This sense of continuity is not *necessarily* contingent on the external stability of place, people, and security or support. But for the working class these concrete, external resources and the experience of stability, availability, and familiarity which they provide are essential for a meaningful sense of continuity. Thus, dislocation and the loss of the residential area represent a fragmentation of some of the essential components of the sense of continuity in the working class.

It is in the light of these observations and conclusions that we must consider problems of social planning which are associated with the changes induced by physical planning for relocation. Urban planning cannot be limited to "bricks and mortar." While these data tell us little about the importance of housing or the aspects of housing which are important, they indicate that considerations of a nonhousing nature are critical. There is evidence, for example, that the frequency of the grief response is not affected by such housing factors as increase or decrease in apartment size or home ownership. But physical factors may be of great importance when related to the subjective significance of different spatial and physical arrangements, or to their capacity for gratifying different sociocultural groups. For the present, we can only stress the importance of local areas as *spatial and social* arrangements which are central to the lives of working-class people. And, in view of the enormous importance of such local areas, we are led to consider the convergence of familiar people and familiar places as a focal consideration in formulating planning decisions.

We can learn to deal with these problems only through research, through exploratory and imaginative service programs, and through a more careful consideration of the place of residential stability in salvaging the precarious thread of continuity. The outcomes of crises are always manifold and, just as there is an increase in strain and difficulty, so also there is an increase in opportunities for adapting at a more satisfying level of functioning. The judicious use of minimal resources of counseling and assistance may permit many working-class people to reorganize and integrate a meaningful sense of spatial and group identity under the challenge of social change. Only a relatively small group of those whose functioning has always been marginal and who cannot cope with the added strain of adjusting to wholly new problems are likely to require major forms of intervention.

In general, our results would imply the necessity for providing increased opportunities for maintaining a sense of continuity for those people, mainly from the working class, whose residential areas are being renewed. This may involve several factors: (1) diminishing the amount of drastic redevelopment and the consequent mass demolition of property and mass dislocation from homes; (2) providing more frequently for people to move within their former residential areas during and after the renewal; and (3) when dislocation and relocation are unavoidable, planning the relocation possibilities in order to provide new areas which can be assimilated to old objectives. A closer examination of slum areas may even provide some concrete information regarding specific physical variables, the physical and spatial arrangements typical of slum areas and slum housing, which offer considerable gratification to the residents. These may often be translated into effective modern architectural and areal design. And, in conjunction with planning decisions which take more careful account of the human consequences of urban physical change, it is possible to utilize social, psychological, and psychiatric services. The use of highly skilled resources, including opportunities for the education of professional and even lay personnel in largely unfamiliar problems and methods, can minimize some of the more destructive and widespread effects of relocation; and, for some families, can offer constructive experiences in dealing with new adaptational possibilities. The problem is large. But only by assuring the integrity of some of the external bases for the sense of continuity in the working class, and by maximizing the opportunities for meaningful adaptation, can we accomplish planned urban change without serious hazard to human welfare.

PART V

Animal Studies

Introduction

THE INVESTIGATION OF ANIMALS IN THEIR NATURAL HABITAT has been a recent focus of ethological studies that have yielded a number of observations about the nature of animal behavior and its relationship to human behavior. This work points to many of the biological and evolutionary origins of human group behavior heretofore considered exclusively human. Reasons for this anthropocentric bias are suggested in the first article in this section.

Colter Rule reviews much data on certain behavior patterns shared by man and nonhuman primates. These include infant-maternal behavior, peer play, sexual courtship, the spacing or the development of a certain amount of distance between members of the social group, territorial behavior and dominant behavior. According to Rule, these behaviors have not disappeared in man, although they seem to have because of man's ability to speak.

While the main function of speech grew out of a need for better expression of one's self in a more differentiated manner, it has developed accompanied by a gradual dropping of non-verbal aspects of communication such as gesture, posture, etc., which actually contributed to understanding. With the absence of physical gesture and reliance on verbalization, came an increase in the covertness of motives and behavior. It is Rule's view that speech in essence "subserves the function of non-communication," and that oftentimes, that which is not said is most significant. Therefore it is in the covertness of speech that the basic primate behaviors are hidden.

The work of the ethologist has much value for psychiatry as Elliot Slater notes in his review of Lorenz's *On Aggression.* In particular, the work of the ethologists has underlined the firm biological or instinctual basis for aggression in man, emphasizing how it is not necessarily dependent upon appropriate stimuli. Furthermore, while the damming up of aggression is more dangerous in groups having "close" members, phylogenetic processes "have mobilized the aggression drive into being the instinctual basis of the bond which unites animals by ties that at the highest level are those of love and friendship." A recognition of some of these "biological givens" is particularly important today for, as Slater observes, attempts to breed out aggression, suppress it by moral vetoes, or starve it by depriving it of appropriate stimuli are "doomed to failure."

At the same time, it is important to note the value of the ecological approach that can help to clarify how the level of functional organization and the changing environmental requirements they must meet influence the way in which animals and humans behave. While Lorenz and Tinbergen have made signal contributions, it is important to keep in mind the species specific character of behavior and the possibility that early learned behavior may not be so fixed as the notion of imprinting suggests, environmental influences being of considerable significance at later stages.

Animal studies are also of special value in that they permit ready experimental manipulation of environmental and experiential variables also thought to be important in human behavior. Like man, the rhesus monkey goes through rather distinctive phases of emotional growth characterized by phases of strong maternal, peer group, and mature heterosexual attachments.

Harlow examined the peer affectional system and the heterosexual affectional system development in the maturing process through age, mate, play, and interaction in peer systems leading to heterosexual behavior in adolescent and adult monkeys. The maternal-paternal affectional systems are thought to be based on early experiences, particularly the peer affectional stage.

Harlow then analyzed variables underlying these affectional systems by studying monkeys in conditions of social isolation. With this isolation it was noted that intense fear of strangeness existed. The majority of socially isolated monkeys exhibited violent aggressive tendencies as socially maladaptive types and, in particular, displayed these actions against young defenseless juveniles.

The author concludes that when considering the developmental sequence of the emotional bases of socialization in primates, namely those of affection, fear, and aggression, the development of affection for members of one's social group by normal process of affectional systems, leads to a socially better adjusted member of the group. The aggressive forces then are turned towards the enemy, and not at, as in the case of the socially isolated monkeys, an in-group member. As Harlow notes, "Failure to develop in-group affection before aggression is fully matured leaves the animal a deviate, a delinquent, and a social outcast."

Chapter 16

Theory of Human Behavior Based on Studies of Nonhuman Primates

COLTER RULE

THROUGHOUT THE MIDDLE AGES, MAN, UNDER THE GUIDANCE of theological leaders, was preoccupied with his immortal soul, with life hereafter, and with the types of ethical behaviors that would win a favored position in the next world. The Age of Reason, the industrial and scientific revolutions, and materialist philosophies offset all this and replaced it with the conviction that, since man could triumph over nature and toil, he could, in effect, have his heaven here on earth. This belief, too, is running its course, and enthusiasm over technological advances has begun to fade. Man the toolmaker excites us less and less. (A telecast of a recent Gemini mission in space shared the screen with a college football game!)

Philosophers decry sterile mechanistic advances by stating that they have failed mankind. This disenchantment stimulates us to reappraise man's relatedness to nature and the animal world. Such an endeavor is made feasible by an ever increasing flood of data arriving anywhere from *A* to *Z*, anthropology to zoology, and much of this data bears directly on behavior. Less than two decades ago, a leading psychologist discussing research in behavior could define psychology as "the study of learning in white rats and college sophomores."[1] Today, the "information explosion" has destroyed the boundaries of the academic disciplines; the multidisciplinary study is the rule rather than the exception. Many fields and many studies contribute to knowledge of behavior whether at a cellular, physiological, psychological, or social level. Archeological discoveries have illuminated crucial areas in the origins of early man.* The controversy between the ethologists on the one hand and the classical learning theorists (and Pavlovians) on the other has given rise to the somewhat contentious but productive science of animal behavior that exists today.[3] But there are many other contributors. Behavioral genetics, neurophysiology, neuroendocrinology, enzyme chemistry, brain and computer circuitry, communications and information theory, all have been deeply involved.[4] Additional crucial and fruitful areas are the studies on circadian rhythms, sensory deprivation, physiology of dreaming, psychopharmacology, the behavioral basis of perception, figure-ground phenomena, etc.

One of the newest additions to the family of multidisciplinary specialties is primatology, barely a decade old. Ten years ago there existed only two centers for the study of primate behavior. Now there are many in both universities and government institutions; the number of field investigators has quadrupled and continues to increase, and the volume of literature is already unwieldy. Two surveys in book form, one mainly of field studies, the other reporting on laboratory research, were published in 1965.[5] One section of the annual convention of the American Association for the Advancement of Science two years ago was devoted entirely to primate behavior. In spite of accelerated effort, most primate studies raise more questions than they answer. Of the approximately 240 living species of nonhuman primates, reliable field studies are available for less than two dozen. Much work lies ahead. The absence of a solid foundation of reliable data has led a profes-

* Primarily, that he was truly bipedal and a tool user with a brain volume not greatly exceeding that of present day apes.[2]

sional primatologist to remark that the amount of interest in primatology shown by scientists in general is out of all proportion to the amount of information available.[6] A possible explanation for this unusual degree of interest may be a rising ground swell of suspicion that in primatology the beginnings of human behaviors may be revealed. While the behaviors observed in nonhuman primates may be little more than seedlings when contrasted with the fully evolved behaviors as revealed in man, they seem, nevertheless, to be identifiable and to demonstrate crucial bridges between biological, psychological, and social man. For clinical psychiatrists, enough data has accumulated about primate social behaviors, about the ways their small societies (usually between fourteen and thirty individuals) are organized, and about dyadic behaviors (behaviors between any two individuals) to speculate about human behavior. Admittedly, the medical profession has never let the paucity of data interfere with its determination to build theories, however fanciful. Perhaps this privilege is justified by the ancient and awful responsibility medicine accepted from society, but another good reason for attempting to theorize about human behavior is the muddled, if not desperate, state of present-day psychiatric theory. Psychiatry was recently described by one of its leading thinkers as a kind of gaggle of cults exhibiting rituals and dialects, isolated from one another, none possessing a broad, integrated, and scientific view of man.[7]

Several phenomena often described under "population statistics" are fundamental to understanding animal behavior, although their precise application to man is not yet known.

Localization.—Perhaps as fundamental to his being a social animal, man is primarily an organism that is attached, and remains attached, to a particular geographical spot near which he was most likely born and for which he formed a firm attachment early in life.* Regardless of the excitement created by the

* If his social nature stems from psychological phenomena classified under "figure," this might be classified under "ground."

conquest of space—regardless of wars, migrations, and modern transportation—the vast majority of the world's people are born and die within the radius of a few miles. Compared to nonhuman primates, of course, the range over which early man traveled was great, hundreds as compared to a few dozen square miles. But man is no nomad, that is, he is not an animal born to wander. Indeed, in the whole animal world nomads are a rarity; much of what was thought to represent nomadism turns out to be migration between primary and secondary localization, for example, summer and winter migration.

Man differs from other animals in having overcome most barriers to free movement, much of this, of course, the result of the accumulated gadgetry of the past few decades. No limitation of bodily equipment now holds him back. Few physical obstacles, no insurmountable food shortages, and no hostile alien species contest his advance into new territory. Indeed, the main barriers to unrestricted movement may be those deep in his own nature, concepts as vague and yet as powerful as "home and mother," or "my people, my land, my country."*

Population size.—Man, though not a nomad, is surely a colonizer, and this has enabled him to multiply in vast numbers. The Malthus theory, with which Darwin concurred, stated that starvation, disease, and war were the sole factors operating to restrict the unlimited multiplication of individuals, including man. Such a formulation was grossly misleading and has required modification. Animals do not blindly reproduce themselves. Rather, animals organize themselves into orderly populations and societies which have various and characteristic ways of controlling population growth. Just what natural laws operate and whether man follows them is one of the most important questions confronting society today.[8] Current scientific studies are seeking to uncover the determinants, not only of total populations, but of the lesser units of population, such as societies, colonies, groups. For such studies, nonhuman primate societies

* Implications of such concepts may have importance for space exploration.

offer helpful material; for behavioral studies seeking to uncover other natural laws, primate societies are excellent. They are composed of small numbers of individuals. Many occupy habitats where visibility is good so that recognition of individuals is possible. Wide choice of environments, often for the same species, offers an unusual opportunity to study the relationship of behavior and environment.

Group size of nonhuman primates under natural conditions is not great, usually not much above thirty individuals. Group size, the differences between birth and death rates, is a vector of various forces, for example, food supply, predator, and other pressures. The limited data-processing capacity of nonhuman primates seems to preclude the maintenance of well-integrated groups much above the figure of thirty mentioned above. Aggregations up to several hundred animals have been described, but these may represent temporary associations of several groups coming together at night or congregating because of food supplies or other factors. The loose structure of certain chimpanzee groups, with individuals, mother-infant-juvenile, and adult male subgroups wandering at considerable distances from one another, has not yet been fully studied but may represent decreasing danger from predation and an increase in sociality rather than the opposite. The frequent intermingling of more than one group without agonistic behavior seems to bear this out.[9] Under captive or semicaptive conditions, as at Cayo Santiago or in certain of the Japanese primate centers where central provision stations have been installed, larger groups and different behaviors from those occurring under natural conditions are described.

Population density.—Like localization and population size, the density of a population cannot properly be called a "behavior." Indeed, it may be viewed as the result of behavior. At the same time, like environmental factors, it determines behavior.

Although multiple variables related to birth and death rates enter into the determination of population density, the number of individuals in a given unit of space, that is, density, is an index of sociality. The psychological counterpart of density has been called "cohesiveness" and represents the final balance between positive and negative social responses. It is also a figure that is the final average of "spacing," the social behavior regulating one's distance from other individuals of the group; spacing will be defined later. The various primate species have distinctive densities and scatter patterns under natural conditions. Howler monkeys are characteristically closely knit and cohesive.[10] Capuchins and baboons scatter widely during the daytime but gather closely together at night. The patas male (a swift-running, savannah-dwelling monkey) remains at a considerable distance from the main body of the group during the day and chooses a distant sleeping tree at night as well.

The patas male also thrashes around and makes much more noise than the rest of the group, indicating that the behavior relates to his drawing predator pressure toward himself and away from the group.[11] The scatter pattern of the chimpanzee was touched on previously. With hundreds of species still unstudied, indeed barely known, much needs to be learned about spacing, cohesiveness, density, intergroup mixing, etc.

The Fundamental Primate Social Behaviors (Including Man)

Primates are social animals. The social group is the unit, and the individual is a fragment of that unity. Separated from the group, the individual neither develops nor long survives; in the vast majority of primate species, the individual is born, lives, and dies never once out of sight or earshot of his social group. While this is not strictly true of the more evolved species, real exceptions are, even for man, rare and trivial. Separateness is an artificial condition; studies of the individual (or of two individuals or, indeed, of any fractions of the totality) are, hence, studies of artifacts, however defended—for example, in psychotherapy—as practical and necessary.

The bias we acquire as members of a society that stresses "individualism" renders this rather simple concept difficult to grasp and retain. We tend to feel that our individualism, which was secondary to our break with the rigid political-economic-religious dominances of Europe, is a fundamental and independent fact of human nature. This individualism entertains such fictions as survival of the individual separated from the group when clearly, except for short intervals after maturity, separateness is impossible. Even the hermit has had years of human tutelage, and his world is probably peopled with imaginary people anyway. Such concepts remain implicit in much of our thinking. The terms "antisocial" and "asocial" are really misnomers since, like separateness, they are not compatible, except temporarily, with development or survival. Relative terms like "dyssocial" or "disharmonious social behavior" are more precise.

A. Infant-Maternal Behavior

The individual at birth is totally dependent upon mothering behavior from one or more individuals for survival and growth. This dependence decreases gradually with growth into and through the peer-play period of behavior and tends to disappear with the attainment of physical maturity.

B. Peer-Play Behavior

The individual after infancy embarks on a prolonged period of peer-play behavior. This phase of physical and intellectual growth is devoted to practicing and mastering social behaviors appropriate to each sex and establishing social rank.

C. Courtship-Sexual Behavior

The individual, using components developed during the peer-play phase, develops the capacity for integrated courtship-sexual behavior. This initiates the period of maturity along with dominance behavior, leadership-follower behavior, maternal behavior, all of which continue until the period of aging and decline.

D. Spacing Behavior

The individual under natural conditions of social life maintains a specific distance between himself and every other member of his social group. This distance, corrected for known variables and averaged over time, indicates the strength and the nature of the social bond existing between any two individuals.

This behavior has been referred to as "spatial equilibration" and is easily demonstrated for mature males, especially during the breeding season. The breakdown of spacing behavior into its many components, e.g., operational, tactile, visual, auditory, and olfactory space, as well as abstract concepts involving time, are a few of the areas for stimulating multidisciplined research. We are concerned here only with the basic "behavioral envelope," which can be clearly differentiated from the other basic "behavioral envelopes."[12]

E. Territorial Behavior

The individual with other members of the social group will defend by threat or fight the territory over which he ranges. He will defend, as well, certain products of that territory—for example, food, tools, trinkets—that he finds, makes, or accumulates.

F. Dominance Behavior

The individual strives throughout life to attain and/or maintain a dominant position in the hierarchy of power and privilege that exists in every primate society.

Alliance behavior.—(This is classified under dominance behavior because as observed in nonhuman primate societies it has thus far been restricted to dominance interactions.) Several forms of behavior involving more than two individuals have been observed. The following are examples:

1. Two individuals may suspend, more or less permanently, dominance interactions between themselves to join forces against a third individual.
2. An individual losing a dominance interaction to a second may forestall this loss by insinuating and ingratiating himself close to a larger or more dominant third individual, who "protects" him.*
3. Dominance rank is accorded the offspring of a high-ranking mother or family group. A female may be accorded dominance rank because she is the consort of a dominant male.

In this paper no detailed description of these behaviors or their ranges and variations will be undertaken. They were described briefly in an earlier paper,[14] and extensive material is available at several levels of detail in the literature.[15] Observing these behaviors, at least on film, is most helpful; seeing is still believing and, in this case, understanding. Further detailed analysis of these six basic categories into their constituents and the determination of the relationships between the categories is an important field for future study. We are concerned here only with an overview and with deriving principles that will help apply these categories to human behaviors. In spite of the range

* This must not be mistaken for philanthropy on the part of the dominant animal. It occurs in nonhuman primates apparently because the third and dominant animal automatically responds to the aggression directed toward himself, not noticing that the aggression is really directed at the ingratiating animal that has come close to him.[13]

and complexity of each behavior category, the fact remains that these behaviors are identifiable, easily distinguishable one from the other, and are basic to all primate groups studied thus far. There is no reason to believe that the same behavioral categories will not extend to all the approximately 240 living species. It is inconceivable that such categories of behavior would not have characterized one additional species, namely, early man. The question becomes, not whether man exhibited these behaviors, but rather what happened to them, and the thesis of this paper is, of course, that they have not disappeared but continue to operate following their own rhythms and can be demonstrated, monitored, and often measured with little difficulty.

The Mystery of Speech

Why did these behaviors seem to disappear? Or perhaps a more blunt question, what blinded us? One thinks immediately of the vast, often glaring, accumulations of human culture and civilization, which distract, preoccupy, fascinate, and often obsess us and which are traceable in almost linear fashion from television and automobiles back to the wheel, fire, and stone-flake weapons.*

But the real, the perennial, stumbling block to understanding is always the mystery of human speech. It is this that blocks the awareness of man's continuity with the animal world (mainly because it illustrates man's abstracting ability, his consciousness of self, and, indirectly, his religiousness). It is this that is always submitted as final proof of the unbridgeable gap between man and beast. This barrier to understanding can disappear only with new concepts of the communications process.[17] When one compares communications in, say, apes with humans, one is tempted to propose that what the ape lacks in speech he makes up for by posture, gesture, facial expression, and vocalizations. Indeed, it has been said that he commu-

* Some human societies do not make fire, they borrow it from neighbors.[16]

nicates about as well as the average excitable human trying to communicate with another human who does not speak the same language. Further, as others have noted, humans equipped with verbal skills ofttimes make a pretty messy business of communication, even at rather low levels of abstraction.

Human verbalization arose out of a communications matrix that once included posture, gesture, facial expression, and vocalization—all more or less undifferentiated.* The origin and development of speech made posture, gesture, facial expression, and some vocal characteristics obsolete for many communications functions, and these nonverbal components tended to drop out. The separation is a tenuous one; in certain emotional states the entire communications complex reappears, and the verbal component becomes relatively small.† The

* The vocabulary of the least evolved human groups, e.g., the natives of the Kalahari Desert, simple food gatherers and hunters, is estimated at eighty words, and their communications system is so embedded in posture and gesture that they have difficulty communicating in the dark. Nonhuman primates have a range of sounds conveying distinguishable meaning, according to some observers, of, perhaps, fifteen to thirty, divisible into five or six groups of calls. There is a fair degree of specificity. A warning call occurring and recorded when a leopard threatens a primate group is not confused with a warning call recorded when the group has spotted a snake. Played back to the primate group, they assume postures and behaviors appropriate to the appearance of these threats. A tape recording taken while it was raining sent chimpanzees scurrying for shelter when it was played back during fair weather. These examples are not submitted to illustrate how close nonhuman primate communications are to human. The Kalahari native has speech, i.e., it is phonetic, a sound substitutes for an idea, and the sounds are formalized statements of relationships between things. The nonhuman primate does not. But the two systems can still be discussed together. This is no commentary on any limitation of the Kalahari's intelligence but reflects the utter and monotonous simplicity of his environment and daily activity.

† The fate of these obsolete or vestigial nonverbal communications forms has been studied.[18] In nonhuman primates they serve as components of display behavior, which probably serve to let off excess "energy emotion." In humans this may apply also, but to the extent that they do not contaminate verbal communications they seem to have funneled off into ritual and ceremony forming the taproot for many of man's cultural pursuits. This is not, of course, to be construed as indicating a superiority of verbal over nonverbal communication. Indeed, the nonverbal is usually the language of beauty and tenderness. Colloquially, pretty is as pretty does.

dropping out of the nonverbal components of communication means that behavior and the underlying motives tend automatically to become covert. Man, of course, discovered the social premium on covertness and has refined it to an infinite degree. In implementing covertness, he naturally used speech. We have for so long thought of speech as serving as a communications vehicle that we have difficulty seeing that it also served the function of furthering covert behavior. Speech may or may not convey something, but it always hides something; it is noteworthy as much for what it conceals as for what it reveals. This is not accidental or incidental; this has been its function. In summary, speech, paradoxically, subserves the function of noncommunication. To understand what a person says, we must fully understand what he does not say or, more practically, what he does not wish to say.* This may help clarify why our clues to the basic primate behaviors were lost in man; they simply became covert. The evidence for the continued operation of these behaviors, therefore, is no longer visual but has to be, primarily, verbal-auditory. Proof for their continued operation requires, furthermore, not only sensitivity and awareness but also an ongoing intimate and unthreatening, possibly even tender, social transaction that permits the communication of such awareness.

Additional difficulty in trying to understand the differences and the similarities between human and nonhuman primates stems from a real lack of understanding and a constant, unscientific exaggeration of the importance of speech, that is, a

* Psychiatrists, of all people, should understand this. Yet, here is an example from a current journal. The author is quoting Freud: ". . . the character of the ego is a precipitate of abandoned object-cathexes and . . . it contains the history of those object-choices." We can launch discussions of this statement in many directions, e.g., the use of the word "object" when referring to human beings, or which individuals or groups in our culture would understand the statement or which would not, etc. But the more interesting point is that the author holds it up as an example of an "elegantly simple statement"! And further, this is from an article dealing with the phenomena of "cultural exclusion."[19] The simple fact is that we all exclude others, and we all hide our meaning, and we all use language to do so.

verbal in contrast to a nonverbal communications system. The written word and all other communications advances that follow the discovery and development of speech are secondary matters. If speech is seen simply as the natural outcome of increasing differentiation and refinement in the evolution of communication—a breakthrough phenomenon at a certain point in the process of cephalization and hierarchization in the evolution of the nervous system—it loses much of its awesome, miraculous uniqueness. More and more evidence is accumulating that this is, in fact, true.

We do not wish to discredit speech. It is given its full role in the subsequent accumulations of man—material, religious, artistic, and otherwise. Overevaluation of the spoken word is characteristic of the primitive-magic stage of development; we can still excuse that in the poet and others. But it has no place in psychiatry, where speech is merely a communications tool and a means to an end. A quote from Sullivan is relevant here: "There are people who seem completely staggered when one talks about nonverbal referential processes—that is, wordless thinking: these people simply seem to have no ability to grasp the idea that a great deal of covert living—living that is not objectively observable but only inferable—can go on without the use of words. The brute fact is, as I see it, that most of living goes on that way."[20]

Speech, "Thought," and Their Relationships

The laws of speech seem to follow the same general laws of the development of the nervous system and of the intelligence. In severe aphasia, for instance, when an individual is unable to say, "yes" or "no," he cannot convey this by shaking or nodding his head either. Nor can he do so with his hands, although muscles of both head and hands work well for other purposes. What was lost is the ability for conceptual thought, and both gesture and speech go with it.[21]

This paper is not the place to discuss abstract, symbolic, conceptual mental activity or, in short, "thought," but certain relevant generalities should be mentioned.

First, the attainment of higher degrees of abstract thought as exemplified in man is the result of three interrelated factors operating over hundreds of thousands of years: (1) the marked increase in size of the cerebral cortex, (2) the prolonged immaturity and dependency on mothering behavior with its extended period of distraction-free learning,* and (3) an increasingly different environment, physical, biological, social.

Second, at a certain point, possibly early to mid-Pleistocene, a symbolic language, namely, speech, arose and by bringing an unusual selective premium to the possessor led to acceleration in each of the three factors mentioned above. Words, because of their great contribution to survival, rapidly supplanted imagery, neuromuscular sensation, and emotion as both the repository and the vehicle of concepts at various levels of generality, for example, Black Beauty, horse, animal, food; or Black Beauty, horse, beast-of-burden, vehicle, status symbol, etc. In general, words and language not only document the distinctions and qualities of the environment—the basic elements of concepts—but permit a great increase in their number, subtlety, and efficiency of storage. It is clear that language multiplies what one sees and, hence, much of what one understands. The discovery of "the word" and the evolution of language gradually gave rise to an increasing complexity of concepts, including such things as the idea of time. Man became a "time-binder." He was taken out of his imbeddedness in immediacy. He acquired a past that he crystallized as history and a future attended with a degree of predictability. As he accumulated concepts, he accumulated material goods (the precipitates of concepts) and even the kinds of material goods,

* Man maintains fetal characteristics throughout life, a biological phenomenon called neoteny. But psychologically, too, he tends to remain immature, and, while we may resent the Peter Pan within us, we also retain for a long time the wonderment and imagination that leads to new things and new ways.

such as dictionaries, libraries, and data-processing and computer machines, that permit the storage and processing of concepts. Words determine man's world, and the worlds in which different language groups live are distinct worlds, not merely the same worlds with different labels.[22] This statement, in essence, applies quite well to a comparison of the communication systems of human and nonhuman primates.

In short, psychologically, speech indicates the arrival at a certain level of conceptual thought. Anatomically, speech indicates the arrival at a certain level of complexity of the developing organism. The term "developing organism" is preferable to the term "developing nervous system" because conceptual or thinking behavior requires the participation of parts of the organism other than just the nervous system. Thinking, at least the form of thinking called for in problem-solving under experimental conditions, is regularly accompanied by an increase in muscle tension (not to mention many other physiological changes), which usually is not visible but is detectable by electrically measured action potentials taken of the muscles themselves. This is true even of the muscles of speech. On occasion, a word used in solving a problem may be identified by the configuration of the electrical potential readings, that is, the experimenter can tell what word the subject had in mind.[23] In deaf people who talk with their hands, the changes in electrical potential during thought occur in the muscles of their hands, not in the muscles of speech. Whether there exist forms of thought involving nervous tissue only will require further study and sharper definitions. Recent studies show that the forms of thought change with sensory deprivation, with variant states of the nervous system as obtained in changes of levels of arousal and dreaming, and, of course, with drugs and with alterations in chemical or metabolic states. The relationship of speech and other aspects of the symbolic-conceptual processes to the metabolic and endocrine phenomena ongoing in the organism is a crucial and very large field for continuing study. At this time, we can assert only that all forms of conceptual thought require a relatively intact organism, certainly for most of the time involved in the process.

Hopefully, it is clear at this juncture why comparisons of the intelligence of man and of the nonhuman primate as exemplified in laboratory studies are unfruitful. What distinguishes man from other primates, and one man from another, is not the laboratory kind of intelligence but the kind he accumulates and uses for social purposes.[24] It is this failure to measure and appreciate social intelligence as it operates under natural conditions that made the gap appear so vast, so unbridgeable, and that has interfered with valid studies. The potential for accumulation, for sharing, for collaboration, and for sociality, this —not intelligence per se—is the area where we have outdistanced the nonhuman primate.* One cannot help but observe that we are still short of the sociality imperative for today's world.

Man's Modifications of Fundamental Behavioral Categories

The foregoing, it is hoped, has made clear that neither the fact of human speech nor the increased capacity of man to be guided by abstract concepts has removed man from the six vast categories of behavior that characterize all primate societies.

* Not that laboratory studies have been misleading; indeed, it is the reciprocity that exists between laboratory and field study that has made modern primatology the science it is. Laboratory studies established the fact that the chimpanzee is for a number of years more intelligent than the human infant of the same age, as measured by learning and by tests of problem solving. These years cover that period of development that is crucial for future socialization and psychological well-being.

An anecdote that leaked out of a government research laboratory has it that a well-conditioned (and obviously well-motivated) chimpanzee defeated a visiting general in a game of tic-tac-toe; since then, the number of challengers has dwindled. This, too, indicates a certain sharpness of intelligence, even in a laboratory setting. But true intelligence is best estimated under natural conditions whenever possible.

Future studies will refine our knowledge of these categories, their relationship to one another, and the laws governing the rhythms of their operation, particularly in their relationship to environment. Indeed, much has been done and is now being done that we cannot go into here. The affectional maternal-infant system, its components, and its reciprocal relations with the peer-play affectional system has been much studied, particularly in the laboratory.[25] The varieties of territorial behavior as well as variations in dominance behavior open wide vistas of endeavor. But in this paper we can state only generalities, namely, that these behaviors are as fundamental to human existence as such short-rhythm phenomena as respiration and the heart beat; intermediate (circadian) rhythms like sleeping, waking, eating, drinking; and longer rhythms like sexuality and seasonal changes.

The development of man is characterized by the ongoing process—now having operated for millennia—of refinement and elaboration, and it is this process that has so altered the six primate behavioral categories as to account for their being ignored. The study of how they have been elaborated and refined is now open to all and should provide for stimulating investigation and speculation. Toolmaking, for instance, can give us a clue to what happens as elaboration and refinement operate over great lengths of time. Regardless of ups and downs of history or circumstance, there is an unbroken line of tool development in which the tool becomes complex and specialized and the toolmaker becomes an ever larger multimembered team, with each team member having a function and an area of endeavor. The chimpanzee toolmaker fashions a probe by stripping leaves from a small branch or a twig and uses it to explore a termite hill, hopefully to extract termites.[26] Man organizes a vast complex team of toolmakers to make a tool to explore space. The same holds true for each of the basic categories of behavior. Take mothering. Mothering behavior is defined as "Care given with satisfaction if not joy and leading to growth and maturity in the one receiving the care. Care is understood to include every nuance of giving from nursing and physical support to protection, teaching, encouragement, etc."[27] Since these must lead to growth, each must be given in appropriate quantities ending in cessation (or a stronger term, rejection). This definition is broad but is well supported by observation of nonhuman primates; it is also definitive in that there is little blurring or overlapping with the other five categories. Man has refined and elaborated this category much as he has toolmaking. Mothering is no longer the province of one individual, the biologic mother, but is the province of a team, and the composition of this team varies widely with history and culture. In our society, the biologic father usually plays the second most important role on the team, although such team functions may be assumed by older siblings, other relatives, or paid employees.* But, most important, the extended team includes teachers, ministers, doctors (and the personnel of institutionalized forms: church, YMCA, Girl Scouts, etc.), ad infinitum. All occupy a place on this team whether they are fully aware of it or not. Sometimes the biologic mother plays no role to speak of, and sometimes, tragically, there is nothing that could even be called a team, and the child exhibits the manifold, often pathetic, distortions of conflict and unguided growth. Fathering, it is clear, is best defined as "mothering behavior learned and performed by a male."[29] The father, theoretically capable of every mothering chore except breast feeding, is often associated for historical and other reasons with the late stages of peer-play behavior, namely, puberty rites in the male child or the introduction to formal courtship behavior in the female child. In view of male domination of the female throughout history, the mental gymnastics the acceptance of the concept of the "mothering male" will call for can be appreciated. This

* The question of the adult male's interest in and protection of the young varies widely among various species of nonhuman primates. It will require much more study.[28]

is a challenge to every male, whether husband or lover or psychiatrist. Many males resist this simple formulation possibly because they feel it reflects on their maleness, whatever that is. Certainly, it need not be confused with sexual potency. It is difficult for the human male, who throughout history has so generally dominated the female, to appreciate fully how much he has learned by observing and mimicking her.

The Relationship of Psychiatry to the Six Behavioral Categories

It is clear that no matter what the theory or technique espoused by the psychiatrist, and by now even the most rigid of us admit that many theories and therapies are helpful, we are, from the standpoint of primatology, society's "specialists in corrective foster mothering." Whether we are shocked or honored by this label, we cannot remove it without losing our real identity. It should be clear that the behavior of the psychiatrist cannot possibly be stretched to fit into any of the other categories. To establish this beyond doubt, we would have to explore in detail what the endless processes of elaboration and refinement have done to the categories we cannot cover in this paper. The processes of elaboration and refinement work largely outside of awareness, which makes the tracing of each category into the past difficult. But we all have a pretty good idea of what dominance behavior is, and unraveling its history and operation is by no means impossible. The same is true of territorial behavior, which appears to be the taproot of property rights. Spacing behavior in the human is of particular interest because it swings back and forth between the literal and the abstract (figurative) so constantly. Our language forms, of course, reflect many of these abstractions, for example, I feel close to him. Fortunately, since there are only six categories, the task of getting to the essence of a disjunctive social transaction is generally easy. To take a simple example, for instance, prostitution becomes essentially a social transaction in which one party is involved in territorial behavior (money and property) and the other, not without exception, is involved in courtship-sexual behavior.

The above should add to the clarification of the psychiatrists's role. How commonly it is significantly contaminated unknowingly by the intrusion of the other behaviors, overtly or covertly! A stimulating controversy arises when it is argued that classical psychoanalysis is by no stretch of the imagination an example of "corrective foster mothering." It is, nevertheless. That it exhibits only one of the many facets of mothering behavior is not significant; mothering permits of wide variations. Mothering of a newborn monkey, for example, is accomplished by a wire frame covered with terry cloth,[30] and good results often seem to be accomplished by "terry-cloth-covered" psychoanalysts. The miracle, however, lies in the monkey or the patient, not in the wire frame. It is clear, on the other hand, that classical analysis can level many charges at other therapies, usually in the category of poorly conceived activity on the part of the therapist. The mother, for instance, strictly speaking does not play with her child but, rather, teaches it to play. Play is with peers. And so it is with psychiatry. The psychiatrist may or may not be friendly, but he is not a friend of the patient. (Personally, I feel he should be friendly to the extent that it is unthreatening to himself or his patient.) The psychiatric transaction ends with the development in the patient of the capacity for true friendship. Whether the psychiatrist ever becomes a friend is incidental or coincidental.

Certain of the disjunctive sequences that take place in the psychiatric transaction are due to distorted definitions of mothering. The essence of mothering is not total acceptance, contrary to much psychiatric opinion. Even the "Pietà" cannot be conceived of as symbolic of this essence, as moving as it may be. The "Pietà" symbolizes mothering only under extremely heroic circumstances. This, fortunately, occurs but rarely in the therapeutic transaction, although the patient often claims otherwise. Mothering is that artful combination of acceptance and rejection which stimulates growth leading to maturity by way of full peer-play behavior.*

Other disjunctive possibilities in therapy derive from the basic categories. Sexual-courtship behavior is probably a common contaminant to the ongoing foster mothering with persons of the opposite sex, as well as dominance behavior (in the form of professionalism) and territorial behavior (in the form of money matters). With surprisingly little effort, these behaviors can be monitored by the psychiatrist once he "gets the hang of it." Further, since these are the precise behaviors the patient is involved with in his outside life, there is no particular harm in the psychiatrist's sharing his knowledge of their operation if he does not force it upon the patient or interfere with the full development of the patient's capacity for self-assertion and self-discovery. Nice distinctions are called for and sometimes difficult ones. However, this is characteristic of most worthwhile endeavors. But a new freedom and a new spontaneity enter the transaction. For the first time, the psychiatrist can dip freely into the reservoir of experience and intuition that he possesses and can shift his responses as quickly and over as wide a range as any sensitive mother. Passivity and activity are variables routinely available to any mother in changing her tactics from one type of child to the next or for the same child at different times. To deny this principle is to restrict sharply the applications and dimensions of therapy. Another way of stating this is to say that the psychiatrist's role as foster mother, that is, an important member of the mothering team, is far more fundamental to the patient's growth than the psychiatrist's role as scientist (Freud) or professional selling a service (Sullivan); as the "I" in the "I-thou" concepts of the Existentialists; or,

* Erich Fromm, for instance, has written much on the acceptance quality of "love," not spelling out the skilled and imaginative forms of rejection, which are growth-provoking.

presumably, as Zen master in the Zen Buddhist views of recent years.*

This implies no disrespect for Existential or Zen Buddhistic or other modes of nondualistic experience. As these have been presented in Western psychiatry, however, they seem little more than intellectual baubles. Even in the Orient, Zen Buddhism is not submitted as the answer to "behavioral-emotional-social" breakdown. Zen (and a number of philosophies invading psychiatry) may represent the cutoff point where psychiatry ends, i.e., when the "mothering job" has been finished and the choice of a mature philosophy is faced.

History, Philosophy, Science: Relationship to This Theory

It would be tempting to dismiss this presentation by stating that the difficulty is semantic, but that is precisely not the case. The term "mothering," or "mothering behavior," is not chosen arbitrarily, nor are the other category headings. They are chosen in spite of alleged vague or controversial aspects, instead of words like "dependency" and "counseling." The word "mothering" is a term used and understood by biologists, by psychologists, and by sociologists and is by no means a vague, bulky, or nebulous term. It is subject to analysis and measurement by each of these disciplines. This term, along with the other five, offers a way out of the private language problem, which reaches Tower of Babel proportions in present-day psychiatry.

In view of the possibilities claimed for the present theory, it may be helpful to take another look into the past. It was the scientist who pointed out the great similarity in structure and physiology of man and animal. The burden of proof should

* My psychiatric training required the study of a number of distinct psychiatric languages, e.g., Meyerian, Freudian, Sullivanian, Jungian, Adlerian. Few terms or concepts are interchangeable even within psychiatry; they are virtually useless for other scientific disciplines.

be on the psychiatric scientist to demonstrate the animal nature of human behavior. But psychiatric theories stubbornly assert how unlike are man and animal.

The doctrine of evolution established the fundamental tenet that, while evolution is irrevocable, never returning to an earlier state, neither does it eliminate all traces of earlier states. No psychiatric theory ever effectively embodied this as part of its structure; all were concerned, not with what and how animal behaviors operate in man, but if they operated at all.*

From the evolutionist's point of view, the gap between nonhuman and human primates is small and is limited mainly to minor changes in the skeletal structure and to increase in size and area of the cerebral cortex. These are small when compared to other evolutionary changes, for example, the change from sea to land, or from land to air, or a number of other evolutionary advances. The change from nonhuman primate to human, though small, was critical and, operating over years, accounts for the accumulations of culture and civilization.† Since structure determines function, that is, behavior, minor structural changes indicate minor behavioral changes, a principle that should hold good in comparing man to the nonhuman primate. Indeed, theorists readily accept the data of the fossil record and the data of comparative anatomy, which confirm the close structural relationship of all primates. The same holds true for all the data on physiological functions. But this open-mindedness is blocked when the question of comparative behaviors is raised. Actually, what lies at the root of the inability to resolve the question is the phenomenon of covertness discussed previously. Man's evolving cortex made it possible for him to inhibit, camouflage, and modify the basic primate be-

* Freud insisted upon a biological orientation supported more by stubborn intuition than by data. It is a shame that he coined a language unusable by biologists.

† One can hear the call "vive la différence" and agree, but these differences must not blind us to the similarities between human and nonhuman primates, which are crucial for psychiatry.

haviors far beyond the ability of any other primate, and the ability increased steadily. This gave rise over the years to the thesis that man does not have basic primate behaviors. The explanation given was that evolution is, periodically, "emergent" and that man was the sole recipient among millions of species of this wonderful gift. Such a view, of course, is closely related to the phenomenon of transcendence, the theological roots of which are more easily identified.

The error is easy to spot. We have conceptualized man as the top of a pyramid representing the animal world (viz., primate), and this conception with roots in animism and primitive religion has contaminated scientific thought, denials to the contrary. A better conceptual schema would be concentric circles, with man being represented by the outer layers, thus indicating that man does not obliterate animal behaviors but simply extends their dimensions, including the ability to inhibit. Such a schema explains why man can be more "beastly" than the animal. Neither torture nor cannibalism, for instance, exists in nonhuman primates; either they are unable to conceive it or unable to carry it out.*

Theorists—both philosophers and psychiatrists—faced with the task of constructing nonanimal behavioral models have been given to all kinds of imaginative pursuits. Usually, however, they have selected such models as gods; heroes; saints; philosophers; artists; scientists; or, latterly and modestly, the product of men's minds, such as mechanical or electronic gadgets. Actually, none of these is a behavioral model; they have no blood and guts, so to speak.† Rather, they represent a succession of man's preoccupations in his evolution from protocultures through savagery and barbarism to the religious and scientific attitudes of later times. They may actually be things

* Further study is required. A baboon did not eat the carcass of an infant baboon killed by a predator, though baboons are known to kill and devour small animals they happen across. They do not hunt.[31]

† The untenability of disembodied "cognitive" behavior to a physician or anyone well grounded in physiology can be appreciated.[32]

he is not, that is, they are rationalizations to cover tabooed behaviors, probably of a sexual or agonistic nature.

One could, perhaps, classify these models as examples of "ruminative" or "investigative" or "appetitive" behaviors, although these are not strictly behavioral entities. Appetitive behaviors are best conceived of as vague "restlessnesses" out of which more definitive behavior arises. Indeed, thought, meditation, and curiosity, particularly, can be imagined as forms of "appetitive" behavior carried to a peculiar length in man and, hence, most difficult to trace to the particular behavioral entities they give rise to. In other words, man focusing with exquisite refinement on a state of being we can call sentience came up with an image of himself as godlike, heroic, or whatever. The only difficulty is that he was wrong and that these images probably had much to do with defenses against his feeling the opposite.

While any behavior is ongoing, other behaviors, covert or inhibited, are building up, largely outside of awareness, preparatory to overt manifestation. We are faced with the problem of dealing with behaviors that are not yet manifest. Hopefully, the study of circadian rhythms and other biologic rhythms will give us clues to understanding these. For this, the human furnishes a good subject because verbal clues may be the earliest available in spotting incipient behavior, at least until better chemical or electrical methods are developed. And we can understand a communication, as with any form of behavior, only when we understand what is not being communicated as well as what is. A communication is simply a wave in a vast sea, and we cannot understand that wave without understanding non-waves, i.e., swells, tides, currents, winds, shorelines, all of which determine that wave which is part of "the sea around us."

We know so little about the substrates of cognition and concept formation that theories remain idiosyncratic, even if artistic and delightful. This paper does not, therefore, recommend that as a theory it be accepted. It recommends that the data be processed again and again.

Final Remarks

Having ventured so far in speculation, it would seem abrupt to end this paper without at least a few remarks concerning the specific theories that determined the course of psychiatry. Earlier theories have now become institutions, but when launched they were often directed against institutions if only for the reason that the beliefs they challenged were held by institutions. Institutions in primate terminology represent alliance behavior, the beginnings of which we identified in nonhuman primate societies and which have been carried forth with the expected elaboration and refinement by man.

Freud's views, regardless of any stated intent, were clearly directed against the institution, the church. Since neither the scientific nor the business institutions have any direct interest in determining moral or ethical practices, if and when they attack Freudian doctrines, they do so simply as allies of the church.* Both the doctrine of a dynamic unconscious and the doctrine of the ubiquity of childhood sexuality were challenges to the territory of the church rather than any other segment of the community. Why Freud selected theses that were primarily antagonistic to the church, long since deposed from the seats of power, poses an interesting question. All ethical and moral considerations involving sex and violence had, long since, been the province of the church. This is what Freud preempted, and the cry of outrage clearly came from the direction of the church, already restless and overzealous to protect its shrinking territory. Business, in essence, is amoral, but it does keep its eye on every other segment of the community. It took a

* We emphasize "doctrine" rather than secondary professional or status considerations.

neutral position in the interminable controversy that raged between science (as represented by Freud) and religion. Indeed, if our reasoning based on observation of nonhuman primates is correct, the controversy, if anything, was helpful to business, since it allowed the business community to pursue its own course of growth free from any moral restraints from the otherwise preoccupied church.

What has been responsible for the continued existence of the Freudian cult? The reason lies in several areas. First, it is a profession, and second, it is a business, and the laws of survival of these entities continue to operate. It continues also to thrive on the original controversy set up with the church and has enlisted as adherents and customers many of those whose quarrel was with the church.

In retrospect, one sometimes wonders why the controversy over sex would ever have been taken so seriously. Primate studies show that under natural conditions sexual behavior follows the rhythms of the days and the seasons. Under conditions of capture, restraint, and crowding, it becomes a frantic preoccupation and a cause for vicious fighting. Embedded in his time, it was impossible for Freud to sense this simple truth. The few who challenged him were accused of lacking the courage to face facts.

Thinkers who took issue with Freud were rebuffed with most unscientific intensity. Both Jung and Adler pointed out the Freudian bias but submitted biased views of their own. Jung's mysticism found an excellent market among those whose lives had been dry and prosaic. Adler's doctrines of power found a comparable market among the socially impotent, namely, the teachers, who have struggled constantly to extricate themselves from the onus of being society's baby-sitters.

Once the factors involved in dominance or status struggles (professional considerations) and territorial behavior (business and market aspects) are cleared away, it can be seen that there is much truth in all three points of view. They were the

Niña, the Pinta, and the Santa Maria of the voyage to "a far country." Each described important facets of many-faceted man.*

The pell-mell, crowded, distracting, struggling, competitive nature of man's evolving social life does do a number of things to man, and it does distort his natural bent. We can actually measure the rather dreadful things that crowding and restriction do to our primate cousins. It destroys and perverts natural sex, motherhood, and peaceful living together. Sex becomes a nervous preoccupation, ofttimes an obsession, sometimes a perversion, and tragically gets hooked up with violence. Motherhood can turn to murder. Peace can turn to carnage. And so it is with man.

Freud noted and documented man's preoccupation with sex, Jung noted man's desire to experience relief by meditation and fantasy, and Adler noted man's tendency to react to being "low man on the totem pole" by dominance struggles.†

* This paper has tried to keep theory as its sole target, not psychiatrists or psychiatry.

† Space forbids dealing with (1) the splinter movements of latter-day psychiatry and (2) with methodology of therapy.

1. The main splinter group after Freud, Jung, and Adler were the "social-cultural-interpersonal theorists" who pointed out that all of the earlier "individualistic" theories overlooked the social (interpersonal) nature of man. But in so doing, they made the error of discounting man's biologic roots and cut themselves off from vast areas of scientific endeavor, including the medical profession itself. H. S. Sullivan, an outstanding theorist of the social-interpersonal group, illustrates this. In a passage from his fundamental book,[33] under a section headed "One-Genus Postulate," he states that the human, no matter how badly damaged or abnormal, is still much more like a human than he is like the nearest animal genus and that the only worthwhile study for psychiatry is of things ubiquitously human.

This is a conceptual error, unusual and curious in a man of Sullivan's brilliance. The "mental patient" has long been subject to humiliation,[34] and one of many forms of this has been classing him with the beast, e.g., being beastly, or his agreeing (desperately) to the friendly suggestion of the psychiatrist that he must feel "beastly." Sullivan's desire to remove him from this category is, of course, praiseworthy. The fact is, however, that the "normal" person in our society in much more "beastlike" than is the "abnormal" person. The beast though unevolved is integrated. Our "patient" though evolved is un- or disintegrated. Integration, not evolvement, is the key. We are not seeing animal behavior in our "distintegrated patients." We are seeing jagged, fragmented human behavior.

They all raised questions that sent us scurrying to the clinic, to the laboratory, and to the library. And in these places we have found answers to some of the questions. This paper has suggested one more place to go, the field and forest.

It is time we paid homage to all of the early theorists as we have to the Pasteurs, the Claude Bernards, the Pavlovs. It is time we dropped controversies that now have only historical validity. The best refutation of the theory presented in this paper is not to point out flaws in the data or the reasoning but to stand quietly and look at a beautiful cathedral, or listen to Brahm's Second Symphony, to immerse one's self, that is, in the creativity that is man. To know the dimensions of man's heroism and sacrifice and to lose one's self in the moving greatness of man at his best—then the data of this theory and the theory itself recede into insignificance.

But if we are concerned with man broken—if we are concerned with collective man in his agonies and antagonisms, with his disintegrating roles as father and mother, brother and sister, lover, leader and follower—then we must use this theory, we must sharpen and tighten it, or forge another of comparable dimensions to take its place.

---

2. As for methodology, the future of Freudian therapies, i.e., therapies that are dyadic and essentially nonresponsive ("projective"), is still pretty much up in the air. Their futility for severe behavioral disturbances, as Freud predicted, has been well established. They are prohibitively impractical for extensive use in even the less serious disorders. In a purely research setting, however (freed, i.e., of status and commercial contaminants), they may serve as a continuing source of meaningful data (incidentally, this also is a prediction by Freud).

Most confusing of all, of course, has been the ever extending range of the responsive ("nonprojective, reactive, suggestive, counseling") therapies. The medical profession, including psychiatry, understandably has been bewildered. It senses something is wrong, almost out of hand, yet it has had no theory to serve as a criteria to describe, much less to criticize, the rapid influx of a wide variety of nonprofessionals into the field of therapy. Under this heading are listed psychologists, marriage counselors, social-service caseworkers, hypnotists, and spiritual counselors in ever increasing numbers. Such phenomena become understandable in the light of present theory.

Chapter 17

Konrad Lorenz—On Aggression

A Review*

ELIOT SLATER

THIS IS A VERY REMARKABLE WORK. LORENZ IS FAMOUS AS AN expert on the behaviour of animals; he is also an extraordinarily gifted observer and in prose that conveys a vivid picture of what he has seen in an underwater world and in the life of reptiles, mammals and birds. He expounds the insights he has derived from these observations, as penetrating as any that psychiatrists have based on the study of humankind. Distance and objectivity are combined with warmth and empathy. One finds to one's astonishment and delight how relevant an understanding of animal behaviour is to an understanding of man, and how many and how important are the lessons which one may derive from it. This particularly relates to the universal primary drive of aggression, perhaps the motivational field which in our own kind we understand least of all, with potentially the most dreadful consequences.

Lorenz contracts intraspecific aggression with the aggression shown between members of different species; in animal economy the latter plays much the lesser role. By and large, mem-

* *On Aggression*. By KONRAD LORENZ, translated by Marjorie Latzke, with a foreword by Sir Julian Huxley, London: Methuen, 1966. Price 30*s*. Pp. xiv+273.

bers of different species can live contentedly together. Even when one species lives by preying on another, the relationship, though it is one of occasional hunting and killing, does not mobilize in the predator an aggressive mood; expression and behaviour are much nearer to those of aggression in the prey that turns at bay to defend itself. In general, members of different species do not compete in a struggle for survival; predator and prey live in equilibrium. What threatens a species is not its "enemies" but its competitors: the mammalian dingo has ousted the marsupial wolf from Australia.

On the other hand intraspecific aggression, the instinctive hostility that springs up, though perhaps only in narrowly definable circumstances, between two members of the same species, has an enormous role in nature's economy. Thus a stretch of coral reef, which harbours perhaps thousands of species living in amity, may be able to support one only of any given species of coral fish. Endowed with brilliant colours to warn the stranger off, the little fish attacks and tries to ram at its first appearance only a similarly coloured member of its own kind. One wonders how these creatures are able to mate. Some of them live permanently in pairs, and then the pair of mates is likely to be even more aggressive than single fish are. In other species at spawning time the fish lose their brilliant colours and become dull, permitting mutual approach. Colouring, aggressiveness and sedentary territorial habits all go together. In such species intraspecific aggression plays a useful survival role: the territorial animal that drives off his rivals helps to spread them around the countryside and so helps towards a wider and a balanced distribution.

Lorenz demonstrates most convincingly that aggression is instinctive and wells up spontaneously; it is not primarily reactive, and for its appearance it does not depend finally on appropriate stimuli. Lorenz illustrates this principle by describing a common error of aquarium keepers who find, after putting a number of young fish into a large aquarium to give them a chance of pairing naturally, that when one couple have paired they become set on driving out all the others.

> Since these unfortunates cannot escape, they swim round nervously in the corners near the surface, their fins tattered, or, having been frightened out of their hiding places, they race wildly round the aquarium. The humane aquarium keeper, pitying not only the hunted fish but also the couple which, having perhaps spawned in the meanwhile, is anxious about its brood, removes the fugitives and leaves the couple in sole possession of the tank. Thinking he has done his duty, he ceases to worry about the aquarium and its contents for the time being, but after a few days he sees, to his horror, that the female is floating dead on the surface, torn to ribbons, while there is nothing more to be seen of the eggs and the young.

This error may be avoided by providing a tank big enough for two pairs and dividing it in half by a glass partition, putting a pair on each side.

> Then each fish can discharge its healthy anger on the neighbour of the same sex—it is nearly always male against male and female against female—and neither of them thinks of attacking its own mate. It may sound funny, but we were often made aware of a blurring of the partition, because of a growth of weed, by the fact that a cichlid male was starting to be rude to his wife. As soon as the partition separating the "apartments" was cleaned, there was at once a furious but inevitably harmless clash with the neighbours and the atmosphere was cleared inside each of the two compartments.

A general principle can be formulated, that the damming up of aggression will be the more dangerous the better the members of the group know, understand and like each other. The validity of this is appreciated by men living in isolation, e.g., in Arctic exploration.

Lorenz notes, somewhat sardonically, that this principle has been forgotten by educationists.

> It was supposed that children would grow up less neurotic, better adapted to their social environment and less aggressive if they were spared all disappointments and indulged in every way. An American method of education, based on these surmises, only showed that the aggressive drive, like many other instincts, springs spontaneously from the inner human being, and the results of this method of upbringing were countless unbearably rude children who were anything but non-aggressive.

Social animals, who have to live together, have to find some way of surmounting the dangerous effects of intraspecific aggression, which still has its part to play (as in the solitary territorial animal) in securing advantages for survival. The fighting of rivals for a mate advances the selection of the strongest; parental aggression serves for the defence of the young against a careless or hungry neighbour, or against the predator; and within the society aggression leads to the working out of a ranking order on which peace depends. Lorenz has a warning for the youthful rebel and for those who tend to see only the evil side of "the Establishment," to the effect that without rank order every turn of the social machinery would grate against friction and resistance.

Species after species in the process of phylogenetic development has worked out its own ways of guiding aggression into harmless channels. Within the species the manifestations of aggression are ritualized; mock battles take the place of real ones; submissive gestures, perhaps based on infantile behaviour patterns, or on the soliciting behaviour patterns of the female, have at once an inhibiting effect on the aggressor. The gesture, as in the wolf who turns his unprotected throat towards the aggressor, may in effect put one animal completely at the mercy of the other. The more dangerous the animal is, the more effective and absolute are the prohibitions imposed by the appeasing gesture; and the most bloodthirsty predators have the most reliable killing inhibitions. It is unfortunately in the animals who are but weakly endowed with natural weapons of offence that these inhibitions are weakest. However, mankind, who can only with difficulty kill his fellow with his bare hands, has invented for himself tools to do so, and moreover ones that, by acting at a distance, have a much reduced effect in awaking such inhibition of a murderous attack as nature has given him.

Lorenz discusses the different means that have been taken by different species towards the aim of keeping intraspecific aggression within bounds. In some species of social animals aggression is reduced to a minimum; but then one finds that the flock is a very loose structure with little internal organization. The shoal of fishes has no structure at all. In general, the ethologist does not know of a single species that is capable of friendship and that lacks aggression. On the other hand, aggression may dominate intraspecific relationships too far when the inhibiting stimuli are confined to, say, the immediate group or clan. Rats are biologically an extremely successful species, tough, courageous, adaptable in their ways, and (one of the few species who can do so) able to pass on information from one generation to the next. But intraspecific aggression constitutes a major danger for them.

Rats living together recognize their common allegiance by smell, and the stranger rat who exhibits the wrong smell is attacked and destroyed as soon as he is recognized. When two clans of rats are living in proximity they are constantly at war; and such warfare must exert a huge selection pressure in the direction of ever-increasing ability to fight. A parallel in man is offered in Sydney Margolin's studies of Prairie Indians, particularly the Utes, who suffer from an excess of aggression drive that under the ordered social conditions of today in the North American Indian reservations they are unable to discharge. At one time Prairie Indians led a life almost entirely of war and raids, when selective pressures must have favoured an extreme aggressiveness. Ute Indians are said to suffer from neuroses more than any other human group, the cause of the trouble being undischarged aggression.

A section of the book, of a strangely attractive and indeed moving kind, is given to the phylogenetic processes that have mobilized the aggression drive into being the instinctual basis of the bond that unites animals by ties that, at the highest level, are those of love and friendship. A very detailed account is given of the triumph rite of geese, which forms the bond between members of the same family and also between the pair when a young male goose falls in love with a young female. Mistakes can be made, and then the triumph rite may unite by accident two males; despite the fact that copulatory attempts prove vain, their relationship becomes as close and as intense as the normal lifelong heterosexual one. The prestige of the male pair in the total society of geese is just as high as that of a married pair. Following on this, a female may fall in love with one of the males. With great patience and assiduity she may eventually seduce him into coitus, after which he immediately flies back to his partner to go through the triumph rite with him. Bit by bit the female may become the sexual partner of both males; and then there is happiness for all. No other couple in the flock can stand up to such a united trio; they are always at the top of the ranking order, they are never driven out of their nesting territories, and they are highly successful parents.

It does not seem that Lorenz goes beyond the support available from biological observations when he applies his theories to man. Human behaviour is not rational, but it is understandable as phylogenetically adapted instinctive behaviour. The nature of the laws that control such behavior can be learned from studying animals. Present-day civilized man suffers from insufficient discharge of his aggressive drive. Lorenz considers that intraspecific selection is still working today in the direction of increasing aggressivity. Aggression is to be controlled by ritualizations and by redirected activity. Hitting the table instead of the other man's jaw, would be a simple example, and another more complex one is what Grzimek has called "bicycling": the "bicyclist" is the man who bows to his superior and treads on his inferior. Every culture has its own ways of channelling aggression. Cultural rites and social norms are indispensable. It is highly dangerous to mix cultures. To kill a culture it is often sufficient to bring it into contact with another, particularly if the other is higher or has a higher prestige. In aping the "higher" culture, the people of the subdued side may lose an invaluable heritage.

On this basis, at the present time, with races and cultures in the melting-pot, we are facing grave dangers. Lorenz points to the coinciding factors that threaten the continuity of Western culture: diminishing cohesion of the family group, decreasing contact between the generations, the greatly diminished tolerance of the young for the values held in honor by their seniors.

What preventive measures can we take? A number are suggested: the ethological investigation of ways and possibilities of discharging aggression on substitute objects: the psychoanalytic study of sublimation; the encouragement of personal friendships between members of different ideologies or nations; the intelligent channelling of militant enthusiasm. Remedies doomed to failure would be any attempt to breed out aggression, the attempt to suppress it by moral vetoes, or to starve it by depriving it of appropriate stimuli. But a simple principle offers an apposite line of approach. Aggression can find complete satisfaction by the use of substitute objects, in fair fighting, in sport, and in dangerous undertakings. The race for space flight may be indeed an inestimable safety valve.

There are points in this book where one would wish to part company with the author. The reviewer, for instance, would demand more evidence before he would accept the view that in civilized societies aggressiveness, that may admittedly tend towards worldly success, tends also to a higher differential survival rate. Nevertheless, the unspoken claim that ethology has an enormous contribution to make to human psychology must be conceded. This book should be read. It is full of magic, full of profound concepts and vivid illustrations, full of wisdom.

Chapter 18

The Primate Socialization Motives

HARRY F. HARLOW

THE VARIOUS SPECIES OF THE PRIMATE ORDER, WHICH includes monkeys, apes, and men, have shown relatively direct, progressive capabilities of socialization throughout the course of evolutionary development, with the result that it is easy to conceptualize the human being as the most social animal ever to be created. However, it should be recognized that primates, both human and simian, are animals endowed with many motives more suited to individual survival than to group living. Such basic motives as hunger, thirst, fear, and rage elicit, or tend to elicit, responses of self-survival so that man and his next of kin are inherently a very different type of social animal from, for example, the social insects, which suffer little conflict between motives for personal survival and motives for social survival.

The primates' capacity for socialization stems from the fact that in addition to the individual motives of survival they also possess complex motives that endow them, both innately and through learning, with strong, positive feelings toward members of their social group. In all primates the self-survival motives and the social motives are often in conflict. In well-run monkey societies there are personal quarrels leading to psychic and physical pain and occasionally to injury and mayhem. In well-run human societies there are also individual or intragroup quarrels and conflicts, and these can have tragic consequences. Whether or not these conflicts and quarrels are more serious in groups of men or monkeys is an open question. However, primate social motives have triumphed over individual-survival motives in all existent simian societies so far.

We have broadly defined the socialization motives as the affectional systems and have presented the position that within, and probably even without, the primate order there are at least five affectional systems.[1] These are: the mother-infant or maternal affectional system, the closely related and complementary infant-mother affectional system, the age-mate or peer affectional system, the heterosexual affectional system, and the paternal affectional system.

During the last several years we have directed our primary research emphasis toward the analysis of individual affectional systems, including the developmental or growth stages through which each progresses and the determination of the relative roles of the various stimulus variables, including the experiential, which elicit, regulate, and order them. The data obtained from a family of researches led us to the conclusion that in all probability the age-mate or peer affectional system, rather than the maternal affectional system, was the primary intraspecies socialization mechanism determining subsequent successful heterosexual adjustment and maternal behavior.[2] This position is supported in a recent study by Alexander and Harlow[3] that showed that baby monkeys raised with cloth surrogate mothers while being denied any opportunity to interact with peers during the first six months of life had greater difficulty in making effective social adjustments during preadolescence and adolescence than did baby monkeys raised by adequate mothers, brutal mothers, or no mothers whatsoever but permitted ample opportunity to establish affectional relationships with their age-mates during the first half-year.

Although research techniques designed to analyze the individual affectional systems and to ascertain their relative importance throughout the total socialization process are justifiable and even meritorious, it is obvious that the various affectional systems do not operate independently and exclusively during the course of socialization in the primate animal. The various affectional systems must appear and elaborate in an orderly and integrated manner and in such sequences that the normal development of the early affectional patterns prepares the animal for the kind of social adjustment that will transpire as each of the subsequent affectional patterns appears.

Mother-Infant Affectional Relationships

By definition the primary affectional systems in terms of ontogenesis, if not of importance, are those of the interacting maternal affectional system and the reciprocal infant-mother affectional system. The initial stage of the mother-infant affectional interaction in the rhesus monkey transpires during the infant's first four or five months of life, and an analogous affectional stage persists in the human being for four to five times as long. During this early developmental stage, the normal monkey mother responds to her infant almost totally positively, giving it tender, loving care and punishing it only infrequently and then but mildly.

During the early stage of mother-infant interaction the normal mother effectively and efficiently carries out three primary functions: (a) she satisfies her infant's physiological requirements, including food and warmth, (b) she meets her infant's psychological needs of intimate bodily contact and comfort, and (c) she protects her infant from the animate and inanimate threats in the external environment. The protective function is very broad, including guarding the baby from predators or hostile monkeys, guiding the infant in the selection of appropriate and inappropriate responses to physical and social environmental stimuli, and comforting the infant when it is frightened or hurt. Thus the protective functions are, in fact, closely allied to the maternal bodily contact and comfort behaviors.

During this early stage of affectional development, the infant's responses to the mother are essentially reciprocal. The infant monkey's reflex clasping, clinging, and climbing responses aid and abet nutritional needs, since they position the baby ventrally on the mother's ventral surface and thereby insure oral nipple contact, one component of the infant monkey's maternal contactual pattern. The infant rhesus also shows a strong propensity toward imitation of maternal responses directed toward the external environment, a mechanism that facilitates early maternal guidance.

The human neonate is so physically immature that it cannot clasp, cling, and feed back to the mother as effectively as the neonatal monkey, but this does not mean that its early affectional requirements are basically different. The human neonate has the same contactual, nutritional, and protective needs as the monkey, but its immaturity places a heavier burden of responsibility upon the human mother and prolongs the period of dependency.

The product of this primordial mother-infant affectional interrelationship from the point of view of the infant's social development is the formation within the infant of strong feelings of safety and security in the physical presence of the maternal figure. All three of the described maternal functions doubtless play a role although our own researches on the surrogate mothers indicated that bodily contact with the mother superceded nursing and calmed the frightened animal. The development of infantile feelings of safety and security are essential since within this period the primate infant has itself matured to the point that strangeness has become a fear stimulus in and of itself, and the infant requires the maternal haven of protection if it is to operate effectively in adjusting to the outside world. Thus, the development in the infant of security and trust in its contact with the mother prepares it for the second stage of mother-infant affectional relationships.

The second stage of mother-infant affectional relationships is one in which the infant gradually emancipates itself from the pervading need of physical maternal attachment, and if this stage is blocked either by infantile or maternal incapacity, the infant will be socially crippled. From the infant's point of view, the basic mechanisms of maternal emancipation are the strong motivations of curiosity and exploration which lead the infant to investigate the physical environment that surrounds it even though this of necessity means the temporary severance of maternal contact. Exploration of the physical world takes two forms: exploration of nearby physical objects and exploration of nearby animate objects, and the most important of these objects are other infants, preferably infants of similar ages.

It is our firm belief that maternal emancipation is not only achieved through the operation of the infant's curiosity and exploratory responses but that it is abetted by simultaneous changes in the mother's behavior which take the form of discouraging continuous bodily contact by mild rejection from time to time. We have described this second maternal stage as that of ambivalence or transition. Although the mother throughout this second stage exhibits strong protective functions whenever these are required, the physiological needs, particularly the nutritional needs, of the infant are gradually waning as other food sources become available and the compelling needs of intimate bodily contact and comfort are also declining or possibly merely being superceded by the incompatible needs for exploration and broadened social contacts. Thus, the effective primate mother in this second period is one that not only gradually accepts infantile separation, but also even encourages it. During this second mother-infant developmental stage the normal monkey mother shows a decreasing tendency to restrain its infant's explorations and also an increasing frequency and severity of punishment responses directed against her infant even though these responses are seldom, if ever, cruel or abusive. Whatever the mechanisms eliciting these maternal punishment responses may be, we strongly suspect that they serve a useful function in supporting the infant's own tendencies to emancipate itself.

The Age-Mate or Peer Affectional System

If the monkey infant achieves maternal independence and is afforded opportunity to interact with age-mates, the age-mate affectional system will inevitably develop. The primary mechanism producing these effective age-mate adjustments is that of physically interactive play, and social play between monkey infants goes through a threefold developmental process, progressing from rough-and-tumble play, to approach-withdrawal or noncontact play, and culminating in aggressive play. Rough-and-tumble play, illustrated in Fig. 1, is characterized by vigorous wrestling, rolling, and sham-biting responses which involve little or no physical discomfort. Noncontact play is characterized by back-and-forth chasing responses by two or more animals with actual physical contact being kept to a minimum. During the latter part of the first year of life the two patterns may become intermixed, and we have sometimes given this alternating and relatively violent pattern of play sequences the special name of interactive or mixed play.

Aggressive play, which develops shortly before or after the first year of life, is similar in form to rough-and-tumble play but the bouts are now characterized by aversive components. The manual contact and release may now be physically painful, and the biting responses may evoke cries of distress and anguish from the victim. Normal rhesus infants are seldom injured during these aggressive play encounters, but firm peer relations establishing dominance position and social status

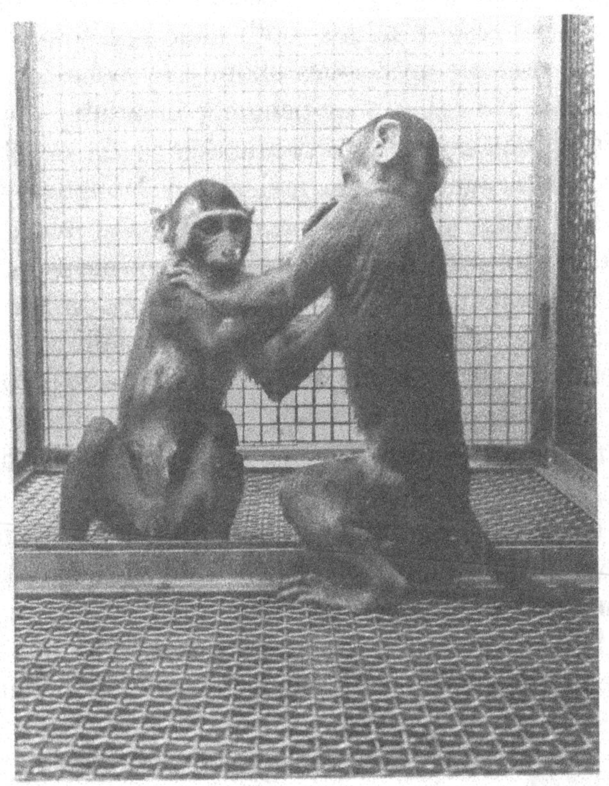

FIGURE 1.

develop both between and among the masculine and feminine infants. Thus we conceive of aggressive play as having an important, positive social role in which the monkeys learn through early experience to try, test, and accept the differential and changing status positions they will occupy during adolescence and adulthood.

Out of the early age-mate affectional interactions the monkey learns the techniques by which it expresses dominance when dominance is appropriate, and submission when submission is required. Thus early play experience trains the monkey to meet the ever increasingly complex patterns of social ordering in monkey societies composed not only of other age-mates, but also of adults, both male and female.

There is nothing mysterious about play behavior. If infant associates are available, play behavior invariably appears and follows a sequence almost as predictable as the developmental sequences of locomotion and prehension. Doubtless play does prepare the infant to assume later adult roles, but so also do locomotion and prehension, and there is no need to assume a teleological explanation. The play sequence is the complex resultant of the maturing of motor and intellectual abilities, the satisfaction of emerging and developing needs for activity and exploration, and, eventually, of the affectional ties that spring from and, in turn, become strengthened by the playful interactions.

Just as the maternal and infantile affectional patterns prepare the monkey infant for entrance into the stage of peer attachment, so does the age-mate affectional system prepare the older infant or juvenile for entering successfully into the complex social requirements of the heterosexual, maternal, and paternal affectional systems.

The Heterosexual Affectional System

The heterosexual affectional system has a long ontogenetic developmental history starting with reflex pelvic thrusting in the neonatal period to any soft, warm surface, such as the mother's body, and progressing in infancy to differential sex behaviors commonly characterized in the male by threatening and following behaviors, and in the female by passivity and rigidity responses. Thus, from early infancy onward there is a tendency, when playful physical interactions take place between male and female, for these interactions to be broken off by the female, which in turn retreats and assumes either a passive or rigid body posture with head averted, and a tendency for the male to follow and make physical contact. These physical interactions by their basic nature lead the male to achieve dorsoventral contact with the female, and probably through some learned process which has not been adequately analyzed, male and female infants show ever increasing frequency of play behaviors which mimic the adult-type male and female sexual postures basic to normal adult heterosexual interactions. However, normal adult heterosexuality involves more than the formation of appropriate postures and motor skills. Both males and females must be willing to accept physical contact by age-mates if normal adult heterosexuality is to be accomplished, and we believe that the acceptance of physical contact is also achieved through age-mate play behaviors. Furthermore, normal heterosexual behavior cannot be attained if the aggressive responses that mature from the second year of life onward are not ameliorated and modulated by the earlier intraspecies affectional responses that also develop out of the early stages of interactive play. Just as the normal operation of the maternal affectional system in association with the normal development of the infant-mother affectional system prepares the organism for age-mate or peer affectional relationships, so do the complicated interactions involved in the age-mate or peer affectional system prepare the monkeys, both male and female, for the adolescent and adult expressions of normal heterosexual behavior.

The Maternal Affectional System

Maternal behavior is in turn based on a family of early-experience variables. At least from late infancy onward the female monkeys show far more interest in baby monkeys than do equal-aged males, and this female interest expresses itself as if the female had a specific need to make positive contactual responses to young monkeys. Thus, before motherhood is normally achieved the female monkey is a highly baby-oriented animal predisposed to welcome or initiate intimate contactuality with infants and, through this contactuality, achieve the complete pattern of normal maternal responses. The same factors that predispose the female to be contactually responsive may also be responsible for the greater frequency of grooming behavior engaged in by females as contrasted with males.

However, we have a wealth of data that show that any innate maternal propensities are not adequate in and of themselves to endow the rhesus mother with normal maternal capabilities. In those cases in which we have impregnated by dark and devious means, female monkeys that had been denied opportunity to form age-mate affectional relationships during the first year of life we have produced mother monsters that were either indifferent to their newborn infants or cruel, brutal, and even lethal. Thus it is obvious that early age-mate association is as essential to the fruition of the later maternal affectional system as it is to the heterosexual affectional system.

We are convinced that the playful interactions that characterize the development of the age-mate affectional system are the basic mechanisms through which monkeys, and probably people, develop generalized feelings of affection for other members of their species. Monkey mothers that have been denied age-mate affection treat their infants with no more concern than they would treat inanimate objects, and those mothers that are aggressive vent their aggression against their own babies in a manner totally devoid of any restraint.

Paternal Affectional System

Laboratory and field studies, particularly field studies, clearly demonstrate that the mature adult male is a highly social animal protecting all members of his group or clan and showing particularly intense protective responses toward young infants, even to the point of occasionally adopting infants for a considerable period of time when these infants have become separated from their mothers, probably because of the advent of a second baby or the death of a mother. Little or nothing is known of the variables, innate or acquired, which lead the adult monkey male to assume these protective functions, although the phenomenon has been demonstrated time and time again. It is, however, inconceivable to us that an adult male monkey would ever adopt an effective paternal role if he had not gone through the peer affectional stage. Indeed, males raised in social isolation for the first or second six months of life subsequently, as adolescents, show aggression toward younger monkeys in contrast with the friendly behavior of socially raised males of the same age.[4]

Effects of Social Isolation

A basic method that we have used to analyze the variables underlying the development of the affectional systems is that of social isolation, in which monkeys are denied any opportunity to form affectional relationships with any other member of their species for predetermined periods of time. We have described one of our isolation techniques as partial social isolation, and it is achieved by raising monkey from birth onward in individual wire cages, as illustrated in Fig. 2 in which the isolates can see and hear other monkeys but cannot make any physical contact with them. This technique makes it impossible for the infants to form any mother-child relationships, and it also makes it impossible for them to form adequate age-mate or peer affectional patterns because any opportunity for interactive play is excluded.

We have raised groups of rhesus monkeys under partial social isolation for periods ranging from a few months to more

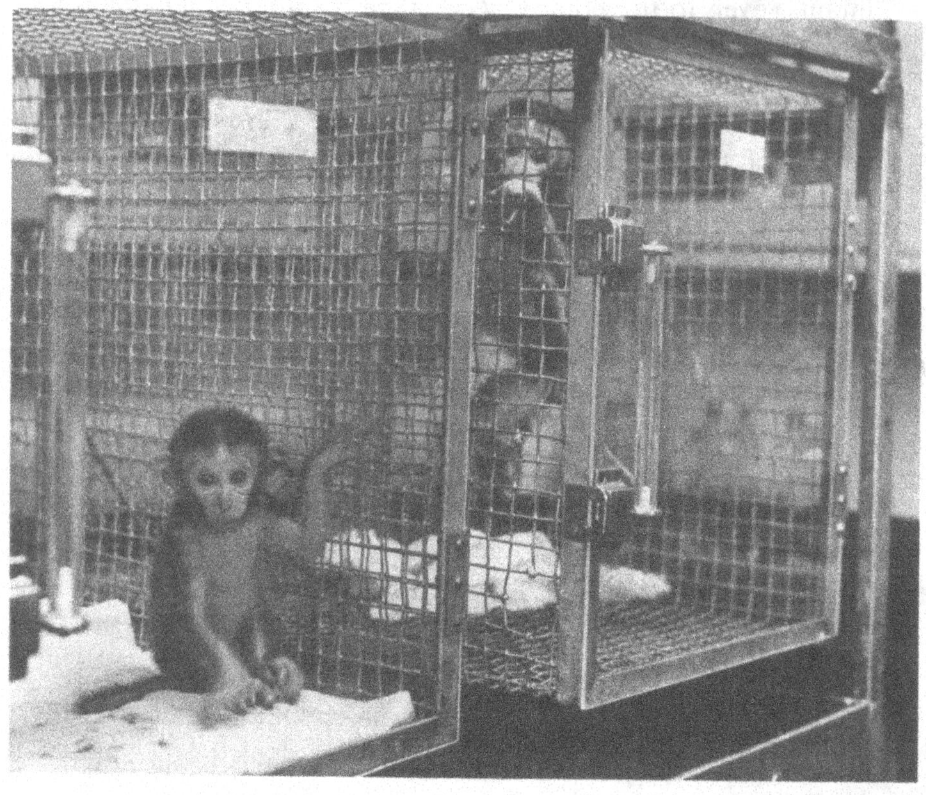

FIGURE 2.

than seven years and have traced the development of abnormal personal behaviors that appear under this condition.[5] Early in life there is a high incidence of diffuse disturbance patterns that include nonnutritional orality, self-clutching, and convulsive jerking. An extreme form of the self-clutching pattern is illustrated in Fig. 3, and we have referred to it as an autistic pattern of response, recognizing that the human autistic pattern is more complex and more variable. These behaviors tend to decrease with time as the animal matures and/or adjusts to its restricted environment, but other dramatic abnormal pat-

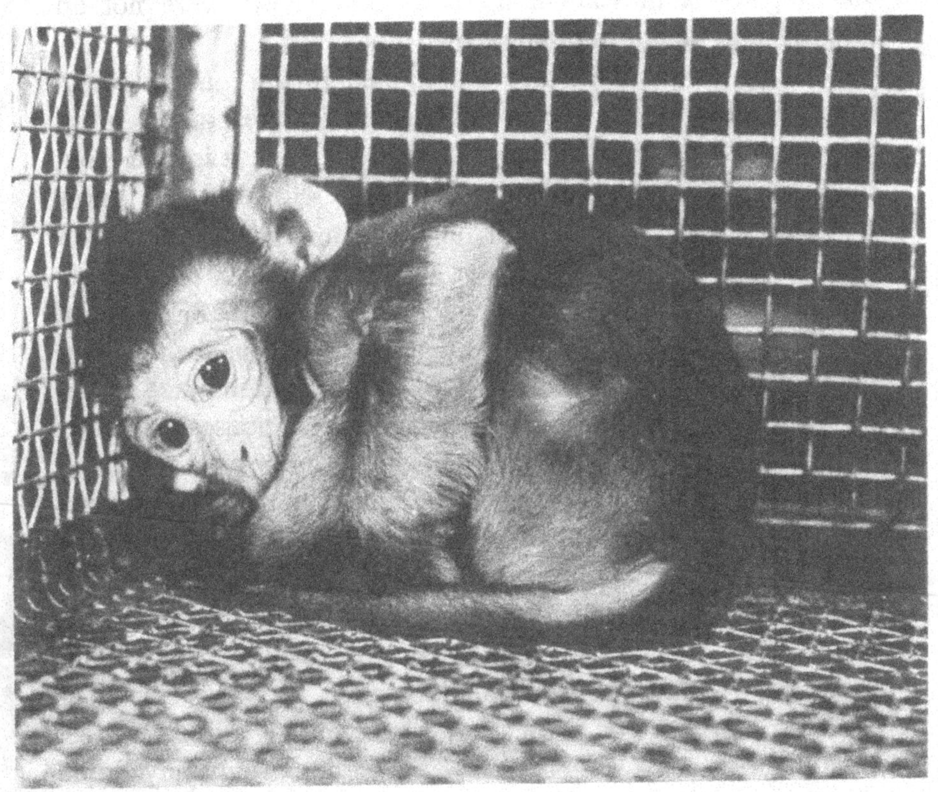

FIGURE 3.

terns take their place. One of these is repetitive stereotyped movements, such as repetitively pacing back and forth across or around the cage, or circling compulsively from the top to bottom of the cage, and these abnormal individual patterns are more persisting than those of nonnutritional sucking or autistic posturing. A third dramatic abnormal pattern that we have observed is one to which we have given the name "catatonic contracture," and it may appear within the first two years of partial social isolation. While the monkey sits in a quiescent state, often staring blankly into space, an arm slowly and gradually floats upward with concurrent flexion of the wrist and fingers—a movement made as if the limb were not an integral part of the monkey's own body.

As long as monkeys are maintained in our partial social isolation situation we see no increase in fear responses, probably because the animal learns that in the cage it is safe from the threats of animals in adjacent cages. However, we know that animals so raised exhibit intense fear of each other or of more normally raised age-mates if they are placed in a social test situation with them after enduring six months or more of partial social isolation. Thus, though we do not see the development of social fears as long as the animal is maintained in the partial isolation situation, these social fear responses are ready to be manifested outside the home cage.

The phenomena relating to the development of aggression are much more striking. The developmental trends may be measured by the simple technique of observing the animal while one experimenter slowly runs his hand, covered by a large black laboratory glove, over the subject's cage. This black glove is familiar to all the laboratory monkeys since it is used by handlers for protection when making direct contact with the animals. Two patterns of aggression are displayed and show progressive increase in frequency under this condition. One pattern is aggression directed toward the observer. This behavior attains near maximal frequency in the second year of life for the male and by the fifth year of life for the female. The second pattern is that of aggression by the animal against its own body, characterized by biting its own hand, arm, foot, or leg. This pattern has a relatively high level of frequency by the fourth year of life in the male and by the sixth year of life in the female. Sex differences in the development of the aggressive patterns are interesting in that aggression is one of the few behavioral patterns to mature earlier in the male than in the female.

We now have a large body of data on the effects of partial social isolation on the animal's subsequent ability to adjust socially to age-mates. Prolonged partial social isolation progressively depresses any capability of social interaction, probably heightens aggression or perhaps only appears to because it prevents learning of restraints in expressing aggression, and inhibits or destroys heterosexual interaction and maternal capabilities. Actually partial social isolation is almost as socially destructive as total social isolation, but in the following pages we shall limit our presentation to the effect of early, complete social isolation because of our greater abundance of long-term total isolation test data.

Total social isolation was achieved by raising various groups of rhesus monkeys in a stainless-steel chamber, from a few hours after birth until 3, 6, or 12 months of age. In addition, one group of monkeys was raised for the first six months in individual cages in the nursery, then subjected to total social isolation for six months. During the period of confinement the monkeys had no social contact with any animal whatsoever. Sensory deprivation was held to a minimum since the chamber was constantly illuminated, transmitted sounds, and afforded limited opportunities for cutaneous-proprioceptive expression and exploration.

The effects of total social isolation were appraised by comparing the interactions of social isolates with the interactions of control animals exposed to our playroom situation[6] as stable groups of four composed of two isolates and two control animals. In each instance the controls were not normally raised animals but monkeys of the same age raised in partial social isolation. Macaque monkeys raised in total isolation for three months are terrified when they are released from the isolation chamber and placed in standard laboratory cages. However, when the period of initial shock subsides, the three-month total social isolate monkeys make a surprisingly good adjustment to the control age-mates, and as we see no indication of any differential frequency in social threats in the members of the experimental and control groups and find no differential incidence that is statistically significant in the frequency of contact play in the isolate and control groups. Thus, rhesus monkeys show a rather surprising capacity to recover from this relatively brief period of total social isolation although we are by no means convinced that there are not some long-term residual effects, at least in some of these subjects.

A far different picture, one of social devastation, is found in the case of macaque monkeys that have undergone six or twelve months of total social isolation and have then been tested with pairs of control age-mates in the social playroom. Contact play is high in the control animals and almost nonexistent in the six-month isolate animals. The slight increase in play that the isolate monkeys show from 24 weeks onward is limited entirely to play with one another; the isolate monkeys have never exhibited any form of positive social interaction with the controls. The controls themselves are retarded in social interactions as compared with monkeys given social experience with peers from at least three months of age onward.

Although six months of total social isolation obviously resulted in drastic curtailment of social activity, the monkeys subjected to twelve months of isolation were even less active. Even activity play—self-play not involving social interaction—is essentially nonexistent in the twelve-month isolates, and these twelve-month isolate monkeys are the only animals we have ever seen in which autoerotic sex behavior was almost nonexistent. The experiment was concluded at the end of ten weeks. This action was taken because the year-old controls were exhibiting progressively greater violent aggression against the totally helpless isolate monkeys, and we were convinced that the isolate monkeys would have been killed had we continued testing for a longer period of time. Probably a more socialized control group would have been less aggressive toward the isolates, but none was available. There were also two pairs of animals isolated between six and twelve months of age. Upon release and exposure to the social playroom one pair was markedly hyperaggressive and abused the control animals, and the other pair held its own with the controls but was not ascendant.

These combined data strongly suggest that rhesus monkeys can recover from a limited period of social isolation beyond which there results a progressive social incapacitation until a point is achieved from which there is probably no recovery. If we interpret our data in terms of a critical period or critical stage hypothesis, it would appear that the first three months of life is not the critical period or the most critical period for the development of socialization in these animals. However, the following three months represents a very critical stage, and in all probability every succeeding month is progressively more devastating and, at least statistically speaking, dramatically lowers any possibility of social rehabilitation until the likelihood of social rehabilitation becomes for practical purposes nonexistent. Not surprising is the qualitatively different effect of total isolation coming after an early period of only limited restriction. Although no human infant could survive the kind of total isolation to which the monkeys were subjected, human infants are sometimes reared under conditions of partial social isolation in institutions. The data suggest that they may suffer damage in the last quarter of their first year of life but may recover if removed. After 12 months in an unstimulating institution the probability for recovery decreases, and after 24 months, the human being raised under social restrictions is a very poor risk for future adjustment in a normal environment.

Mechanisms of Socialization

Psychologists, anthropologists, and sociologists have placed great emphasis on the importance of learning in the development of socialization. No one will deny the importance of social learning or deny that learning variables play progressively greater roles as primate social organizations become progressively more complex. However, the fixation on the role of learning by many socially minded theorists obscures the fact that success or failure of primate social learning is dependent upon many basic, complex, unlearned behaviors that progressively mature long after birth. In rhesus monkeys masculine and feminine behaviors are relatively undifferentiated during the first 90 days of life but are progressively more differentiated thereafter, and learning is in no sense the variable of primary importance. Maternal behavior changes during the periods of gestation and parturition and the sequential development of primate play patterns are not to be explained by learning alone. However, above and beyond the maturation of these relatively specific social behaviors the natural and orderly sequential development of three major categories of behavior determines in large part the success or failure of primate socialization.

Affection, Fear, and Aggression

In all primate species, in all mammalian species, and in many or most vertebrate species there is an orderly development of affection, regardless of the specific form it takes, of fear, and of aggression. One or more forms of affection precede the appearance of specific environmental fears, and fear in turn precedes the development of intraspecies aggression. Thus in the macaque monkey intense mother-infant affectional responses are formed in the first days of the infant's life and have become deep and enduring during the first month. Fear of strange external stimuli, even though they may be of low physical intensity, are first evident between 60 to 90 days of age, and as we have already indicated, intraspecies aggressive responses play no important social role until the macaque monkey is approximately one year old.

In the human being infant-mother affectional ties are established during the first half-year of life, fear of strangeness, characterized by Spitz as eight-months' anxiety, typically develops in the second half-year of life, and aggression between human children attains social importance between the third and fourth year.

Puppies form warm relationships to their mothers during the first few hours or days of life, show fear of unfamiliar objects by the sixth or seventh week,[7] and develop intraspecies aggressive responses at some later period of time.

Below the class of mammals are the data on many species of nidifugous birds. The imprinting process which we will include as an avian infant-mother affectional mechanism normally develops at birth or shortly thereafter. Fear of external stimuli develops after the sensitive period of imprinting, and if imprinting is not achieved before these external fears develop, the very process of imprinting may be difficult or impossible.[8] The development of social aggressive responses has not been traced in birds, but it clearly follows the appearance of fear and is definitely present in the courtship and mating patterns. In those fish that lack parental ties, the first positive bonds would be with peers. Fear must appear early if the fry are to survive at all, but aggression presumably appears much later. For guppies we have a few informal observations that support the principle of delayed appearance of aggression for this species. Guppies removed from a tank with adults soon after birth very quickly show no avoidance of peers. Placed with larger but immature guppies, they avoid the larger fish. Three- to four-month-old guppies approaching maturity do not attack two-week-old guppies, but mature guppies immediately attack two-week-old guppies and even incapacitated mature guppies.

Social isolation is a technique making it possible to eliminate all opportunities for affectional formation until fear of external stimuli or of strangeness and until socially aggressive responses have developed. Fear of strangeness appears in monkeys by 90 days of age, and all rhesus monkeys subjected to total social isolation for three months or more show intense fear to strange environmental stimuli, animate or inanimate. Indeed, this period of panic may be so extreme as to be lethal. Our own data indicate that this fear of strangeness becomes more pervasive and prolonged the greater the period of social isolation, but this may be an artifact of our test situation. The older our isolated monkeys are when they are introduced into the playroom with pairs of strangers, the older and more aggressive are the strangers, and the progressively increasing fear of the isolates may consequently be the result of being confronted by more and more ominous social stimuli and more and more abuse.

Macaque monkeys subjected to total social isolation for the first year of life show no aggressive tendencies when paired in the playroom with control age-mates. We attribute this to the fact that their aggressive tendencies are hidden by their overwhelming social terror. Two of the monkeys subjected to total social isolation during the second half-year of life, contrariwise, turned out to be extremely hyperaggressive, and the other two were a match for the controls. We assume that while they had no opportunity to form affectional attachments in their first six months, they did have a chance to adjust to fear of strange situations, including other monkeys, leaving delayed aggression to flourish without tempering by affectional attachments after their release from isolation and introduction to social stimuli.

We also have long-term follow-up data on the monkeys subjected to total social isolation for both the early social isolates (first six months of life) and the late social isolates (second six months of life). When these monkeys were approaching or had reached adolescence they were subjected to social tests with stranger adults, stranger age-mates, and one-year-old juveniles. Theoretically by this time aggression has had ample opportunity to reach or approach its maturational peak.

Most of the monkeys in both the early and late social isolation groups exhibited violent aggressive tendencies of strange, bizarre, and socially maladaptive types. Frequently the social isolates would engage in a single act of aggression against a stranger adult, a suicidal act that no socially experienced adolescent would ever attempt. In all cases social learning was rapid. Furthermore, the social isolates, both male and female, would frequently aggress against defenseless young juveniles, a social transgression not seen in normal adolescent monkeys.

The developmental sequence of the emotional trilogy of affection, fear, and aggression provides a basis for primate socialization and doubtless for the socialization of many other species. The early affectional bonds between mother and child and the subsequent peer affectional bonds provide basic social security before external fear can arise. Members of one's own species, particularly one's own social group, are external objects that do not induce terror, indeed, they become security-providing objects. If, however, no opporunity has been afforded for the formation of affectional alliances with members of one's own species until after fear of strangers has developed, the capability of subsequent socialization will be seriously impaired.

If affection for members of one's social group has developed through normal mother-infant relationships and normal peer relationships before full-fledged aggression has matured, the later expression of aggression toward in-group members will be greatly ameliorated, and the full force of aggression can be turned against external enemies and predators instead of in-group associates. Failure to develop in-group affection before aggression is fully matured leaves the animal a deviate, a delinquent, and a social outcast. Both the self-survival motives of fear and aggression become effective social forces if they operate within useful social bonds, but if they operate against useful social alliances they convert the individual into a scapegoat on the one hand or a social menace on the other that cannot and will not be tolerated by his society.

Notes

INTRODUCTION

1. Hagnell, Olle: *A Prospective Study of the Incidence of Mental Disorder,* Lund: Berlingska Boktryckerist, 1966.

2. Bahn, A. K.: "Diagnostic and Demographic Characteristics of Patients Seen in Out Patient Psychiatric Clinics for an Entire State (Maryland), *American Journal of Psychiatry,* 117:769-778, 1961. Gardner, E. A.: "The Use of a Psychiatric Case Register in the Planning and Evaluation of a Mental Health Program," *Psychiatric Epidemiology and Mental Health Planning,* Monroe, R. R., Klee, G. D. and Brody, E. B., eds., Psychiatric Research Report #22, American Psychiatric Association.

3. Hare, E. H. and Shaw, G. K.: *Mental Health on a New Housing Estate: A Comparative Study of Health in the Two Districts of Croyden:* Oxford University Press, 1965.

4. Shepherd, M., Cooper, B., Brown, A. C., Kalton, G. W.: *Psychiatric Illness in General Practice:* Oxford University Press, 1966.

5. National Health Survey: "Appendix III Current Estimates from the Health Interview Survey," *Vital and Health Statistics: Public Health Service Publication No. 1000*-Series, 10, No. 37, 1967.

6. Leighton, A.: "Is Social Environment a Cause of Psychiatric Disorder?," *Psychiatric Epidemiology and Mental Health Planning,* Monroe, R., et. al., eds., Psychiatric Research Report #22: American Psychiatric Association.

7. Kiev, Ari: *Psychiatry in the Communist World,* New York: Science House, in press.

8. Lambo, T. A.: "Patterns of Psychiatric Care in Developing African Countries," *Magic, Faith and Healing,* Kiev, A., ed.: Free Press, 1964.

9. Querido, A.: "Mental Health Program in Public Health Planning," *International Trends in Mental Health,* David, H. P., ed., New York: McGraw-Hill, 1966.

10. Bellak, L.: *Handbook of Community Psychiatry,* New York: Gruen & Stratton, 1964.

11. Brown, G. W., Bone, M., Dalison, B. and Wing, J. K.: *Schizophrenia and Social Care, A Comparative Follow-up Study of 339 Schizophrenic Patients,* London: Oxford University Press, 1966.

12. Grad, J. and Sainsbury, P.: "Evaluating the Community Psychiatric Service in Chichester: Results, *Milbank Memorial Fund Quarterly,* 44, 1966.

13. Pasamanick, B., Scarpitti, F. R. and Dinitz, S.: *Schizophrenics in the Community, An Experimental Study in the Prevention of Hospitalization,* New York: Appleton-Century-Crofts, 1967.

14. Rogler, L. H. and Hollingshead, A. B.: *Trapped Families and Schizophrenia,* New York: John Wiley & Sons, 1965.

15. *Ibid.*

16. Carstairs, G. M., Brown, G. W. and Topping, G. G.: "The Post-Hospital Adjustment of Chronic Mental Patients," *Lancet,* II:685, 1958. Freeman, H. E. and Simmons, O. G.: *The Mental Patient Comes Home,* New York: John Wiley & Sons, 1963. Schooler, N. R., Goldberg, S. C., Boothe, H. and Cole, J. O.: "One Year After Discharge: Community Adjustment of Schizophrenic Patients," *American Journal of Psychiatry,* 123:8, 1967.

17. Program Area Committee on Mental Health, American Public Health Association: *Mental Disorders: A Guide to Control Methods,* New York: American Public Health Association, 1962. Zusman, J.: "Some Explanations of the Changing Appearance of Psychotic Patients: Antecedents of the Social Breakdown Syndrome Concept: *Milbank Memorial Fund Quarterly,* 44:363, 1966.

18. Wittkower, E. D., Murphy, H. B. M. and Chance, N. A.: "Cross-cultural Inquiry into the Symptomatology of Depression: A Preliminary Report," Montreal: *Proceedings of the Third World Congress of Psychiatry,* 1961.

19. Harlow, H. F.: "The Primate Socialization Motives," *Transactions and Studies of the College of Physicians of Philadelphia,* 4 Ser., 33:No. 4, 1966. Calhoun, J.B.: "Ecological Factors in the Development of Behavioral Anomalies," *Comparative Psychopathology, Animal and Human,* Zubin, J. and Hunt, H. F., eds., New York: Grune & Stratton, 1967.

20. Lorenz, K.: *On Aggression,* London: Methuen, 1966.

CHAPTER I

1. Jaspers, K.: *General Psychopathology,* Chicago: University of Chicago Press, 1963.

2. Hoselitz, B. F., ed.: *Reader's Guide to the Social Sciences,* Glencoe, Illinois: Free Press, a division of the Macmillan Co., 1959.

3. Handy, R. and Kurtz, P.: *Current Appraisal of Behavioral Sciences,* Great Barrington, Mass.: Behavioral Research Council, 1964.

4. Bellak, L., ed.: *Community Psychiatry and Community Mental Health,* Grune & Stratton, Inc., 1964. Hoch, P. H.: "Social Psychiatry," in *Soziale und Angewandte Psychiatrie:* Vol. 3 of *Psychiatrie der Gegenwart:* Forschung and Praxis, Berlin: Springer-Verlag, 1961, pp. 9-35. Hoch, P. H. and Zubin, J., eds.: *Future of Psychiatry,* New York: Grune & Stratton, Inc., 1962.

5. Leighton, A. H.; Clausen, J. A.; and Wilson, R. N., eds.: *Explorations in Social Psychiatry,* New York: Basic Books Inc., Pub, 1957.

6. Davidson, H. A.: *Forensic Psychiatry,* New York: Ronald Press, 1952.

7. Ahrenfeldt, R. H.: *Psychiatry in British Army in Second World War,* New York: Columbia University Press, 1958.

8. Funkenstein, D. H., ed.: *Student and Mental Health: International View,* International Conference on Student Mental Health, Princeton, N.J., 1956.

9. McLean, A. A., and Taylor, G. C.: *Mental Health in Industry,* New York: McGraw-Hill Book Co., Inc., 1958.

10. Group for Advancement of Psychiatry, Committee on Governmental Agencies: *Preventive Psychiatry in Armed Forces: With Some Implications for Civilian Use,* New York: GAP Report No. 47, 1960.

11. Group for Advancement of Psychiatry, Committee on Psychiatry and Religion: *Psychiatry and Religion: Some Steps Toward Mutual Understanding and Usefulness,* New York: GAP Report No. 48, 1960.

12. Stanton, A. H. and Schwartz, M. S.: *The Mental Hospital,* New York: Basic Books, Inc., Pub., 1954.

13. Hoch, P. H.: "Social Psychiatry," *op. cit.*, see reference 4.

14. Apple, D., ed.: *Sociological Studies of Health and Sickness,* New York: McGraw-Hill Book Co., Inc., 1960. Bellak, L., *op. cit.,* see reference No. 4. Birren, J. E., ed.: *Handbook of Aging and the Individual: Psychological and Biological Aspects,* Chicago: University of Chicago Press, 1959. Freeman, H. E.; Levine, S.; and Reeder, L. G., eds.: *Handbook of Medical Sociology,* Englewood Cliffs, N.J.: Prentice-Hall, 1963. Goffman, E.: *Asylums,* Garden City, N.Y.: Doubleday Anchor Books, 1961. Hawkins, N. G.: *Medical Sociology,* Springfield, Ill.: Charles C. Thomas, Pub., 1958. Hollander, E. P., and Hunt, R. G., eds.: *Current Perspectives in Social Psychology,* New York: Oxford University Press, 1963. Hollingshead, A. B., and Redlich, F. C.: *Social*

Class and Mental Illness, New York: John Wiley & Sons, Inc., 1958. Jaco, E. G., ed.: *Patients, Physicians, and Illness,* Glencoe, Ill.: Free Press, a division of the Macmillan Co., 1958. Kleemeier, R. W., ed.: *Aging and Leisure,* New York: Oxford University Press, 1961. Merton, R. K.: *Social Theory and Social Structure,* Glencoe, Ill.: The Free Press, a division of the Macmillan Co., 1957. Murphy, H. B. M.: "Social Change and Mental Health," in *Causes of Mental Disorders,* New York: Milbank Memorial Fund, 1961, pp. 280-329. Opler, M. K., ed.: *Culture and Mental Health,* New York: Macmillan Co., 1959. Rubin, V., et al: *Culture, Society, and Health, Ann NY Acad Sci* (84), 17:783-1060, 1960. Rushing, W. A.: *Psychiatric Professions,* Chapel Hill, N.C.: University of North Carolina Press, 1964. Seward, G.: *Psychotherapy and Culture Conflict,* New York: Ronald Press, 1956. Seward, G. ed.: *Clinical Studies in Culture Conflict,* New York: Ronald Press, 1958. Simmons, L. W., and Wolff, H. G.: *Social Science in Medicine,* New York: Russell Sage Foundation, 1954, Simmons, O. G.: *Social Status and Public Health,* New York: Social Science Research Council, pamphlet No. 13, 1958. Society for Psychological Study of Social Issues: *Readings in Social Psychology,* ed. 3, New York, Holt, Rinehart & Winston, 1958. Srole, L., et al: *Mental Health in Metropolis: The Midtown Manhattan Study,* in Thomas A. C. Rennie Series in Social Psychiatry, New York: McGraw-Hill Book Co., Inc., 1962, vol. 1. Stanton, A. H. and Schwartz, M. S.: *op. cit.,* see reference No. 12. Stirling County Studies of Psychiatric Disorder and Sociocultural Environment, New York: Basic Books, Inc., Pub., 1959-1963, 3 vol.

15. American Psychiatric Association: "Epidemiology of Mental Disorder," in *Symposium cosponsored by the APA and the American Public Health Association,* December 1956, B. Pasamanick, ed., Washington: American Assoc. Advancement of Science, Publication No. 60, 1959. Dunham, H. W.: *Sociological Theory and Mental Disorders,* Detroit: Wayne State University Press, 1959. Hoch, P. H., and Zubin, J., eds.: *Comparative Epidemiology of Mental Disorders,* New York: Grune & Stratton, Inc., 1961. Jaco, E. G.: *Social Epidemiology of Mental Disorders,* New York: Russell Sage Foundation, 1960. Malzberg, B., and Lee, E. S.: *Migration and Mental Disease,* New York: Social Science Research Council, 1956. Milbank Memorial Fund: *Epidemiology of Mental Disorder,* New York: Milbank Memorial Fund, 1950. Milbank Memorial Fund: *Interrelations Between Social Environment and Psychiatric Disorders,* New York: Milbank Memorial Fund, 1953. Milbank Memorial Fund: *Causes of Mental Disorders,*

New York: Milbank Memorial Fund, 1961. Norris, V.: *Mental Illness in London,* London: Chapman & Hall, for the Institute of Psychiatry, 1959. Shepherd, M.: *Study of Major Psychoses in an English County,* London: Chapman & Hall, for the Institute of Psychiatry, 1957. World Health Organization, Expert Committee on Mental Health: *Epidemiology of Mental Disorders,* eighth report of committee, WHO Technical Report Series, No. 185, Geneva, 1960.

16. Caplan, G.: *Principles of Preventive Psychiatry,* New York: Basic Books Inc., Pub., 1964. Lemkau, P. V.: *Basic Issues in Psychiatry,* Springfield, Ill.: Charles C. Thomas, Pub., 1959. McLean, A. A., and Taylor, G. C.: *op. cit.,* see reference No. 9. Ross, W. D.: *Practical Psychiatry for Industrial Physicians,* Springfield, Ill.: Charles C. Thomas, Pub., 1956. *Symposium on Preventive and Social Psychiatry,* April 15-17, 1957, Washington, D.C.: Walter Reed Army Medical Center and the National Research Council, 1958. World Health Organization, Expert Committee on Mental Health: *Social Psychiatry and Community Attitudes,* seventh report of committee, WHO Technical Report Series No. 177, Geneva, 1959.

17. Ackerman, N. W., et al: *Exporing Base for Family Therapy,* New York: Family Service Association, 1961. Bell, J. E.: *Family Group Therapy,* Washington: Public Health Monograph No. 64, 1961. Epps, R. L., and Hanes, L. D., eds.: *National Day Hospital Workshop: Day Care of Psychiatric Patients,* Springfield, Ill.: Charles C. Thomas, Pub., 1963. Grotjahn, M.: *Psychoanalysis and Family Neurosis,* New York: W. W. Norton & Co., 1960. Howells, J. G.: *Family Psychiatry,* London: Oliver & Boyd, 1963. Jones M.: *Therapeutic Community,* New York: Basic Books Inc., Pub., 1953. Jones, M.: *Social Psychiatry,* Springfield, Ill.: Charles C. Thomas, Pub., 1962. Querido, A.: Efficiency of Medical Care, Leiden: H. E. Stenfert Krose N. V., 1963. Raker, J. W., et al: *Emergency Medical Care in Disasters, a Summary of Recorded Experience,* publication No. 457, Washington: National Academy of Sciences—National Research Council, 1956. Ruesch, J.: *Therapeutic Communication,* New York: W. W. Norton & Co., 1957. Ruesch, J., Brodsky, C. M. and Fischer, A.: *Psychiatric Care,* New York: Grune & Stratton, Inc., 1964. Slavson, S. R.: *Textbook in Analytic Group Psychotherapy,* New York: International Universities Press, 1964. Wilmer, H. A.: *Social Psychiatry in Action,* Springfield, Ill.: Charles C. Thomas, Pub., 1958.

18. Ruesch, J., and Bateson, G.: *Communication: Social Matrix of Psychiatry,* New York: W. W. Norton & Co., 1951.

19. Ruesch, J.: *Therapeutic Communication, op. cit.*, see Reference 17.

20. Neiman, L. J., and Hughes, J. W.: *Problem of Concept of Role: Re-Survey of Literature,* Soc. Forces 30:141-149, 1951. Sarbin, T. R.: "Role Theory," in *Handbook of Social Psychology: Theory and Method,* G. Lindzey, ed., Reading, Mass.: Addison-Wesley Press, 1954, Vol. 1, pp. 223-258.

21. Ruesch, J.: Research and Training in Social Psychiatry in United States, *Int. J. Soc. Psychiat.* 7:87-96, 1961.

22. Hall, E. T.: *Silent Language,* Garden City, N.Y.: Doubleday & Co., Inc., 1959. Symposium on Preventive and Social Psychiatry, April 15-17, *op. cit.*, see Reference No. 16.

23. Morris, C.: *Varieties of Human Value,* Chicago: University of Chicago Press, 1956.

24. Seward, G.: *op. cit.*, see Reference 14.

25. Hollingshead, A. B., and Redlich, F. C., *op. cit.*, Reference 14. Seward, G.: *op. cit.*, see Reference 14.

26. Institute of Social and Historical Medicine: *Man's Image In Medicine and Anthropology,* I. Galdston, ed., New York: International Universities Press, 1963.

27. Birren, J. E., ed., *op. cit.*, Reference 14. Lowenthal, M. F.: *Lives in Distress,* New York: Basic Books, Inc., Pub., 1964.

28. Ross, W. D., *op. cit.*, see Reference 16. Slavson, S. R., *op. cit.*, Reference 17.

29. Birren, J. E., ed., *op. cit.*, Reference 14. Rosow, I.: *Housing and Social Integration of Aged,* mimeographed, final report of study submitted to Cleveland Welfare Federation and the Ford Foundation, Cleveland, Western Reserve University, 1964. Williams, R. H.; Tibbits, C.; and Donahue, W., eds.: *Processes of Aging: Social and Psychological Perspectives,* New York: Atherton Press, 1963. Vol. 2.

30. Berlin, I. N.: *Bibliography of Child Psychiatry,* Washington, D.C.: American Psychiatric Association, 1963. Szurek, S. A., and Boatman, M. J.: "Clinical Study of Childhood Schizophrenia," in *Etiology of Schizophrenia,* D. D. Jackson, ed., New York: Basic Books Inc., Pub., 1960, pp. 389-440.

31. Glueck, S. and Glueck, E.: *Unraveling Juvenile Delinquency,* New York: Commonwealth Fund, 1950.

32. Merton, R. K., *op. cit.*, Reference 14.

33. Jaco, E. G., ed., *op. cit.*, Reference 14.

34. Milbank Memorial Fund, *Epidemiology of Mental Disorder,* see Reference 15. Milbank Memorial Fund, *Causes of Mental Disorders,* see Reference 15.

35. Moore, W. E.: *Social Change,* Englewood Cliffs, N.J.: Prentice-Hall, Inc., 1963. Murphy, H. B. M., *op. cit.,* see Reference 14.

36. Malzberg, B., and Lee, E. S., *op. cit.,* see Reference 15.

37. Hollingshead, A. B., and Redlich, F. C., *op cit.,* see Reference 14.

38. Seward, G., *op. cit.,* see Reference 14.

39. Dunham, H. W., *op. cit.,* see Reference 15.

40. Caudill, W.: *Effects of Social and Cultural Systems in Reactions to Stress,* New York: Social Science Research Council, Pamphlet No. 14, 1958.

41. World Health Organization, Expert Committee on Mental Health, *op. cit.,* see Reference 16.

42. Freeman, H. E.; Levine, S.; and Reeder, L. G., eds., *op. cit.,* Reference 14. Hawkins, N. G., *op cit,* see Reference 14. Hollander, E. P., and Hunt, R. G., eds., *op. cit.,* see Reference 14.

43. Berne, E.: *Games People Play,* New York: Grove Press, Inc., 1964.

44. Grotjahn, M., *op. cit.,* see Reference 17. Lidz, T.: *Family and Human Adaptation,* New York: International Universities Press, 1963.

45. Ginsberg, E., et al.: "Breakdown and Recovery," in *Ineffective Soldier,* New York: Columbia University Press, 1959, Vol. 2.

46. Schwartz, M. S., et al: *Social Approaches to Mental Patient Care,* New York: Columbia University Press, 1964. *Symposium on Stress,* March 16-18, 1953, Washington, D.C.: Army Medical Service Graduate School, 1953.

47. Freeman, H. E. and Simmons, O. G.: *Mental Patient Comes Home,* New York: John Wiley & Sons, 1963. Greenblatt, M.; Levinson, D. J., and Klerman, G. L., eds.: *Mental Patients in Transition,* Springfield, Ill.: Charles C. Thomas, Pub., 1961. Epps, R. L., and Hanes, L. D., eds., *op. cit.,* see Reference 17.

48 Goffman, E., *op. cit.,* see Reference 14. Stanton, A. H., and Schwartz, M. S., *op. cit.,* see Reference 12.

49. Cressey, D. R., ed.: *Prison,* New York: Holt, Rinehart & Winston, 1961. Jones, M., *op. cit.,* Reference 17.

50. McLean, A. A., and Taylor, G. C., *op. cit.,* Reference 9. Ross, W. D., *op. cit.,* Reference 16.

51. Kleemeier, R. W., ed., *op. cit.,* see Reference 14.

52. Huntington, E.: *Mainsprings of Civilization,* New York: John Wiley & Sons, Inc., 1945.

53. Baker, G. W., and Chapman, D. W., eds.: *Man and Society in Disaster,* New York: Basic Books Inc., Pub., 1962.

54. Malmo, R. B., and Surwillo, W. W.: *Sleep Deprivation: Changes*

in Performance and Physiological Indicants of Activation, Psychol. Monogr. Gen. Appl. (74) 15:1-24, 1960. Solomon, P., et al, ed.: *Sensory Deprivation,* Cambridge, Mass.: Harvard University Press, 1961.

55. Group for Advancement of Psychiatry, Committee on Governmental Agencies, *op. cit.,* see Reference 10. *Symposium on Stress,* March 16-18, 1953, *op. cit.,* see Reference 46.

56. Raker, J. W., et al., *op. cit.,* Reference 17.

57. Lifton, R. J.: *Thought Reform and Psychology of Totalism,* New York: W. W. Norton & Co., Inc., 1961. Meerloo, J. A. M.: *Rape of Mind,* New York: World Publishing Co., 1956. Sargant, W.: *Battle for the Mind,* New York: Doubleday & Co., Inc., 1957.

58. Ruesch, J.: *Disturbed Communication,* New York: W. W. Norton & Co., 1957.

59. Oliver, R. T.: *Culture and Communication,* Springfield, Ill.: Charles C. Thomas, Pub., 1962.

60. Ruesch, J., and Kees, W.: *Nonverbal Communication,* Berkeley, Calif.: University of California Press, 1956.

61. Ruesch, J., *Disturbed Communication, op. cit.,* see Reference 58.

62. Glueck, S. and Glueck, E., *op. cit.,* Reference 31. Group for Advancement of Psychiatry, Committee on Public Education: *Psychiatrist's Interest in Leisure-Time Activities,* New York: GAP Report No. 39, 1958.

63. American Psychiatric Association, *op. cit.,* Reference 15. Dunham, H. W., *op. cit.,* see Reference 15. Hawley, A. H.: *Human Ecology, Theory of Community Structure,* New York: Ronald Press, 1950. Hoch, P. H., and Zubin, J., eds.: *op. cit.,* see Reference 15. Leighton, A. H.; Clausen, J. A.; and Wilson, R. N., eds.: *Explorations in Social Psychiatry,* New York: Basic Books Inc., Pub., 1957. Norris, V., *op. cit.,* Reference 15. Rose, A. M., ed.: *Mental Health and Mental Disorder,* New York: W. W. Norton & Co., 1955. Rubin, W. D., *op cit.,* Reference 14. Shepherd, M., *op. cit.,* see Reference 15. Simmons, L. W. and Wolff, H. G., *op. cit.,* see Reference 14. Simmons, O. G., *op. cit.,* Reference 14. Srole, L., et al., *op. cit.,* see Reference 14. *Stirling County Study of Psychiatric Disorder and Sociocultural Environment, op. cit.,* see Reference 14. World Health Organization, Expert Committee on Mental Health, *op. cit.,* Reference 15.

64. Leighton, A. H., *op. cit.,* see Reference 5.

65. American Psychiatric Association: *Rehabilitation of Mentally Ill—Social and Economic Aspects,* M. Greenblatt and B. Simon, eds., Washington, D.C., AAAS Publication No. 58, 1959. Apple, D., ed.,

op. cit., see Reference 14. Caudill, W.: *Psychiatric Hospital as Small Society*, Cambridge: Harvard University Press, 1958. Goffman, E., *op. cit.*, see Reference 14. Querido, A., *op. cit.*, see Reference 17. Ruesch, J., *Disturbed Communication, op. cit.*, Reference 17. Ruesch, J.; Brodsky, C. M.; and Fisher, A., *op. cit.*, Reference 17. Rushing, W. A., *op. cit.*, see Reference 14. Schwartz, M. S., et al., *op. cit.*, see Reference 46. Szasz, T. S.: *Myth of Mental Illness*, New York: Paul B. Hoeber, medical division of Harper & Row, Pub., Inc., 1961. Watts, A. W.: *Psychotherapy East and West*, New York: Pantheon Books, 1961.

66. Bellak, L., ed.: *op. cit.*, see Reference 4. Harvard Medical School and Psychiatric Service, Massachusetts General Hospital: *Community Mental Health and Social Psychiatry:* Reference Guide, Cambridge, Mass.: Harvard University Press, 1962.

67. Williams, R. H., ed.: *Prevention of Disability in Mental Disorders*, Washington, D. C., Public Health Service, publication No. 924, 1962.

68. Jones, M., *op. cit.*, see Reference 17.

69. Slavson, S. R., *op. cit.*, see Reference 17.

70. Ackerman, N. W., et al, *op. cit.*, see Reference 17.

71. Bell, J. E., *op. cit.*, Reference 17. Howells, J. G., *op. cit.*, see Reference 17.

72. Fidler, G. S. and Fidler, J. W.: *Occupational Therapy*, New York: Macmillan Co., 1963.

73. Ruesch, J., *Therapeutic Communication*, see Reference 17.

74. Spitz, R. A.: *No and Yes*, New York: International Universities Press, 1957.

75. Macfarlane, J. W.: "Life-Career Approach to Study of Personality Development," in *Conference on Personality Development*, Berkeley, Calif., May 4-6, 1960.

76. Birren, J. E., ed., *op. cit.*, Reference 14.

77. Rosow, I., *op. cit.*, Reference 29. Williams, R. H., *op. cit.*, Reference 29.

Chapter 2

1. Hippocrates: "On Airs, Waters, and Places," *Med. Classics*, 3:19-42, (Sept.) 1938.

2. Southard, E. E.: "Alienists and Psychiatrists," *Ment. Hyg.*, 1:567-571, 1917.

3. *Ibid.*

4. *Ibid.*, p. 569.

5. Southard, E. E.,: "Mental Hygiene and Social Work: Notes on a Course in Social Psychiatry for Social Workers," *Ment. Hyg.*, 2:388-406, 1918.

6. *Ibid.*

7. *Ibid.*, p. 398.

8. Spaulding, E. R.: "The Course in Social Psychiatry in the Training School of Psychiatric Social Work at Smith College," *Ment. Hyg.*, 2 (pt. 3):582-594, 1918.

9. "Sociological Significance of Psychoanalytic Psychology," *Publications Amer. Sociol. Soc.*, 15:203-216, 1921.

10. Southard, E. E., and Jarrett, M. C.: *The Kingdom of Evils*, New York: Macmillan Co., 1924, p. 523.

11. Group for the Advancement of Psychiatry: *Urban America and the Planning of Mental Health Services*, Symposium No. 10, 1964, New York, and *The Community Mental Health Center: An Analysis of Existing Models*, Washington, D.C.: The Joint Information Service, 1964.

12. McCord, C. P.: "Social Psychiatry—Its Significance as a Specialty," *Amer. J. Psychiat.*, 5:233-240, 1925.

13. Plant, J. S.: "Sociological Factors Challenging the Practice of Psychiatry in a Metropolitan District," *Amer. J. Psychiat.*, 8:712, 1929.

14. Groves, E. R.: "The Development of Social Psychiatry," *Publications Amer. Social Soc.*, 27:143-144, 1932.

15. *Ibid.*, p. 143.

16. Brown, L. G.: "Social Psychiatry," in Bernard, L. L., (ed.): *The Field and Methods of Sociology*, New York: Long and Smith, Inc., 1934, p. 129.

17. *Ibid.*, p. 142.

18. Folsom, J. K.: "The Sources and Methods of Social Psychiatry," in Bernard, L. L., (ed.): *The Field and Methods of Sociology*, New York: Long and Smith, Inc., 1934.

19. Dunham, H. W.: "The Field of Social Psychiatry" reprinted in Rose, A. M., (ed.): *Mental Health and Mental Disorder*, New York: W. W. Norton & Co., Inc., 1955, Chap. 4, pp. 61-86.

20. Folsom, J. K.: *The Family: Its Sociology and Social Psychiatry*, New York: John Wiley & Sons, Inc., 1934.

21. Folsom, J. K.: *Social Psychology*, New York: Harper & Brothers, 1931.

22. Hartwell, S. W.: "Social Psychiatry—Our Task or a New Profession," *Amer. J. Psychiat.*, 96:1089-1098, 1940.

23. *Ibid.*, p. 1089.

24. Rennie, T. A. C.: "Social Psychiatry—A Definition," *Int. J. Soc. Psychiat.*, 1:5-13, 1955.

25. *Ibid.* p. 10.

26. *Ibid.*, p. 12.

27. *Ibid.*, p. 13.

28. Leighton, A. H.; Clausen, J. A.; and Wilson, R. N., eds.: *Explorations in Social Psychiatry,* New York: Basic Books, Inc., 1957.

29. *Ibid.*, p. vii.

30. Spiegel, J. P., and Bell, N. W.: "The Family of the Psychiatric Patients," in Arieti, S., (ed.): *American Handbook of Psychiatry,* New York: Basic Books, Inc., 1959, pp. 139-143 and references.

CHAPTER 3

1. Hollingshead, A. B., and Redlich, F. C.: *Social Class and Mental Illness,* New York: John Wiley & Sons, Inc., 1958, p. 236, Table 17.

2. Riessman, F., and Miller, S. M.: "Social Class and Projective Tests," in Riessman, F.; Cohen, J.; and Pearl, A., (ed.): *Mental Health of the Poor,* New York: Free Press of Glencoe, Inc., a division of the Macmillan Co., 1964, p. 248.

3. Avnet, H.: *Psychiatric Insurance,* New York: Group Health Insurance, 1962, p. 147.

4. Mental Health Research Unit, New York State Department of Mental Hygiene: *A Mental Health Survey of Older People,* Utica, N.Y.: State Hospital Press, 1961.

5. Casriel, D.: *So Fair a House,* Englewood Cliffs, N.J.: Prentice-Hall, Inc., 1963.

6. Gellman, I. P.: *The Sober Alcoholic,* New Haven, Conn.: College and University Press, 1964.

7. Essien-Udom, E. V.: *Black Nationalism,* New York: Dell Publishing Co., 1964.

8. Branch, C. H. H.: "Therapy Sine Psychiatry," in Masserman, J., (ed.): *Current Psychiatric Therapies,* New York: Grune & Stratton, Inc., 2:1, 1962.

9. Pullinger, W. F.: "Remotivation," *Ment. Hosp.*, 9:14-17, 1958. Kantor, D. and Greenblatt, M.: Wellmet: Halfway to Community Rehabilitation, *Ment. Hosp.*, 13:146-152, 1962.

10. Rioch, M.; Elkes, C.; and Flint, A.: *Pilot Project in Training Mental Health Counselors,* Washington, D.C.: Public Health Service Publication No. 1254.

11. Sigerist, H.: *Civilization and Disease,* Chicago: University of Chicago Press, 1962, p. 70.

12. Parsons, T.: "Illness and the Role of the Physician," *Amer. J. Orthopsychiat.,* 21:452, 1951.

13. Artiss, K. L.: "The Symptom During Therapy," in Artiss, K. L., (ed.): *The Symptom as Communication in Schizophrenia,* New York: Grune & Stratton, Inc., 1959, p. 226.

14. Berne, E.: *Transactional Analysis in Psychotherapy,* New York: Grove Press, Inc., 1961, p. 110.

15. Jackson, D. D., and Waltzlawick, P.: "The Acute Psychosis as a Manifestation of Growth Experience," in Mendel, W., and Epstein, L., (ed.): *Acute Psychotic Reaction,* Psychiatric Research Report 16, Washington, D.C.: American Psychiatric Association, May, 1963, pp. 88-99.

16. Barton, R.: *Institutional Neurosis,* Bristol: John Wright and Sons, Ltd., 1959.

17. Metcalf, G.: *The English Open Mental Hospital,* Milbank Memorial Fund Quart., 39:579-593, 1961. Clark, D.: "Background and Present Day Status of Industrial and Occupational Therapy Program in English Hospitals," *Amer. Arch. Rehabilitation Therapy,* 11:35-44, 1963.

18. Hunt, R. C.: "Ingredients of a Rehabilitation Program," in *An Approach to the Prevention of Disability From Chronic Psychoses,* New York: Milbank Memorial Fund, 1958.

19. Gruenberg, E. M., and Zusman, J.: "The Natural History of Schizophrenia," *Int. Psychi. Clin.,* 1:699-710, 1964, pp. 706-707.

20. Greenblatt, M.: "Perspectives on Rehabilitation Within the Hospital," in *Proceedings of the Institute on Rehabilitation of the Mentally Ill,* New York: Altro Health and Rehabilitation Services (April 4-6), 1962, p. 16. Wilmer, H.: *Social Psychiatry in Action,* Springfield, Ill.: Charles C. Thomas Publishers, 1958, p. 325.

21. Proceedings of the Workshop "Compensated Work as Therapy" held at the Institute of Pennsylvania Hospital, Nov. 1, 1963, Philadelphia: Institute of Pennsylvania Hospital, 1963. McGrath, V., and Burke, B.: "Compensated Work Therapy in the New York State Department of Mental Hygiene," *Amer. Arch. Rehabilitation Therapy,* 11:48-50, 1963.

22. Banen, D. M.: Proceedings of the Workshop, "Compensated

Work as Therapy" held at the Institute of Pennsylvania Nov. 1, 1963, Philadelphia: University of Pennsylvania Press, 1963.

23. Miller, M. D.: "The Mobile Psychiatric Team," *Amer. J. Psychiat.*, 121:1 (suppl), 1965.

24. Satir, V.: *Conjoint Family Therapy*, Palo Alto, Calif.: Science and Behavior Books, Inc., 1964, pp. 27-44.

25. Goffman, E.: "The Characteristics of Total Institutions," in *Symposium on Preventive and Social Psychiatry*, Washington, D.C.: Walter Reed Army Institute of Research, 1957. Dunham, H. W. and Weinberg, S. K.: *The Culture of the State Mental Hospital*, Detroit: Wayne State University Press, 1960.

26. Brown, C.: *Manchild in the Promised Land*, New York: Macmillan Co., 1965.

27. Paul, L.: "The Extended Analytic Situation in a Psychoanalytic Ward Milieu," *J. Nerv. Ment. Dis.*, 139:313, 1964. Simmel, E.: "Psychoanalytic Treatment in a Sanatorium," *Int. J. Psychoanal.*, 10:70, 1929.

28. Greenblatt, M.; York, R. H.; and Brown, E. L.: *From Custodial to Therapeutic Care in Mental Hospitals*, New York: Russell Sage Foundation, 1955.

29. Michelson, E.: "Volunteers Work for Mental Patients," *J. Vocational Rehabilitatiion*, 30:14, 1964. Umbarger, C. C., et al: *College Students in a Mental Hospital*, New York: Grune and Stratton Inc., 1962.

30. Berelson, B., and Steiner, G.: *Human Behavior*, New York: Harcourt, Brace and World, Inc., 1964, p. 331.

31. Wing, J. K.: "Institutionalism in Mental Hospitals," *Brit. J. Soc. Clin. Psychol.*, 1:38, 1962.

32. Program Area Committee on Mental Health: *Mental Disorders: A Guide to Control Methods*, New York: American Public Health Assoc., 1962, pp. 1-3.

33. Orne, M. T.: "Psychotherapy and Hypnosis: Implications From Research," in Masserman, J., (ed.): *Current Psychiatric Therapies*, New York: Grune & Stratton, Inc., 2:75, 1962.

34. Goffman, E.: "The Characteristics of Total Institutions," in *Symposium on Preventive and Social Psychiatry*, Washington, D.C.: Walter Reed Army Institute of Research, 1957, *op. cit.*, see reference 25, p. 50.

35. Berelson, B., and Steiner, G.: *Human Behavior*, New York: Harcourt, Brace and World, Inc., 1964, pp. 374-376. Katz, D., and Kahn, R.: "Leadership Practices in Relation to Productivity and Morale," in Cartwright, D., and Zander, A., (eds.): *Group Dynamics:*

Research and Theory, Evanston, Ill.: Row, Peterson & Co., 1960, pp. 612-628. Clark, D. H.: *Administrative Therapy,* London: Tavistock Publications Ltd., 1964.

36. Szasz, T. S.: *Law, Liberty and Psychiatry,* New York: Macmillan Co., 1963.

37. Durkheim, E.: *Suicide,* Glencoe, Ill.: Free Press of Glencoe, Inc., 1951.

38. Merton, R. K.: *Social Theory and Social Structure,* New York: Free Press of Glencoe, Inc., 1949, Chap. 5. Cloward, R. A., and Ohlin, L. E.: *Delinquency and Opportunity,* New York: Free Press of Glencoe, Inc., a division of the Macmillan Co., 1960.

39. Faris, R. E. L., and Dunham, H. W.: *Mental Disorders in Urban Areas,* New York: Hafner Publishing Co., Inc., 1960. Cleveland, E. J., and Longaker, W. D.: "Neurotic Patterns in the Family," in Leighton, A. A.; Clausen, J. H.; and Wilson, R. N.: *Explorations in Social Psychiatry,* New York: Basic Books Inc., 1957. "Social Structures and Mental Disorders," in *Causes of Mental Disorders: A Review of Epidemiological Knowledge,* 1959, New York: Milbank Memorial Fund, 1961.

40. Cloward, R. A., and Ohlin, L. E.: *Delinquency and Opportunity,* New York: Free Press of Glencoe, Inc., a division of the Macmillan Co., 1960.

41. Mobilization for Youth, Inc.: *A Proposal for the Prevention and Control of Delinquency by Expanding Opportunities,* New York: Mobilization for Youth, Inc., 1961.

42. *Ibid.*

CHAPTER 4

1. Milbank Memorial Fund: *Epidemiology of Mental Disorder,* New York: 1950.

2. Rawnsley, K.: M. R. C. Committee on the Epidemiology of Psychiatric Illness, Unpublished, 1963.

3. Lin, T. -Y., and Standley, C. C.: *The Scope of Epidemiology in Psychiatry,* Geneva: W. H. O., Public Health Papers, No. 16, 1962.

4. Lewis, A. J.: *Yale Journal of Biological Medicine,* 35:62, 1962.

5. Frost, W. H.: in *Public Health and Preventive Medicine,* London: Nelson, 2:163, 1927.

6. *Ibid.*

7. Meyer, A.: *Journal of the American Medical Association,* 58:911, 1912.

8. Greenwood, M.: *Epidemics and Crowd-Disease,* London: Williams & Norgate, 1935, p. 133.

9. Leighton, A. H.: *Bulletin of Johns Hopkins Hospital,* 89:73, 1951.

10. Trotter, W.: *Instincts of the Herd in Peace and War* (2nd ed.), London: Scientific Book Club, 1942.

11. Freud, S.: "Group Psychology and the Analysis of the Ego," in *Complete Psychological Works,* London: Hogarth Press, 18:69, 1955.

12. Brown, J. A. C.: *Freud and the Post-Freudians,* London: Penguin Books, 1961, p. 124.

13. Zilboorg, G.: *American Journal of Psychiatry,* 92:1347, 1963.

14. Lewis, E. O.: "Board of Education and Board of Control Mental Deficiency Committee Report," Pt. 4, London: H.M.S.O., 1929. Brugger, C.: *Z. Ges. Neurol. Psych.,* 133:352, 1931. Rosanoff, A.: *Psychiatric Bulletin,* 2:109, 1917.

15. Strömgren, E.: *Congres International de Psychiatrie: VI. Psychiatrie Sociale,* Paris: Hermann, 1950.

16. Malzberg, B.: *Social and Biological Aspects of Mental Disease,* Utica, New York: State Hospital Press, 1940. Pollock, H. M.: *State Hospital Quarterly,* 10:1934, 1925.

17. Faris, R. E. L. and Dunham, H. W.: *Mental Disorders in Urban Areas: an Ecological Study of Schizophrenia and Other Psychoses,* Chicago: University of Chicago Press, 1939. Robinson, W. S.: *American Sociological Review,* 15:351, 1950.

18. Ryle, J. A.: *Changing Disciplines,* London: Oxford University Press, 1948.

19. Ginsberg, M.: *On the Diversity of Morals,* London: Heinemann, 1956, p. 157.

20. Reid, D. D.: "Epidemiological Methods in the Study of Mental Disorders," Geneva: W.H.O., Public Health Papers No. 2, 1960, pp. 8 and 15.

21. World Health Organization: "Eighth Report of the Expert Committee on Mental Health," *World Health Organization Technical Report Series* No. 185, 1960.

22. Gruenberg, E. M.: *Explorations in Social Psychiatry,* A. H. Leighton, J. A. Clausen, and R. N. Wilson, (eds.), London: Tavistock, 1957.

23. Penrose, L. S.: *On the Objective Study of Crowd Behaviour,* London: Lewis, 1952.

24. Hecker, J. F. C.: *The Epidemics of the Middle Ages,* Translated by B. G. Babington (3rd ed.), London: Trubner, 1859.

25. Durkheim, E.: *Suicide: A Study in Sociology,* Translated by J. A. Spaulding and G. Simpson, Glencoe, Illinois: Free Press, 1951.

26. Kräupl-Taylor, F., and Hunter, R. C. A.: *Psychiatric Quarterly,* 32:821, 1958.

27. Böök, J. A.: *Causes of Mental Disorders: A Review of Epidemiological Knowledge,* New York: Milbank Memorial Fund, 1959.

28. Marshall, T. H.: *Sociology at the Crossroads and Other Essays,* London: Heinemann, 1963, p. 41.

29. Kreitman, N.: *Journal Ment. Science,* 107:876, 1961.

30. Kessel, N., and Shepherd, M.: *Journal Ment. Science,* 108:159, 1962.

31. Crombie, D. L.: *Lancet,* i:1205, 1961.

32. Zubin, J.: Unpublished manuscript, 1963.

33. Blum, R. H.: *Milbank Memorial Fund Quarterly,* 40:253, 1962.

34. Hinkle, L. E., and Wolff, H. G.: *Explorations in Social Psychiatry,* Leighton, A. H.; Clausen, J. A.; and Wilson, R. N. (eds.), London: Tavistock, 1957.

35. Morris, J. N.: *Uses of Epidemiology,* Edinburgh: Livingstone, 1957.

36. Siler, J. F.; Garrison, P. E.; and MacNeal, W. J.: "Third Report of the Robert M. Thompson Pellagra Commission of the New York Postgraduate Medical School and Hospital," New York, 1917.

37. Goldberger, J.: *De Lamar Lectures,* New York: Williams & Wilkins, 1927, p. 128.

38. Goldberger, J.: *Public Health Rep. Washington,* 29:1683, 1914.

39. Goldberger, J.; Wheeler, G. A.; and Sydenstricker, E.: *Public Health Rep. Washington,* 35:2673, 1920.

40. Hersov, L. A., and Rodnight, R.: *Journal Neurol. Neurosurg. Psychiat.,* 23:40, 1960.

41. Parsons, R. P.: *Trail of Light,* Indianapolis: Bobbs-Merrill, 1943.

42. Milbank Memorial Fund: *Causes of Mental Disorders: A Review of Epidemiological Knowledge, 1959,* New York, 1961.

43. Rawnsley, K., and Loudon, J. B.: *British Journal of Psychiatry,* 110:830, 1964.

44. Thomas, C. L., and Gordon, J. E.: *American Journal Med. Sci.,* 238:363, 1959.

45. Paffenbarger, R. S.: *Journal of Chronic Disease,* 13:161, 1961.

46. Knobloch, H., and Pasamanick, B.: *Mental Retardation,* "Proceedings of the 1st International Conference on Mental Retardation," P. W. Bowman, and H. V. Mautner, (eds.), New York: Grune & Stratton, 1960a.

47. Knobloch, H., and Pasamanick, B.: *Pediatrics,* 26:210, 1960b.

48. Douglas, J. W. B., and Mulligan, D. G.: *Proc. Roy. Soc. Med.,* 54:885, 1961.

49. Mangus, A. R., and Dager, E. Z.: *Epidemiology of Mental Disorder,* B. Pasamanick, (ed.), Washington, D.C.: American Association for the Advancement of Scientific Publications, No. 60, 1959.

50. Shepherd, M.; Oppenheim, A. N.; and Mitchell, S.: *Proc. Roy. Soc. Med.,* 59:379, 1966.

51. Cohen, B. H.; Lilienfeld, A. M.; and Sigler, A. T.: *American Journal of Public Health,* 53:223, 1963.

52. Fremming, K. H.: *The Expectation of Mental Infirmity in a Sample of the Danish Population* (Occasional Papers on Eugenics, No. 7) London: Cassell, 1951, p. 12.

53. Greenwood, M., and Woods, H. M.: "Industrial Fatigue Research Board Report," No. 4, London: H.M.S.O., 1919.

54. Farmer, E., and Chambers, E. G.: "Industrial Fatigue Research Board Report," No. 38, London: H.M.S.O., 1926.

55. Adelstein, A. M.: *J. Roy. Stat. Soc. A.,* 115:354, 1952.

56. Smart, R. G., and Schmidt, W. S.: *Journal of Psychosomatic Research,* 6:191, 1962.

57. Kesell, N., and Shepherd, M., *op. cit.,* see reference 30.

58. Querido, A.: *British Journal of Preventive Soc. Med.,* 13:33, 1959.

59. Rutter, M.: *Journal of Psychosomatic Research,* 7:45, 1963.

60. Penrose, L. S.: *The Biology of Mental Defect,* London: Sidgwick & Jackson, 1949.

61. Arieti, S., and Meth, J. M.: *American Handbook of Psychiatry,* S. Arieti, (ed.), New York: Basic Books, 1959.

62. Murphy, H. B. M.: Unpublished manuscript, 1955.

63. World Health Organization, *op. cit.,* see reference 21.

64. Lewis, A. J.: *Comparative Epidemiology of the Mental Disorders,* Hoch, P. H. and Zubin, J., eds., New York: Grune & Stratton, 1961.

65. Brodman, K.; Erdmann, A. J.; Lorge, I.; Deutschberger, J.; and Wolff, H. G.: *American Journal of Psychiatry,* 111:37, 1954.

66. MacMillan, A. M.: *Psychol. Rep.,* Southern Universities Press, 111:325, Monograph Suppl. 7, 1957.

67. Shepherd, M.; Oppenheim, A. N.; and Mitchell, S., *op. cit.,* see reference 50.

68. Lewis, E. O., *op. cit.,* see reference 14.

69. Medical Research Council: *British Medical Journal,* 2:1691, 1963.

70. Shepherd, M.; Cooper, B.; Brown, A. C.; and Kalton, G.: *British Medical Journal,* ii:1359, 1964.

71. Martin, F. M.; Brotherston, J. H. F.; and Chave, S. P. W.: *British Journal of Preventive Soc. Med.,* 11:196, 1957.

72. Srole, L.; Langner, T. S.; Michael, S. T.; Opler, M. K.; and Rennie, T. A. C.: *Mental Health in the Metropolis: The Midtown Manhattan Study,* New York: McGraw-Hill, 1962.

73. Wittson, C. L., and Hunt, W. A.: *American Journal of Psychiatry,* 107:582, 1951.

74. Leighton, A. H.: *My Name is Legion,* New York: Basic Books, 1959.

75. Essen-Möller, E.: *Comparative Epidemiology of the Mental Disorders,* P. H. Hoch, and J. Zubin, (eds.), New York: Grune & Stratton, 1961, p. 1.

76. Wilner, D. M.; Walkley, R. P.; Pinkerton, T. C.; and Tayback, H.: *The Housing Environment and Family Life,* Baltimore: Johns Hopkins Press, 1962.

77. Hare, E. H.: *Journal Ment. Sci.,* 105:594, 1959.

78. Goldhamer, H., and Marshall, A.: *Psychosis and Civilization* (2nd ed.), Glencoe, Illinois: Free Press, 1953.

79. Halliday, J. L.: *Psychosocial Medicine,* London: Heinemann, 1949.

80. Maclay, W. S.: *American Journal of Psychiatry,* 120:209, 1963.

81. Shepherd, M.; Goodman, N.; and Watt, D. C.: *Comprehensive Psychiatry,* 2:11, 1961.

82. Lawrence, A. R. Le V.: *Ph.D. Thesis,* University of London, 1963.

83. Pasamanick, B.: *The Future of Psychiatry* (Proc. 51st. Meeting American Psychopathological Association, 1961), P. H. Hoch, and J. Zubin, (eds.), New York: Grune & Stratton, 1962.

84. Spence, J.: *Lect. Sci. Basis Med.* 2:5, 1954.

85. Odegaard, O.: *Proc. Roy. Soc. Med.,* 55:831, 1962.

Chapter 5

1. Tsung-Yi Lin: "A Study of the Incidence of Mental Disorder in Chinese and Other Cultures," *Psychiatry,* 16:313-336, 1953.

2. Leighton, A. H.: *My Name is Legion: Foundations for A Theory of Man in Relation to Culture,* New York: Basic Books, 1959. Hughes, C. C. with Tremblay, M.; Rapoport, R. N.; and Leighton, A. H.:

People of Cove and Woodlot: Communities from the Viewpoint of Social Psychiatry, New York: Basic Books, 1960. Leighton, D. C. with Harding, J. S.; Macklin, D. B.; Macmillan, A. M.; and Leighton, A. H.: *The Character of Danger,* New York: Basic Books, 1963.

3. Leighton, A. H.; Lambo, T. A.; Hughes, C. C.; Leighton, D. C.; Murphy, J. M.; and Macklin, D. B.: *Psychiatric Disorder Among the Yoruba,* Ithaca: Cornell University Press, 1963. "Psychiatric Disorder in West Africa," *American Journal of Psychiatry,* 120:521-527, December, 1963.

4. Eaton, J. W., and Weil, R. J.: *Culture and Mental Disorders, An Epidemiological Approach,* Glencoe, Illinois: Free Press, 1955.

5. Goldhammer, H., and Marshall, A. W.: *Psychosis and Civilization,* Glencoe, Illinois: Free Press, 1953.

6. Rosenthal, D.: "Problems of Sampling and Diagnosis in the Major Twin Studies of Schizophrenia," *Journal of Psychiatric Research,* 1:116-134.

7. Tienari, P.: "Psychiatric Illness in Identical Twins," *Acta Psychiatrica Scandinavica,* 39: Suppl. 169, 1963.

8. Kringlen, E.: "Disordance with Respect to Schizophrenia in Monozygotic Twins: Some Genetic Aspects," *Journal of Nervous and Mental Disease,* 138:26-31, Jan. 1964. Kringlen, E.: *Schizophrenia in Male Monozygotic Twins,* Oslo: Universitetsforlaget, 1964.

9. Kety, S.: "Recent Biochemical Theories of Schizophrenia," Jackson, D. D., (ed.), *The Etiology of Schizophrenia,* New York: Basic Books, 1960.

10. Faris, R. E. L., and Dunham, H. W.: *Mental Disorders in Urban Areas: An Ecological Study of Schizophrenia and Other Psychoses,* Chicago: University of Chicago Press, 1939.

11. Clark, R. E.: "Psychoses, Income, and Occupational Prestige," *American Journal of Sociology,* LIV:433-440, March, 1949.

12. Faris, R. E. I., and Dunham, H. W., *op. cit.,* see reference 10. Schroeder, C. W.: "Mental Disorders in Cities," *American Journal of Sociology,* 48:40-48, July, 1942.

13. Sundby, P., and Nyhus, P.: "Major and Minor Psychiatric Disorders in Males in Oslo: An Epidemiological Study," *Acta Psychiatrica Scandinavica,* 39:519-547, 1963.

14. Hollingshead, A. B., and Redlich, F. C.: *Social Class and Mental Illness,* New York: John Wiley, 1957.

15. Srole, L.; Langner, T. S.; Michael, S. T.; Opler, M. K.; and Rennie, T. A. C.: *Mental Health in the Metropolis: The Midtown Manhattan Study,* Vol. I, New York: McGraw-Hill, 1962.

16. Frumkin, R. M.: "Occupation and Major Mental Disorders," in A. Rose, (ed.), *Mental Health and Mental Disorder,* New York: W. W. Norton, 1955.

17. Svalastoga, K.: *Social Differentiation,* in press.

18. Ødegaard, Ø.: "The Incidence of Psychosis in Various Occupations," International Journal of Social Psychiatry, II:85-104, Autumn, 1956. Ødegaard, Ø.: "Psychiatric Epidemiology," *Proceedings of the Royal Society of Medicine,* 55:831-837, October, 1962. Ødegaard, Ø.: "Occupational Incidence of Mental Disease in Single Women," *Living Conditions and Health,* 1:169-180, 1957.

19. Clausen, J. A., and Kohn, M. L.: "Relation of Schizophrenia to the Social Structure of a Small City," in B. Pasamanick, (ed.), *Epidemiology of Mental Disorder,* Washington, D.C.: American Association for the Advancement of Science, 1959.

20. Leighton, D. C. et al: "Psychiatric Findings of the Stirling County Study," *American Journal of Psychiatry,* 119:1021-1026, May, 1963.

21. Hagnell, O.: "A 10-Year Followup of a Psychiatric Fields Study," Mimeographed, 1963. Essen-Möller, E.: "Individual Traits and Morbidity in a Swedish Rural Population," *Acta Psychiatrica et Neurologica Scandinavia,* Suppl. 100:1-160, 1956. Essen-Möller, E.: "A Current Field Study in the Mental Disorders in Sweden," in P. H. Hoch, and J. Zubin, (eds.), *Comparative Epidemiology of the Mental Disorders,* New York: Grune & Stratton, 1961.

22. Owen, M. B.: "Alternative Hypotheses for the Explanation of Some of Faris and Dunham's Results," *American Journal of Sociology,* 47:48-52, July, 1941. Lystad, M. H.: "Social Mobility Among Selected Groups of Schizophrenic Patients," *American Sociological Review,* 22:288-292, June, 1957. Schwartz, M. S.: *The Economic and Spatial Mobility of Paranoid Schizophrenics and Manic Depressives,* Unpublished M. A. Thesis: University of Chicago, 1946. Gerard, D. L., and Houston, L. G.: "Family Setting and the Social Ecology of Schizophrenia," *Psychiatric Quarterly,* XXVII:90-101, January, 1953. Srole, L. et al., *op. cit.,* see reference 15. Clausen, J. A., and Kohn, M. L., *op. cit.,* see reference 19. Hollingshead, A. B., and Redlich, F. C.: "Social Stratification and Schizophrenia," *American Sociological Review,* 19:302-306, June, 1954.

23. Goldberg, E. M., and Morrison, S. L.: "Schizophrenia and Social Class," *British Journal of Psychiatry,* 109:785-802, Nov., 1963.

24. Ødegaard, Ø.: "Emigration and Mental Health," *Mental Hy-*

giene, 20:546-553, 1936. Astrup, C., and Ødegaard, Ø.: "Internal Migration and Disease in Norway," *Psychiatric Quarterly Supplement,* 34:116-130, 1960.

25. Jaco, E. G.: *The Social Epidemiology of Mental Disorders,* New York: Russell Sage Foundation, 1960.

26. Dohrenwend, B. P., and Dohrenwend, B. S.: "The Problem of Validity in Field Studies of Psychological Disorder," *Journal of Abnormal Psychology,* 70:52-69, Feb., 1965.

27. Leighton, D.: "The Distribution of Psychiatric Symptoms in a Small Town," *American Journal of Psychiatry,* 112:716-723, March, 1956.

28. Star, S.: "The Screening of Psychoneurosis in the Army," Stouffer, S. A.; Guttman, L.; Suchman, E. A.; Lazarsfeld, P. F.; Star, S. A.; and Clausen, J. A., (eds.), *Measurement and Prediction,* Princeton, N.J.: Princeton University Press, 1950.

29. Kramer, M.: "A Discussion of the Concepts of Incidence and Prevalence as Related to Epidemiologic Studies of Mental Disorders," *American Journal of Public Health,* 47:826-840, July, 1957.

30. Kohn, M. L., and Clausen, J. A.: "Social Isolation and Schizophrenia," *American Sociological Review,* 20:265-273, June, 1955.

31. Mintz, N. L., and Schwartz, D. T.: *Urban Ecology and Psychosis: Community Factors in the Incidence of Schizophrenia and Manic-Depression Among Italians in Greater Boston,* mimeographed, 1963.

32. Langner, T. S., and Michael, S. T.: *Life Stress and Mental Health,* New York: The Free Press of Glencoe, 1963.

33. Clausen, J. A., and Kohn, M. L.: "Social Relations and Schizophrenia: A Research Report and a Perspective," in D. D. Jackson, (ed.), *The Etiology of Schizophrenia,* New York: Basic Books, 1960.

34. Bateson, G.; Jackson, D.; Haley, J.; and Weakland, J.: "Toward A Theory of Schizophrenia," *Behavioral Science,* 1:251-264, Oct., 1956.

35. Wynne, L. C.; Ryckoff, I. M.; Day, J.; and Hirsch, S. I.: "Pseduo-Mutuality in the Family Relations of Schizophrenics," *Psychiatry,* 22:205-220, May, 1958. Ryckoff, I. with Day, J., and Wynne, L. C.: "Maintenance of Stereotyped Roles in the Families of Schizophrenics," *American Medical Association Archives of Psychiatry,* 1:93-98, July, 1959.

36. Sanua, V. D.: "Sociocultural Factors in Families of Schizophrenics: A Review of the Literature," *Psychiatry,* 24:246-265, 1961.

37. Kohn, M. L., and Clausen, J. A.: "Parental Authority Behavior and Schizophrenia," *American Journal of Orthopsychiatry,* 26:297-313, April, 1956.

38. Kohn, M. L.: "Social Class and Parent-Child Relationships: An Interpretation," *American Journal of Sociology,* LXVIII:471-480, Jan., 1963. Reissman, F. with Cohen, J., and Pearl, A., (eds.): *Mental Health of the Poor,* New York: The Free Press of Glencoe, 1964.

Chapter 6

1. Post, F., and Wardle, J.: "Family Neurosis and Family Psychosis: A Review of the Problem," *J. Ment. Sci.,* 108:147-158, 1962.

2. Ackerman, N. W.: "Towards an Integrative Therapy of the Family," *American Journal of Psychiatry,* 114:727-733, 1958. Bell, J. E.: "Recent Advances in Family Group Therapy," *J. Child Psychol. Psychiat.,* 1:1-15, 1962. Howells, J. G.: *Family Psychiatry,* Edinburgh & London: Oliver and Boyd, 1963. Laing, R. D., and Esterson, A.: "Sanity, Madness, and the Family," in Vol. 1, *Families of Schizophrenics,* London: Tavistock, 1964.

3. Brown, G. W.; Monck, E. M.; Carstairs, G. M.; and Wing, J. K.: "Influence of Family Life on the Course of Schizophrenic Illness," *British Journal of Preventive Social Medicine,* 16:55-68, 1962.

4. Rutter, M.: "Children of Sick Parents: An Environmental and Psychiatric Study," *Maudsley Monograph No. 16* (in press), 1966.

5. Clausen, J. A.: "The Marital Relationship Antecedent to Hospitalization of a Spouse for Mental Illness," unpublished paper, 1959. Clausen, J. A., and Yarrow, M. R.: "Mental Illness and the Family," *Journal of Social Issues,* 11:No. 4, 1955. Sainsbury, P., and Grad, J.: "An Evaluation of Treatment and Services," in *The Burden on the Community: Epidemiology of Mental Disease,* A Symposium, London: Oxford University Press, 1962. Grad, J., and Sainsbury, P.: "Mental Illness and the Family," *Lancet,* 1:544-547, 1963. Wing, J. K.; Monck, E.; Brown, G. W.; and Carstairs, G. M.: "Morbidity in the Community of Schizophrenic Patients Discharged from London Mental Hospitals in 1959," *British Journal of Psychiatry,* 110:10-21, 1964. Brown, G. W., and Rutter, M.: "The Measurement of Family Activities and Relationships: A Methodological Study," *Human Relations,* 19: 1966.

6. Rutter, M., *op. cit.,* see reference 4.

7. Nimkoff, M. F.: "Trends in Family Research," *American Journal of Sociology,* 53:477-482, 1948. Nye, F. I., and Bayer, A. E.: "Some Recent Trends in Family Research," *Social Forces,* 41:290-301, 1963.

8. Hoffman, L. W. and Lippitt, R.: "The Measurement of Family Life Variables," Mussen, P. H., (ed.), *Handbook of Research Methods in Child Development,* New York: Wiley, 1960. Nye, F. I. and Bayer, A. E., *op. cit.,* see reference 7. Yarrow, M. R.: "Problems of Methods in Parent-Child Research," *Child Development,* 34:215-266, 1963.

9. Cumming, E.; Dean, L. R.; and Hewell, D. S.: "What is 'Morale'? A Case History of a Validity Problem," *Human Organization,* 17:3-8, 1958. Dean, J. P. and Whyte, W. F.: "How Do You Know if the Informant Is Telling the Truth," *Human Organization,* 17:34-38, 1958. Hoffman, M. L., and Lippitt, R., *op. cit.,* see reference 8. Vidich, A., and Benson, J.: "The Validity of Field Data," *Human Organization,* 13:20-27, 1954.

10. Ellis, A.: "Questionnaire Versus Interview Methods in the Study of Human Love Relationships," *American Sociological Review,* 12:541-553, 1947. McCord, J., and McCord, W.: "Cultural Stereotypes and the Validity of Interviews for Research in Child Development," *Child Development,* 32:171-185, 1961. Richardson, S. A.; Dohrenwend, B. S.; and Klein, D.: *Interviewing: Its Forms and Functions,* New York: Basic Books, 1965. Smith, H. T.: "A Comparison of Interview and Observation Measures of Mother Behavior," *Journal of Abnormal Social Psychology,* 57:278-282, 1958. Yarrow, M. R., *op. cit.,* see reference 8.

11. Baldwin, A. L.: "The Study of Child Behavior and Development," in Mussen, P. H., (ed.), *Handbook of Research Methods in Child Development,* New York: John Wiley, 1960. Bell, R. Q.: "Retrospective and Prospective Views of Early Personality Development," *Merrill-Palmer Quarterly,* 6:131-144, 1960. Yarrow, M. R., *op. cit.,* see reference 8. Yarrow, M. R.; Campbell, J. D.; and Burton, R. V.: "Reliability of Maternal Retrospection: A Preliminary Report," *Family Process,* 3:207-218, 1964.

12. Clark, A. W., and Sommers, P. V.: "Contradictory Demands in Family Relations and Adjustment to School and Home," *Human Relations,* 14:97-111, 1961.

13. Dean, J. P., and Whyte, W. F., *op. cit.,* see Reference 9. Garrett, A.: *Interviewing: Its Principles and Methods,* New York: Family Service Association of America, 1942. Hoffman, L. W. and Lippitt, R., *op. cit,* see Reference 8.

14. Yaukey, D.; Roberts, B. J.; and Griffiths, W.: "Husbands' vs Wives' Responses to a Fertility Survey," *Population Studies,* 19:29-43, 1965.

15. Dean, J. P., and Whyte, W. F., *op. cit,* see Reference 9.

16. Schaeffer, E. S., and Bell, R. Q.: "Development of a Parental Attitude Research Instrument," *Child Development,* 29:339-361, 1958.

17. Becker, W. C.: *Unpublished Supplemental Analyses of Parent-Child Data,* 1961.

18. Becker, W. C., and Krug, R. S.: "The Parent Attitude Research Instrument—A Research Review," *Child Development,* 36:329-365, 1965.

19. Peterson, D. R.; Becker, W. C.; Shoemaker, D. J.; Luria, Z.; and Hellmer, L. A.: "Child Behaviour Problems and Parental Attitudes," *Child Development,* 32:151-162, 1961.

20. McCord, W.; McCord, J.; and Nerden, P.: "Familial and Behavioural Correlates of Dependency in Male Children," *Child Development,* 33:313-326, 1962.

21. Sears, R. R.; Maccoby, E. E.; and Levin, H.: *Patterns of Child Rearing,* White Plains, New York: Row Peterson & Company, 1957.

22. Becker, W. C.: "The Relationship of Factors in Parental Ratings of Self and Each Other to the Behaviour of Kindergarten Children as Rated by Mothers, Fathers, and Teachers," *Journal of Consulting Psychology,* 24:507-527, 1960. Becker, W. C., *op. cit.,* see Reference 18.

23. Baldwin, A. L.; Kalhorn, J.; and Breese, F. H.: "The Appraisal of Parent Behaviour," *Psychol. Mon.,* 63: No. 4, 1949.

24. Tizard, J., and Grad, J. C.: "The Mentally Handicapped and their Families," *Maudsley Monograph No. 7,* London: Oxford University Press, 1961.

25. Hamburg, D. A.; Sabshin, M. A.; Board, F. A.; Grinker, R. R.; Korchin, S. J.; Basowitz, H.; Heath, H.; and Persky, H.: "Classification and rating of Emotional Experiences," *Archives of Neurological Psychiatry,* 79:415-426, 1958.

26. Bandura, A., and Walters, R. H.: *Adolescent Aggression,* New York: Ronald Press, 1959.

27. Brown, G. W.; Monck, E. M.; Carstairs, G. M.; and Wing, J. K., *op. cit.,* see Reference 3.

28. Harris, A., and Metcalf, M.: "Inappropriate Affect," *Journal of Neurol. Neurosurg. Psychiat.,* 19:308-313, 1956.

29. Ekman, P.: "Body Position, Facial Expression and Verbal Behavior During Interviews," *Journal of Abnormal Social Psychology,* 68:295-301, 1964.

30. Alpert, M.; Kurtzberg, R. L.; and Friedhoff, A. J.: "Transient Voice Changes Associated with Emotional Stimuli," *Archives of General Psychiatry,* 8:362-365, 1963.

31. Starkweather, J. A.: "Content Free Speech as a Source of Information about the Speaker," *Journal of Abnormal Social Psychology*, 52:394-402, 1956.

32. Herbst, P. G.: "The Measurement of Family Relations," *Human Relations*, 5:3-30, 1952.

33. Yamamura, D. S., and Zald, M. N.: "A Note on the Usefulness and Validity of the Herbst Family Questionnaire," *Human Relations*, 9:217-221, 1956.

34. Hoffman, L. W., and Lippitt, R., *op. cit.*, see Reference 8.

35. Tharp, R. G.: "Dimensions of Marriage Roles," *Marriage and Family Living*, 25:389-404, 1963.

36. Hoffman, L. W., and Lippitt, R., *op. cit.*, see Reference 8.

37. Radke, M. J.: "The Relation of Parental Authority to Children's Behavior and Attitudes," *Institute Child. Welf. Monogr. No. 22*, 1946.

38. Cheek, F. E.: "The Father of the Schizophrenic," *Archives of General Psychiatry*, 13:336-345, 1965. Goodrich, D. W., and Boomer, D. S.: "Experimental Assessment of Modes of Conflict Resolution," *Family Process*, 2:15-24, 1963. Ryder, R. G., and Goodrich, D. W.: *Married Couples Responses to Disagreement*, Unpublished manuscript, 1965. Haley, J.: "Research on Family Patterns: An Instrument Measurement," *Family Process*, 3:41-65, 1964. Kenkel, W. F., and Hoffman, D. K.: "Real and Conceived Roles in Family Decision Making," *Marriage and Family Living*, 18:311-316, 1956. Mishler, E.: *Personal Communication*, 1965. Strodbeck, F. L.: "Husband-Wife Interaction over Revealed Differences," *American Sociological Review*, 16:468-473, 1951. Vidich, A. J.: "Methodological Problems in the Observation of Husband-Wife Interaction," *Marriage and Family Living*, 18:234-239, 1956.

39. Goodrich, D. W., and Boomer, D. S., *op. cit.*, see Reference 38. Ryder, R. G. and Goodrich, *op. cit.*, see Reference 38. Mishler, E., *op. cit.*, see Reference 38.

40. Cheek, F. E., *op. cit.*, see Reference 38.

41. O'Rourke, J. F.: "Field and Laboratory: The Decision Making Behaviour of Family Groups in Two Experimental Conditions," *Sociometry*, 26:422-435, 1963.

42. Marshall, H. R.: "Relations Between Home Experiences and Children's Use of Language in Play Interactions with Peers," *Psychology Monograph 75*, No. 5, 1961.

43. Bandura, A., and Walters, R. H., *op. cit.*, see Reference 26.

44. Blood, R. O., and Wolfe, D. M.: *Husbands and Wives: The Dynamics of Married Living*, Illinois: Free Press of Glencoe, 1960.

45. Clark, A. L., and Wallin, P.: "The Accuracy of Husbands' and Wives' Reports of Frequency of Marital Coitus," *Population Studies,* 18:165-173, 1964.

46. *Ibid.*

47. Kohn, M. L., and Carroll, E. E.: "Social Class and the Allocation of Parental Responsibilities," *Sociometry,* 23:372-392, 1960.

48. Andry, R. G.: *Delinquency and Parental Pathology,* London: Methuen, 1960.

49. Eron, L. D.; Banta, T. J.; Walder, L. O.; and Laulight, J. H.: "Comparison of Data Obtained from Mothers and Fathers on Child-Rearing Practices and their Relation to Child Aggression," *Child Development,* 32:457-472, 1961.

50. Young, F. W., and Young, R. C.: "Key Informant Reliability in Rural Mexican Villages," *Human Organization,* 20:141-148, 1961.

51. Yaukey, D. B.; Roberts, B. J.; and Griffiths, W., *op. cit.,* see Reference 14. Kenkel, W. F., and Hoffman, D. K.: "Real and Conceived Roles in Family Decision Making," *Marriage and Family Living,* 18:311-316, 1956.

52. Haggerty, R. J.: "Family Diagnosis: Research Methods and Reliability of Studies of the Medico-Social Unit, The Family," *American Journal of Public Health,* 55:1521-1533, 1965.

53. Bandura, A., and Walters, R. H., *op. cit.,* see Reference 26. Levinger, G.: "Tasks and Social Behaviour in Marriage," *Sociometry,* 27:433-448, 1964.

54. Frumkin, R. M.: "The Kirkpatrick Scale of Family Interests as an Instrument for the Indirect Assessment of Marital Adjustment," *Marriage and Family Living,* 15:35-37, 1953. Hoffman, L. W., and Lippitt, R., *op. cit.,* see Reference 8.

55. Geismar, L. L. and Ayres, B.: *Measuring Family Functioning,* St. Paul, Minnesota: Greater St. Paul Community Chest and Councils, Inc., 1960.

56. Geismar, L. L.: "Family Functioning as an Index of Need for Welfare Services," *Family Process,* 3:99-113, 1964.

57. Robbins, L. C.: "The Accuracy of Parental Recall of Aspects of Child Development and of Child Rearing Practices," *Journal of Abnormal Social Psychology,* 66:261-270, 1963. Yarrow, M. R., *op. cit.,* see Reference 8. Yarrow, M. R.; Campbell, J. D.; and Burton, R. V., *op. cit.,* see Reference 11.

58. Yarrow, M. R., *op. cit.,* see Reference 8.

59. Brown, G. W., and Rutter, M., *op. cit.,* see Reference 5.

60. Richardson, S. A.; Dohrenwend, B. S.; and Kleni, D., *op. cit.*, see Reference 10.

61. *Ibid.*

62. Hoffman, M. L.: "Power Assertion by the Parent and its Impact on the Child," *Child Development*, 31:129-143, 1960.

63. Thomas, A.; Birch, H. G.; Chess, S.; Hertzig, M. E.; and Korn, S.: *Behavioural Individuality in Early Childhood*, New York: New York University Press, 1963.

64. Herbst, P. G., *op. cit.*, see Reference 32.

65. Bandura, A., and Walters, R. H., *op. cit.*, see Reference 26.

66. Hoffman, M. L., *op. cit.*, see Reference 62.

67. Chapple, E. D.: "The Standard Experimental (stress) Interview As Used in Interaction Chronograph Investigations," *Human Organization*, 12:23-32, 1953.

68. Reece, M. M., and Whitman, R. N.: "Expressive Movements, Warmth, and Verbal Reinforcement," *Journal of Abnormal Social Psychology*, 64:234-236, 1962.

69. Salzinger, K., and Pisoni, S.: "Reinforcement of Verbal Affect Responses of Normal Subjects During the Interview," *Journal of Abnormal Social Psychology*, 60:127-130, 1960.

70. Johnson, M. L.: "Observer Error: Its Bearing on Teaching," *Lancet*, 2:422-424, 1955.

71. Bandura, A., and Walter, R. H., *op. cit.*, see Reference 26.

72. Baruch, D.: "A Study of Reported Tension in Interparental Relationships as Co-Existent with Behaviour Adjustment in Young Children," *Journal Exp. Educ.*, 6:187-204, 1937.

73. Hoffman, L. W., and Lippitt, R., *op. cit.*, see Reference 8.

74. Brown, G. W. and Rutter, M., *op. cit.*, see Reference 5.

75. *Ibid.*

76. *Ibid.*

77. Becker, W. C., *op. cit.*, see Reference 22. Becker, W. C., *op. cit.*, see Reference 17.

78. Hoffman, L. W. and Lippitt, R., *op. cit.*, see Reference 8. Richardson, S. A., Dohrnewend, B. S. and Klein, D., *op. cit.*, see Reference 10.

79. Newson, J. and Newson, E.: *Infant Care in an Urban Community*, London: Allen and Unwin, 1963. Richardson, S. A., Dohrenwend, B. S. and Klein, D., *op. cit.*, see Reference 10.

80. Robbins, L. C., *op. cit.*, see Reference 57. Yarrow, M. R., Campbell, J. D. and Burton, R. V., *op. cit.*, see Reference 11.

Chapter 7

1. Halevi, H. S.: *Mental Illness in Israel: Admission to Mental Hospitals and Institutions for In-Patients During 1958,* Jerusalem: Ministry of Health, 1960 (mimeographed).

2. Moses, R., and Shanan, J.: "Psychiatric Outpatient Clinic," *Archives of General Psychiatry,* 4:60-73, 1961.

3. Srole, L. et al.: *Mental Health in the Metropolis: The Midtown Manhattan Study,* New York: McGraw-Hill, 1962.

4. Leighton, D. C.: "Distribution of Psychiatric Symptoms in a Small Town," *American Journal of Psychiatry,* 112:716-726, 1956.

5. Pasamanick, B.: "A Survey of Mental Disease in an Urban Population," *American Journal of Public Health,* 47:923-929, 1957.

6. Kessel, W. I. N.: "Psychiatric Morbidity in a London General Practice," *British Journal of Preventive Social Medicine,* 14:16-22, 1960.

7. Primrose, E. J. R.: *Psychological Illness, A Community Study,* London: Tavistock Publications, 1962.

8. Kessel, W. I. N.: "Conducting a Psychiatric Survey in General Practice," *The Burden on the Community: The Epidemiology of Mental Illness,* London: Oxford University Press, 1962. Ryle, A.: "The Neuroses in a General Practice Population," *J. Coll. Gen. Practice,* 3:313-328, 1960. Primrose, E. J. R., *op. cit.,* see reference 7.

9. Weinberg, A. A.: *Migration and Belonging: A Study of Mental Health and Personal Adjustment in Israel,* The Hague: M. Nyhoff, 1961.

10. Opler, M. K.: "Social and Cultural Backgrounds of Mental Illness," *Culture, Psychiatry and Human Values,* Springfield, Illinois: Charles C. Thomas, 1956.

11. Malzberg, B., and Lee, E. S.: *Migration and Mental Disease,* New York Social Research Council, 1956.

12. Murphy, H. B. M.: "Social Change and Mental Health," *Milbank Memorial Fund Quarterly,* 39:385-445, 1961.

13. Leighton, A. H., and Hughes, J. M.: "Cultures as Causative of Mental Disorder," *Milbank Memorial Fund Quarterly,* 39:446-488, 1961.

14. Ruesch, J., et al., "Acculturation and Illness," *Psychol. Monographs,* 5:1-40, 1948.

15. Kessel, W. I. N., *op. cit.,* see reference 8. Plunkett, R. J., and Gordon, J. E.: *"Epidemiology and Mental Illness,"* Joint Commission

on Mental Illness and Health Monograph Series 6, New York: Basic Books, 1960. Blum, R. H.: "Case Identification in Psychiatric Epidemiology: Methods and Problems," *Milbank Memorial Fund Quarterly,* 40:253-288, 1962.

16. Redlich, F. C.: "The Concept of Health in Psychiatry," in *Explorations in Social Psychiatry,* Leighton, A. H.; Clausen, J. A.; and Wilson, R. N., New York: Basic Books, 1957, pp. 138-166.

17. Ryle, A., *op. cit.,* see reference 8.

18. Kessel, W. I. N., *op. cit.,* see reference 8, p. 15

19. Balint, M.: *The Doctor, His Patient and the Illness,* New York: International Universities Press, 1957.

20. Weinberg, A. A., *op. cit.,* see reference 9, p. 243.

21. Srole, L., et al., *op. cit.,* see reference 3.

22. Stein, L.: " 'Social Class' Gradient in Schizophrenia," *British Journal of Preventive Social Medicine,* 11:181-195, 1957.

23. Srole, L. et al., *op. cit.,* see reference 3, pp. 138-139.

24. Plunkett, R. J. and Gordon, J. E., *op. cit.,* see reference 15.

25. Primrose, E. J. R., *op. cit.,* see reference 7.

26. *Ibid.* See also Ryle, A., *op. cit.,* see reference 8.

CHAPTER 9

1. Bernard, V.: "Some Interrelationships of Training for Community Psychiatry, Community Mental Health Programs and Research in Social Psychiatry," *Proceedings of Third World Congress of Psychiatry,* Montreal, Canada: McGill University and University of Toronto Press, 3:67-71, 1961.

2. Goldston, S. E.: "Training in Community Psychiatry: Survey Report of Medical School Departments of Psychiatry," *American Journal of Psychiatry,* 120:789-792, Feb. 1964.

3. *Ibid.*

4. Duhl, L. J.: "Problems in Training Psychiatric Residents in Community Psychiatry," Paper read before the Institute on Training in Community Psychiatry at University of California, Texas, Columbia, and Chicago, mimeographed, Fall-Winter, 1963-1964, p. 6.

5. *Ibid.*

6. Merton, R. K.: "Social Structure and Anomie," in *Social Theory and Social Structure,* Glencoe, Illinois: The Free Press, 1949, pp. 125-150.

7. Kobrin, S.: "Chicago Area Project—25 Year Assessment," *Ann. Amer. Acad. Political Soc. Sci.,* 322:20-29, March, 1959.

8. *Ibid.*

9. Powers, E., and Witmer, H.: *Experiment in Prevention of Delinquency,* New York: Columbia University Press, 1951.

10. Goldhamer, H., and Marshall, A.: *Psychoses and Civilization,* Glencoe, Illinois: The Free Press, 1953.

11. Plunkett, R. J., and Gordon, J. E.: *Epidemiology and Mental Illness,* New York: Basic Books, Inc., 1960, p. 90.

12. Srole, L. et al.: *Mental Health in the Metropolis: Midtown Manhattan Study,* New York: McGraw-Hill Book Co., Inc., 1962, Vol. 1.

13. Barton, W. E.: "Presidential Address—Psychiatry in Transition," *American Journal of Psychiatry,* 119:1-15, July, 1962.

14. Szasz, T. S.: *Myth of Mental Illness: Foundation of Theory of Personal Conduct,* New York: Paul B. Hoeber, Inc., Medical Division of Harper & Brothers, 1961.

15. See Hoch, P. H.: in "Therapeutic Accomplishments of Mental Health Clinics," *Mental Hygiene News,* June, 1963, p. 1-3.

16. *Ibid.*

17. *Ibid.*

18. Menninger, W.: *Psychiatry in a Troubled World,* New York: The Macmillan Company, 1948, Chap. 13.

19. Thompson, C. B.: "Psychiatry and Social Crisis," *Journal of Clinical Psychopathology,* 7:697-711, April, 1946.

20. Jones, M.: *Therapeutic Community: New Treatment Method in Psychiatry,* New York: Basic Books, Inc., 1953.

21. Stanton, A., and Schwartz, M. S.: *Mental Hospital: Study of Institutional Participation in Psychiatric Illness and Treatment,* New York: Basic Books, Inc., 1954.

22. Dunham, H. W., and Weinberg, S. K.: *Culture of State Mental Hospital,* Detroit: The Wayne State University Press, 1960.

23. Belknap, I.: *Human Problems of State Mental Hospital,* New York: Blakiston, Medical Division of McGraw-Hill Book Co., 1956.

24. Cumming, J., and Cumming, E.: *Closed Ranks: Experiment in Mental Health Education,* Cambridge, Massachusetts: Harvard University Press, Commonwealth Fund, 1957.

25. Caudill, W.: *Psychiatric Hospital as a Small Society,* Cambridge, Massachusetts: Harvard University Press, 1958.

26. Joint Commission on Mental Illness and Health: *Action for Mental Health,* New York: Basic Books, Inc., 1961, p. 338.

27. Kennedy, J. F.: "Message From President of United States

Relative to Mental Illness and Mental Retardation: February 5, 1963," *American Journal of Psychiatry,* 120:729-737, Feb., 1964.

Chapter 10

1. Ellis, J. M.: "Socio-Economic Differentials in Mortality from Chronic Diseases," *Social Problems,* 5:30-36, 1957.

2. Allport, G. W., Perception and Public Health, *Health Education Monographs,* No. 2, 1958.

3. Anderson, O. W.: "Infant Mortality and Social and Cultural Factors: Historical Trends and Current Patterns," in E. G. Jaco, (ed.), *Patients, Physicians and Illness,* New York: The Free Press of Glencoe, 1958, pp. 10-24.

4. Graham, S.: "Social Factors in Relation to Chronic Illnesses," in H. Freeman; S. Levine; and L. Reeder, (eds.), *Handbook of Medical Sociology,* Englewood Cliffs, New Jersey: Prentice-Hall, Inc., 1963, pp. 65-98.

5. Wolff, H. G.: "Disease and the Patterns of Behaviour," in E. G. Jaco (ed.), *Patients, Physicians and Illness,* New York: The Free Press of Glencoe, 1958, pp. 54-60.

6. *Ibid.*

7. Leighton, D. C. et al., *The Character of Danger: Psychiatric Symptoms in Selected Communities,* New York: Basic Books, 1963.

8. Kvaraceus, W. C., and Miller, W. B.: *Delinquent Behavior: Culture and the Individual,* Washington, D.C.: National Education Association, 1959.

9. Kluckhohn, F. R.: "Family Diagnosis: Variations in the Basic Values of Family Systems," *Social Casework,* 1958.

10. Koss, E. L.: *The Health of Regionville,* New York: Columbia University Press, 1954.

11. Parsons, T.: "Definitions of Health and Illness in the Light of American Values and Social Structure," in E. G. Jaco, (ed.), *Patients, Physicians and Illness,* New York: The Free Press of Glencoe, 1958, pp. 165-187.

12. Kaplan, B. and Plaut, T. F. A.: *Personality in a Communal Society: An Analysis of the Mental Health of the Hutterites,* Lawrence, Kansas: University of Kansas Publications, 1956.

13. Zborowski, M.: "Cultural Components in Responses to Pain," *Journal of Social Issues,* 8:16-30, 1952.

14. Rosenstock, I. M.: "What Research in Motivation Suggests for

Public Health Programmes," Paper presented at 86th Annual Meeting of the American Public Health Association, St. Louis, Mo., Oct. 30, 1958.

15. Chafetz, M. et al.: "Establishing Treatment Relations with Alcoholics," *The Journal of Nervous and Mental Disease,* 134:395-409, 1962.

16. Plaut, T. F. A.: "New Dimensions in Public Health," *Proceedings of the Public Health Nursing Conference—Family-Centered Approach to the Control of Alcoholism,* Boston, Massachusetts: Department of Public Health, 1959, pp. 13-21.

17. Saunders, L., and Samora, J.: "A Medical Care Programme in a Colorado County," in B. D. Paul, (ed.), *Health, Culture and Community,* New York: Russell Sage Foundation, pp. 377-400, 1955.

18. Kluckhohn, F. R., *op. cit.,* see Reference 9.

19. Sanders, I. T.: "Public Health in the Community," in H. Froeman, S. Levine, and L. Reeder, eds., *Handbook of Medical Sociology,* Englewood Cliffs, New Jersey: Prentice-Hall, Inc., pp. 369-396, 1963.

20. Freeman, L. C. et al.: "Locating Leaders in Local Communities: A Comparison of Some Alternative Approaches," *American Sociological Review,* 28:791-798, 1963.

21. Banfield, E. C.: *Political Influence,* New York: The Free Press of Glencoe, 1961.

22. *Ibid.*

23. Cumming, E. and Cumming, J.: *Closed Ranks: An Experiment in Mental Health Education,* Cambridge: Harvard University Press, 1957.

24. Cumming, E. and Cumming, J.: "Mental Health Education in a Canadian Community," in B. D. Paul, (ed.), *Health, Culture and Community,* New York: Russell Sage Foundation, 1955, p. 62.

25. *Ibid.,* p. 63.

26. Sanders, I. T., *op. cit.,* see Reference 19.

27. Roemer, M. I.: "Changing Patterns of Health Service: Their Dependence on a Changing World," *The Annals of the American Academy of Political and Social Science,* 346:44-56, 1963.

28. Johns, R. E., and de Marche, D. F.: *Community Organization and Agency Responsibility,* New York: Association Press, 1951.

29. Miller, W. B.: "Inter-Institutional Conflict as a Major Impediment To Delinquency Prevention," *Human Organization,* 17:20-23, 1958.

30. James, G.: "Effective Community Health Services," *Public*

Health Concepts in Social Work Education: Council on Social Work Education, 1962.

CHAPTER 12

1. Querido, A.: *The Efficiency of Medical Care,* H. V. Kroeser, Leiden, 1963.

2. Barton, W. Russell: *Institutional Neurosis,* Bristol, England: John Wright and Sons, 1959.

3. Tooth, G. C. and Brooke, E. M.: "Trends in the Mental Hospital Population and Their Effects on Future Planning," *Lancet,* 1:710, 1961.

4. Jones and Sidebotham, R.: *Mental Hospitals at Work,* London: Routledge & Kegan Paul, Ltd., 1962. *Psychiatric Services in 1975, P.E.P.* (Political and Economic Planning), London, 1963.

5. Sivadon, P.: "Address to the Annual Conference of the International Hospital Federation," Paris, June, 1963.

6. Jones and Sidebotham, *op. cit.*, see Reference 4.

7. Jones, K.: *Lunacy: Law and Conscience, 1744-1845,* London: Routledge & Kegan Paul, Ltd., 1962.

8. *Action for Mental Health: Final Report of the Joint Commission on Mental Illness and Health,* New York: Basic Books, Inc., 1961.

CHAPTER 13

1. Vickers, G.: "The End of Free Fall," mimeographed article, Fall, 1964, p. 21.

2. "Computers: How They're Remaking Companies," *Business Week,* Feb. 29, 1964. Morgello, Clem: "The Challenge of Automation," *Newsweek,* Jan. 25, 1965. "The Cybernated Generation," *Time,* April 2, 1965.

3. Bell, D.: "The Post-Industrial Society," in *Technology and Social Change,* E. Ginzberg, (ed.), New York: Columbia University Press, 1964, pp. 58-59.

4. *The Integrity of Science,* Washington, D.C.: American Association for the Advancement of Science, 1964.

5. Morganthau, H. J.: "Modern Science and Political Power," *Columbia Law Review,* CLIV:1402, 1964.

6. Kraft, J.: "The Politics of the Washington Press Corps," *Harper's Magazine,* June, 1965, pp. 101-102.

7. Fabricant, S.: *Measurement of Technological Change,* Washington, D.C.: Manpower Administration, U.S. Department of Labor, 1965, p. 3.

Chapter 14

1. Grootenboer, E. A.: *American Journal of Psychiatry,* 119:469, 1962.

2. Martin, F. M.: Brotherson, J. H. F.; and Chave, S. P. W.: *British Journal of Preventive Social Medicine,* 11:196, 1957.

3. Logan, W. P. D.: "Studies on Medical and Population Subjects," *General Practitioners Records No. 7,* London: H. M. Stationery Office, 1953.

4. Tyhurst, L.: *American Journal of Psychiatry,* 107:561, 1951.

5. Wilner, D. M.; Walkley, R.; Pinkerton, T. C.; and Tayback, M.: *The Housing Environment and Family Life,* Baltimore: Johns Hopkins Press, 1962, p. 338.

6. Abraham, K.: *Versuch Einer Entwicklungsgeschichte der Libido,* Berlin: Internationaler Psycho-analytischer Verlag, 1924, p. 28.

7. Buck, J. N.: *Journal of Clinical Psychcology,* 4:317, 1948.

8. Langveld, M. J.: "De 'Verborgen Plaats' in het Leven Van het Kind, in *Persoon en Wereld,* Utrecht: Bijleveld, 1953.

9. Buck, J. N., *op. cit.,* see Reference 7.

10. Wilner, D. M.; Walkley, R.; Pinkerton, T. C.; and Tayback, M., *op. cit.,* see Reference 5.

Chapter 15

1. Abraham, K.: "Notes on the Psycho-analytical Investigation and Treatment of Manic-Depressive Insanity and Allied Conditions," 1911, and "A Short Study of the Development of the Libido, Viewed in the Light of Mental Disorders," 1924, in *Selected Papers of Karl Abraham,* Vol. 1, New York: Basic Books, 1953. Bibring, E.: "The Mechanisms of Depression," in P. Greenacre, (ed.), *Affective Disorders,* New York: International Universities Press, 1953. Bowlby, J.: "Processes of Mourning," *International Journal of Psychoanalysis,* 42:317-340, 1961. Freud, S.: "Mourning and Melancholia," *Collected Papers,* 1917, Vol. III, New York: Basic Books, 1959. Hoggart, R.: *The Uses of Literacy: Changing Patterns in English Mass Culture,* New York: Oxford Uni-

versity Press, 1957. Klein, M.: "Mourning in Its Relations to Manic-Depressive States," *International Journal of Psychoanalysis,* 21:125-153, 1940. Lindemann, E.: "Symptomatology and Management of Acute Grief," *American Journal of Psychiatry,* 101:141-148, 1944. Marris, P.: *Widows and Their Families,* London: Routledge and Kegan Paul, 1958. Rochlin, G.: "The Dread of Abandoment," *The Psychoanalytic Study of the Child,* Vol. XVI, New York: International Universities Press, 1961. Volkart, E. H., and Michael, S. T.: "Bereavement and Mental Health," in A. H. Leighton; J. A. Clausen, and R. N. Wilson, (eds.), *Explorations in Social Psychiatry,* New York: Basic Books, 1957.

2. Fried, M. and Gleicher, P.: "Some Sources of Residential Satisfaction in an Urban Slum," *Journal of American Inst. Planners,* 27: 305-315, 1961.

3. Gans, H.: *The Urban Villagers,* New York: The Free Press of Glencoe, 1963. Gans, H.: "The Human Implications of Current Redevelopment and Relocation Planning," *Journal Amer. Inst. Planners,* 25:15-25, 1959. Hoggart, R., *op. cit.,* see Reference 1. Hole, V.: "Social Effects of Planned Rehousing," *Town Planning Rev.,* 30:161-173, 1959. Marris, P.: *Family and Social Change in an African City,* Evanston: Illinois: Northwestern University Press, 1962. Mogey, J. M.: *Family and Neighbourhood,* New York: Oxford University Press, 1956. Seeley, J.: "The Slum: Its Nature, Use, and Users," *Journal Amer. Inst. Planners,* 25:7-14, 1959. Vereker, C. and Mays, J. B.: *Urban Redevelopment and Social Change,* New York: Lounz, 1960. Young, M., and Willmott, P.: *Family and Kinship in East London,* Glencoe, Illinois: The Free Press, 1957.

4. Erikson, E.: "Ego Development and Historical Change," *The Psychoanalytic Study of the Child,* Vol. II, New York: International Universities Press, 1946. Erikson, E.: "The Problem of Ego Identity," *Journal of the American Psychoanalytical Association,* 4:56-121, 1956.

CHAPTER 16

1. Beach, F. A.: *American Psychology,* 5:115, 1950.

2. Oakley, K. P.: "A Definition of Man," *Science News,* No. 20, Baltimore: Penguin, 1951. Washburn, S. L., and Avis, V.: in *Behavior and Evolution,* A. Roe, and G. G. Simpson, (eds.), New Haven, Connecticut: Yale University Press, 1958. Schultz, A. H.: *Z. Morphol. Anthropol.* 50:136, 1960. Oakley, K. P.: *Antiquity,* 31:199, 1957.

3. Schneirla, T. C.: in *Advances in the Study of Behavior,* Vol. 1, D. S. Lehrman, R. Hinde, and E. Shaw, (eds.), New York: Academic Press, 1965. Lorenz, K.: in *Instinctive Behavior, the Development of a Modern Concept,* Part II, Chapters i, ii, iii, v, and vii, C. H. Schiller, (ed.), New York: International Universities Press, 1957. Scott, J. P.: *Science,* 138:949, 1962. Schneirla, T. C. and Rosenblatt, J. S.: in *Readings in Animal Behavior,* T. E. McGill, (ed.), New York: Holt, Rinehart & Winston, 1965, p. 287. Scott, J. P.: in *Readings in Animal Behavior,* T. E. McGill (ed.), New York: Holt, Rinehart, and Winston, 1965, p. 290.

4. Brooks, G. W., and Mueller, E.: *Journal of the American Medical Association,* 195:415, 1966. Orowan, E.: *Nature,* 175:683, 1955.

5. DeVore, I., (ed.): *Primate Behavior, Field Studies of Monkeys and Apes,* New York: Holt, Rinehart & Winston, 1965. Schrier, A. M., Harlow, H. F. and Stollnitz, F.: *Behavior of Non-Human Primates: Modern Research Trends,* New York: Academic Press, 1965.

6. Altmann, S. A.: *Science,* 150:40, 1965.

7. Grinker, Sr., R. G.: *American Journal of Psychiatry,* 122:367, 1965.

8. Wynne-Edwards, V. C.: *Animal Dispersion in Relation to Social Behavior,* Edinburgh: Oliver & Boyd, 1963.

9. Van Lawick Goodall, J.: *National Geographic,* 128:802, 1965.

10. Carpenter, C. R.: *Compar. Psychol. Monog.,* 10:1, 1934.

11. Hall, R. R. L.: Paper read at the American Association for the Advancement of Science Convention, Montreal, December, 1964.

12. Carpenter, C. R.: *Biol. Symp.,* 8:177, 1942. Von Uexkull, J.: in *Instinctive Behavior,* C. H. Schiller, (ed.), New York: International Universities Press, 1957.

13. Kummer, H.: *Beih. Schweiz. Z. Psychol.,* Suppl., 33:1, 1957.

14. Rule, C.: *American Journal of Psychiatry,* 121:344, 1964.

15. DeVore, I., (ed.), *op. cit.,* see Reference 5. Schrier, A. M.; Harlow, H. F.; and Stollnitz, F., *op. cit.,* see Reference 5. Washburn, S. L.: *Social Life of Early Man,* Chicago: Aldine, 1961. Roe, A. and Simpson, G. G. (eds.): *Behavior and Evolution,* New Haven, Connecticut: Yale University Press, 1958. Southwick, C. R.: *Primate Social Behavior,* Princeton, New Jersey: Van Nostrand, 1963.

16. Oakley, K. P.: in *Social Life of Early Man,* S. L. Washburn, (ed.), Chicago: Aldine, 1961.

17. Hockett, C. F.: in *Animal Sounds and Communication,* W. E. Lanyon and W. N. Tavolga, (eds.), Washington, D.C.: American Institute of Biological Sciences, 1960, p. 392.

18. Reusch, J.: *Therapeutic Communication,* New York: Norton, 1961. Reusch, J., and Bateson, G.: *Communication,* New York: Norton, 1951.

19. Brody, R. B.: *American Journal of Psychiatry,* 122:852, 1966.

20. Sullivan, H. S.: *Nonverbal Communication,* quoted in J. Reusch and W. Kees, (eds.), Berkeley: University of California Press, 1956.

21. Penfield, W. and Roberts, L.: *Speech and Brain Mechanisms,* Princeton, New Jersey: Princeton University Press, 1959.

22. Sapir, E.: *Language,* 5:21, 1929.

23. Jacobson, E.: *American Journal of Psychology,* 44:677, 1932.

24. Bastian, J.: in *Primate Behavior, Field Studies of Monkeys and Apes,* I. DeVore, (ed.), New York: Holt, Rinehart & Winston, 1965, chap. xvii.

25. Harlow, H. F.: *American Journal of Orthopsychiatry,* 30:676, 1960.

26. Goodall, J., in *Primate Behavior, Field Studies of Monkeys and Apes,* see Reference 24.

27. Rule, C., *op. cit.,* see Reference 14.

28. Jay, P., *op. cit.,* see Reference 24.

29. Rule, C., *op. cit.,* see Reference 14.

30. Harlow, H. F., *op. cit.,* see Reference 25.

31. Altmann, S. A.: Film and Remarks at American Association for the Advancement of Science Convention, Montreal, December, 1964.

32. Arieti, S.: *American Journal of Psychiatry,* 122:361, 1965.

33. Sullivan, H. S.: *The Interpersonal Theory of Psychiatry,* New York: Norton, 1953.

34. Foucault, M.: *Madness and Civilization, A History of Insanity in the Age of Reason,* New York: Pantheon, 1965.

Chapter 17

1. Harlow, H. F., and Harlow, M. K.: "The Affectional Systems," in *Behavior of Non-Human Primates,* Vol. 2, A. M. Schrier; H. F. Harlow; and F. Stollnitz, (eds.) New York: Academic Press, 1965, pp. 287-334.

2. Harlow, H. F., and Harlow, M. K.: "The Effect of Rearing Conditions on Behavior," *Bulletin of the Menninger Clinic,* 26:213-224, 1962.

3. Alexander, B. K., and Harlow, H. F.: "Social Behavior of Rhesus

Monkeys Subjected to Different Rearing Conditions During the First Six Months of Life," *Zool. Jb. Physiol. Bd.*, 71:489-508, 1965.

4. Harlow, H. F.; Dodsworth, R. O.; and Harlow, M. K.: "Total Social Isolation in Monkeys," *Proc. Nat. Acad. Sci.*, 54:90-97, 1965.

5. Cross, H. A. and Harlow, H. F.: "Prolonged and Progressive Effects of Partial Isolation on the Behavior of Macaque Monkeys," *J. Exp. Res. Pers.*, 1:39-49, 1965.

6. Harlow, H. F., Dodsworth, R. O. and Harlow, M. K., *op. cit.*, see Reference 4.

7. Elliot, O., and Scott, J. P.: "The Development of Emotional Distress Reactions to Separation, in Puppies," *J. Genet. Psychol.*, 99:3-22, 1961.

8. Spalding, D. A.: "Instinct: With Original Observations on Young Animals," *MacMillan's Magazine*, 27:282-293, 1873. Reprinted in *British Journal of Animal Behavior*, 2:2-11, 1954. Hess, E. H.: " 'Imprinting' in Animals," *Scientific American*, 198:81-90, 1958. Fabricus, E.: "Crucial Periods in the Development of the Following Response in Young Nidifugous Birds," *Zeitschrift für Tierpsychologie*, 21:326-337, 1964.

INDEX

For Product Safety Concerns and Information please contact our EU
representative GPSR@taylorandfrancis.com
Taylor & Francis Verlag GmbH, Kaufingerstraße 24, 80331 München, Germany

www.ingramcontent.com/pod-product-compliance
Lightning Source LLC
Chambersburg PA
CBHW050553270326
41926CB00012B/2031

* 9 7 8 1 1 3 8 3 2 0 1 9 2 *